Multidisciplinary Management of Liver Metastases in Colorectal Cancer

Xinyu Qin • Jianmin Xu • Yunshi Zhong
Editors

Multidisciplinary Management of Liver Metastases in Colorectal Cancer

Early Diagnosis and Treatment

PEOPLE'S MEDICAL PUBLISHING HOUSE
Springer

Editors
Xinyu Qin
Department of General Surgery
Zhongshan Hospital, Fudan University
Shanghai
China

Yunshi Zhong
Department of General Surgery
Zhongshan Hospital
Shanghai
China

Jianmin Xu
Department of General Surgery
Zhongshan Hospital, Fudan University
Shanghai
China

ISBN 978-94-017-7753-7 ISBN 978-94-017-7755-1 (eBook)
DOI 10.1007/978-94-017-7755-1

The print edition is not for sale in China Mainland. Customers from China Mainland please order the print book from: People's Medical Publishing House

Library of Congress Control Number: 2016959598

Printed on acid-free paper

This Springer imprint is published by Springer Nature
The registered company is Springer Science+Business Media B.V. Dordrecht
The registered company address is: Van Godewijckstraat 30, 3311 GX Dordrecht, The Netherlands

Contents

Present Situation and Prospect of Diagnosis and Treatment of Colorectal Cancer

1

Jianping Wang

1.1 Epidemiological Trend of Colorectal Cancer

1.1.1 Distribution Rule of Colorectal Cancer in the World

Colorectal cancer (CRC) is one of the most common malignant tumors. The probability of suffering from colorectal cancer in a person's life is 6 %. There are about 1.20 million new colorectal cancer cases in the world each year. Nearly 600,000 people die of colorectal cancer each year. Among all malignant tumors, both incidence and mortality of colorectal cancer are in the third position. In recent years, incidence and mortality of colorectal cancer in western-developed countries have decreased a little, whereas incidence of colorectal cancer in developing countries has still showed a rising trend [1].

1.1.2 Distribution Rule of Colorectal Cancer In China

Among all malignant tumors, incidence and mortality of colorectal cancer are in the third and fifth position, respectively, with a slight difference in different regions. In 2000, there were about 150,000 new colorectal cancer cases in our country, and nearly 80,000 patients died of colorectal cancer, and it showed a rising trend [2]. Over the past 20 years, epidemiological trend of colorectal cancer in our country has changed and showed some new characteristics: (1) Colorectal cancer showed a trend from low to high incidence. As the population base of our country is great, the absolute number of cases suffering from colorectal cancer and cases that die of colorectal cancer have surpassed that in the United States in recent years. (2) Rising trend of incidence of colon cancer is more significant than that of rectal cancer. (3) Low rectal cancer accounts for a high proportion, and early-stage colorectal cancer accounts for a low proportion. (4) Young people (<30 years old) account for a high proportion; average age of rectal cancer cases shows a trend of approaching to the level in developed countries [3].

1.2 Diagnosis of Colorectal Cancer

1.2.1 Significance of Diagnosis of Early-Stage Colorectal Cancer

Radical surgical resection is the only opportunity to cure colorectal cancer confined in the intestinal wall. Therefore, it has 80 % of the opportunity to cure colorectal cancer still confined in the intestinal wall in definite diagnosis and nearly 90 % of 5-year survival rate after

J. Wang
Department of Colorectal Surgery, The Sixth Affiliated Hospital, Sun Yat-sen University, Guangzhou, People's Republic of China
e-mail: wangjply@yahoo.com.cn

X. Qin et al. (eds.), *Multidisciplinary Management of Liver Metastases in Colorectal Cancer*,
DOI 10.1007/978-94-017-7755-1_1

performing radical surgical resection. However, if there is lymph node metastasis, 5-year survival rate will decrease to 60 % or so [4]. In general, earlier stage of colorectal cancer leads to a higher survival rate, and natural prognosis study on colorectal cancer indicates that early discovery is the most important measure to reduce disease-related mortality.

As onset of colorectal cancer is not obvious, clinical manifestation lacks specificity. About 60 % of colorectal cancer cases have had lymph node metastasis or distant metastasis when diagnosed [5]. Therefore, overall prognosis of colorectal cancer is still not optimistic at present. Although pathogeny of colorectal cancer is not clear, there have already been many reports on pathogeny-related risk factors during the course of development in the order of "normal mucosa-adenoma-adenocarcinoma," which provides the possibility of colorectal cancer screening and early diagnosis.

Zheng Shu et al. carried out colorectal cancer screening by adoption of fecal occult blood test (FOBT) combined with sequential screening scheme. Eight-year follow-up results show that case fatality rate of colorectal cancer of screening group is lower than that of control group by 14.7 %, of which that of rectal cancer is reduced by 31.2 %, which indicates that primary prevention may intervene in and prevent the occurrence of colorectal cancer and secondary prevention can still reduce case fatality rate after occurrence of tumor [6]. Data of US National Polyp Study demonstrate that adenoma canceration rate is directly proportional to age and size of adenoma. Resection of adenoma may significantly reduce incidence rate of colorectal cancer [7].

The present study indicates that hereditary colorectal cancer accounts for about 20 % of the total colorectal cancer. The most common hereditary colorectal cancer includes familial adenomatous polyposis (FAP) and hereditary nonpolyposis colorectal cancer (HNPCC). The former relates to APC gene mutation, whose manifestation is more than 100 diffuse adenomatous polyps in the large intestine, or there is definite familial history or hyperplasia occurs in congenital retinal pigment epithelium although the number of polyps is less than 100, while the latter relates to mismatch repair gene (hMLH1, hMSH2, hPMS1, hPMS2, etc.) mutation, whose manifestation is familial aggregation, where tumors are mostly located at the right colon, and extra-colorectal tumors frequently occur. Therefore, mutation detection of the abovementioned genes may provide reference for early discovery of hereditary colorectal cancer [8].

Because of the living standard, hygiene and health consciousness, and technical reasons, even in relatively developed provinces and municipalities in our country, the large-scale survey system including endoscopy for colorectal cancer, as established in European- and American-developed countries, has not been established; early diagnosis rate of colorectal cancer is low in our country. Overall 5-year survival rate is not so satisfactory either. How to establish an effective and convenient survey system to provide intervention and prevention during the course of development in the order of "normal mucosa-adenoma-adenocarcinoma" or realize early diagnosis after tumor is formed, which is a topic that each of us – colorectal surgeons – must consider carefully.

1.2.2 Significance of Digital Rectal Examination in Diagnosis of Colorectal Cancer

Digital rectal examination (DRE), as a simple and important examination method, has great significance in early discovery of anal canal cancer and rectal cancer. As mentioned above, incidence of low rectal cancer is high in our country. About 75 % of rectal cancer may be touched when conducting digital rectal examination. Among the cases where diagnosis of rectal cancer is delayed, about 85 % do not receive digital rectal examination. In addition, DRE may help judge the site and size of rectal tumor and its relation with adjacent tissues, such as prostate, vagina, etc., and if there is pelvic-planted metastatic node of colon cancer, etc., and provide reference for making clinical decisions. Therefore, digital rectal examination has important significance in the diagnosis and treatment of rectal cancer. If a patient has symptoms such as there is blood in his stool or his defecation habit changes or his stool deforms, conventional digital rectal examination should be conducted.

1.2.3 Significance of Endoscopy in Diagnosis of Colorectal Cancer

Endoscopy includes proctoscopy, sigmoidoscopy, and colonoscopy. At present digital rectal examination and colon fiberscopy are the basic means to examine colorectal cancer. Electronic colon fiberscopy is widely used in clinical applications. Endoscopy can examine the total colon, can even examine the pathological changes in the terminal ileum, and may obtain pathological biopsy simultaneously to define the nature of pathological changes. What should be stressed is that when a great colorectal tumor is discovered by colonoscopy, making the intestinal cavity become too narrow to allow the colonoscope body to pass, endoscopy has been unable to examine the total large intestine mucosa before operation. So the intestinal canal that has been examined by preoperative colonoscope should be examined more carefully during operation. When necessary, intraoperative colonoscope may be used for further examination to avoid omission of missed diagnosis of simultaneous multiple primary carcinoma or other adenomas.

It is indubitable that endoscopy is sensitive to the diagnosis of colorectal cancer, whereas such examination method still has some limitation. For example, examination results are affected by examinator's operation level. Study shows that about 13 % of 5–9 mm adenomas and 27 % of less than 5 mm adenomas are missed in diagnosis. Even if the size of tumor mass is greater than 1 cm, the rate of missed diagnosis still reaches nearly 6 % [9]. In addition, such examination may be affected by the blind spot of the endoscope and has such risks as perforation, bleeding, or even death. Despite this, no other examination method can replace the important role of endoscopy in the diagnosis of colorectal cancer at present.

1.2.4 Other Diagnostic Examination

1.2.4.1 Fecal Occult Blood Test

Since Greegor took fecal occult blood test (FOBT) as screening method in 1967, FOBT has still been the main screening method except digital rectal examination and endoscopy up till now. Results of a study that involves 300,000 objects and follows up them more than 18 years show that sequential FOBT may reduce mortality by 13–33 % [5]. However, as colorectal cancer often does not cause bleeding at early stage, sensitivity of FOBT examination of colorectal cancer is only 27–57 %, and that of adenoma is only 8 % [10]. Food containing peroxide may cause false-positive FOBT result. Therefore, positive FOBT result cannot definitely diagnose colorectal cancer or adenoma. It just indicates the possibility. Further examination and confirmation are needed.

1.2.4.2 Double-Contrast Barium Enema

Double-contrast barium enema (DCBE) is one of the important examination methods for colon cancer, with little significance in the diagnosis of low rectal cancer. As sensitivity and specificity of DCBE on the discovery of colorectal cancer are not as good as endoscopy, and endoscopy may conduct pathological biopsy or excise adenoma simultaneously, clinical application of DCBE becomes less and less. However, reoperative tumor localization of DCBE is better than that of endoscopy.

1.2.4.3 CTC and MRC

Sensitivity and accuracy of computed tomography colonography (CTC) to discover colorectal cancer are almost equivalent to that of traditional colon fiberscopy [11]. So it is also called virtual colonoscopy. In addition, CTC can still examine colorectal cancer infiltration and adjacent tissue involvement to a certain degree, especially whether rectal cancer invades the bladder, uterus, and pelvic wall or not, and at the same time examine whether there is lymph node beside the intestine or not, and whether there is lymph node metastasis beside the abdominal aorta or not, which has important significance in the preoperative staging of colorectal cancer and selection of treatment scheme.

Magnetic resonance colonography (MRC) is superior to CTC in the aspects of judgment of rectum and anal canal cancer infiltration and diffusion range, preoperative staging, identification and diagnosis of postoperative recurrence, etc. Both examination methods are noninvasive, but results are greatly affected by machine, X-ray image-reading level, etc.

1.2.4.4 Endorectal Ultrasound Examination

Endorectal ultrasound (ERUS) examination may clearly display five hierarchies of the intestinal wall, i.e., the mucosa, muscularis mucosa, submucosa, muscularis propria, and serosa, and can provide visual judgment on thickness of each hierarchy and homogeneity of echo. It can provide a general judgment on rectal tumor size, infiltration depth, relation with adjacent tissues, etc., and thereby relatively reliable preoperative staging can be determined. Especially when rectal tumor is small and infiltration depth is T1/T2, ERUS has important reference value for selection of treatment scheme of low rectal cancer.

1.2.4.5 Positron Emission Tomography

Positron emission tomography (PET) relies on high metabolism of tumor cells that is different from normal tissues and makes a judgment on whether there is tumor or not after examination of local metabolism of the human body. It has important reference value especially in judgment if there is postoperative local recurrence or distant metastasis of colorectal cancer and reaction of the human body to chemotherapy drugs. It is a noninvasive examination mean with highest sensitivity and specificity at present, which can discover about 5 mm-size pathological changes.

1.3 Present Situation of Treatment of Colorectal Cancer

1.3.1 Selection of Operation Method

Basic principles of colorectal cancer operation are to (1) pay attention to "no-touch isolation technique," (2) appropriate intestinal segment resection, and (3) normative lymphadenectomy. As for simultaneous multiple primary carcinoma, surgical resection should be strictly subject to colorectal cancer operation principles, respectively.

1.3.1.1 Operation Method for Colon Cancer

Determination of operation method for colon cancer depends on the site of tumor and its relation with the peripheral organs, including the right colectomy, transverse colectomy, left colectomy, sigmoid colectomy, and related extended resection. If tumor is big, locally invades peripheral organs, such as colon cancer of hepatic flexure invades gallbladder and right kidney, colon cancer of splenic flexure invades spleen and left kidney, transverse colon cancer invades gastric wall, etc, we can conduct the extended radical resection for colon cancer and internal organs. Complete resection will result in good effect.

Surgical treatment for obstructive colon cancer is aimed at eliminating obstruction, excising tumor, and restoring the smoothness of the intestinal canal. As for the right colon cancer obstruction, there is no dispute on performing first-stage resection and anastomosis. As for the left colon cancer obstruction, whether or not to perform first-stage tumor resection or first-stage anastomosis should depend on systematic status of patient, local infiltration of tumor, and surgeon's technical level. Because of the popularization and application of intraoperative intestinal tract lavage, the progress of nutritional support treatment, and the development of surgical ICU in recent years, more and more scholars prefer to first-stage resection and anastomosis for obstructive left colon cancer patients in feasible conditions.

1.3.1.2 Operation Method for Rectal Cancer

In recent years, discussion on operation method for rectal cancer focuses on how to make patients obtain the highest living quality in the condition of ensuring radical treatment of tumor. Radical treatment of tumor must ensure complete resection of tumor, low local recurrence rate, and long survival time. Improvement of quality is mainly reflected by anal preservation rate, postoperative defecation function, sexual function, etc. Therefore, a great deal of clinical study concentrates on the comparison of advantages and disadvantages between low anterior resection (LAR) and abdominoperineal resection (APR) or discussion on the safety of local resection for rectal cancer.

The study on biological behaviors of low rectal cancer infiltration and metastasis indicates that appropriate distance between the remote resection margin of low rectal cancer and the tumor is 2 cm. This concept causes LAR operation to be widely generalized. Combined with total mesorectal excision (TME), it has preserved most patients' anuses, while those patients had to receive APR operation in the past. There is no significant difference in operative complications, recurrence rate, and survival rate of both operation methods, but living quality of the patients that receive LAR operation is obviously better.

Sexual dysfunction is a common postoperative complication of rectal cancer. Along with the increase in young rectal cancer patients and extension of survival time, their requirement for living quality is also gradually improved. Sexual dysfunction increasingly attracts attention from rectal cancer patients. Pelvic autonomic nerve preservation (PANP) is an operation method that identifies and preserves the pelvic autonomic nerve on the premise of ensuring radical treatment of tumor. PANP plays a significant role in the prevention from postoperative sexual desire disorder of rectal cancer, erectile dysfunction, ejaculation dysfunction, urinary dysfunction, and vagina ache. The author's unit compared male patients' erectile function, ejaculation function, local recurrence rate, and 5-year survival rate between 105 cases that received PANP operation and 110 cases that received no PANP. It discovered that incidence rate of sexual dysfunction among patients that received PANP radical resection of rectal cancer is about 30 %, equivalent to that of patients that received sigmoid colectomy, but obviously lower than that of patients that received conventional Miles – 43–67 %; PANP also plays a significant role in protecting postoperative sexual function of female patients, whereas the effect is not significant in posterior pelvis dissection [12–15].

The key to PANP operation is to get familiar with anatomical characteristics of the pelvic autonomic nerve and lymphatic metastasis rule of each segment of rectal cancer, pay attention to the sense of anatomical hierarchy during operation, and fully expose operative field when conducting operation below the peritoneal reflection. Serious damage to the autonomic nerve is likely to occur at the following sites: (1) the left trunk of the abdominal aortic plexus when cutting the inferior mesenteric vessel, (2) the superior hypogastric plexus and hypogastric nerve in posterior rectal separation, (3) the inferior hypogastric plexus and pelvic autonomic nerve in lateral separation of the rectum, and (4) the erectile nerve in anterior hepatic separation [16]. PANP operation requires the surgeon to have a rich operative experience and anatomical knowledge. In our country, such kind of operations is mainly limited to a few large hospitals, which needs further generalization.

There are more and more study reports related to local resection of rectal cancer. Theoretical basis of such kind of operation is that when pathological change is limited in the mucosa and not beyond the muscularis mucosa, there is almost no lymph node metastasis risk; but when pathological change invades the submucosa, the probability of occurrence of lymph node metastasis is nearly 5 %. So when pathological change is limited in the mucosa or muscularis mucosa, radical treatment can be achieved just by resecting the site of pathological change instead of local lymphadenectomy. After local resection, patients are subject to the risk of postoperative local recurrence and metastasis. So indication of local resection of rectal cancer should be strictly controlled, and overall consideration should be made according to preoperative staging, pathological situation, and systemic status. A scholar had once reported that when pathological change is limited at T1, there is no significant difference in recurrence rate and 5-year survival rate between local resection and traditional APR results [17–19]. Although these study results are encouraging, when pathological change is limited at T2, whether or not local resection is suitable and whether or not auxiliary chemoradiotherapy is needed after local resection operation are the topics not solved yet. Along with in-depth screening work for high-risk population of colorectal cancer, undoubtedly more and more early-stage colorectal cancer will be discovered. As one of the important operation methods, more and more attention will be paid to rectal cancer local resection and it will be more and more widely used. Its safety and effectiveness urgently need demonstration through large-scale multicenter randomized clinical research.

1.3.2 Significance of Total Mesorectal Excision in Rectal Cancer Treatment

1.3.2.1 Definition of Total Mesorectal Excision

Total mesorectal excision (TME) is to conduct sharp separation in the clearance between the visceral pelvic fascia and parietal pelvic fascia of the anterior sacral under direct view during the radical resection of middle and lower-segment rectal cancer so as to completely resect the visceral pelvic fascia as well as fat, connective tissue, blood vessel, and lymphoid tissue at the back side of the rectum that it wraps, making resected part of the mesorectum at the far end of the tumor not less than 5 cm and distance from the intestinal canal resected to lower edge of the tumor not less than 2 cm.

1.3.2.2 Significance of Total Mesorectal Excision

The TME principle, proposed by Heald in 1982, is one of the basic principles that should be observed in the operation of middle and low rectal cancer at present. It has great significance in reducing postoperative local recurrence rate of rectal cancer and improving anal preservation rate. TME places emphasis on sharp separation between the visceral pelvic fascia and parietal pelvic fascia, completeness of the visceral pelvic fascia, avoidance of residual tumor in the mesorectum, and reduction of postoperative local recurrence rate. In 1995, McCall et al. analyzed over 10,000 colorectal cancer cases. Data showed that overall local recurrence rate was 18 %, of which 1033 cases received TME operation; recurrence rate was only 7 % [20]. In 1998, Kockerling et al. also reported 1581 colorectal cancer cases, of which local recurrence rate of rectal cancer of the cases that received no TME was 39 %, while local recurrence rate of the cases that received TME operation was only 10 % [21]. In the past, it was thought that the intestinal canal resected should be 5 cm from lower edge of tumor. But on the premise of TME, a distance of 2 cm has been enough from resection margin at remote end to lower edge of tumor, which makes about 77 % patients obtain radical treatment and preserve their anuses [22]. Furthermore, TME places emphasis on separation between two pelvic fascias under the direct view and realizes PANP operation. It plays an important role in prevention from postoperative micturition dysfunction and sexual dysfunction of rectal cancer patients [12].

But a report showed that compared with the previous operations, TME would increase operation time, intraoperative bleeding amount, incidence rate of anastomotic leakage, and hospitalization time [23, 24]. These are closely associated with surgeon's operating level. A study showed that TME operation carried out by specialist physicians of colorectal cancer can not only shorten operation time, reduce bleeding amount, and reduce operative complications, but also significantly decrease local recurrence rate and increase 5-year survival rate [21, 25–27]. Many European and American countries have realized this problem and implemented colorectal specialist physicians training system. But in our country, there is no standardized training and access system for colorectal specialist physicians.

1.3.3 Dispute on Lateral Pelvic Lymphadenectomy for Rectal Cancer

Eastern and western scholars always have dispute on whether or not conventional lateral pelvic lymphadenectomy (LPLD) should be performed for rectal cancer. Most Japanese scholars believe that lateral lymph node metastasis rate is between 14 and 29 %. Lateral lymphadenectomy may result in reduction of postoperative local recurrence rate by nearly 50 % and increase in 5-year survival rate by about 10 %. Therefore, conventional lateral pelvic lymphadenectomy is recommended. Japanese scholars proposed extended radical resection for rectal cancer by dissection of Clearance A, B, and C of the peripheral connective tissues of the rectum, of which A is the tissue resected by the aforesaid TME, B is the inside dissection of the internal iliac artery of the lateral lymph node, and C is the outside dissection of the internal iliac artery of the lateral lymph node, including obturator lymphadenectomy. Takahashi analyzed 764 rectal cancer cases that received the abovementioned three clearance dissection, of which lateral lymph node metastasis occurred in 66 cases; cases with lateral lymph node metastasis account for 8.6 % of all rectal cancer cases and account for 16.4 % of low rectal cancer cases (less than 5 cm above dentate line). Therefore, the author's opinion is that rectal cancer patients should receive extended dissection [28]. Domestic study carried out by Dong Xinshu et al. showed that among 782 cases of rectal cancer patients, lateral lymph node metastasis occurred in 64 cases; cases with lateral lymph node metastasis account for 8.2 % of all rectal cancer cases, of which lateral lymph node metastasis rate of rectal cancer below the peritoneal reflection is 12.5 %, while lateral lymph node metastasis rate of rectal cancer above the peritoneal reflection is 1.3 %. Based on this, the author thinks that upper metastasis and lateral metastasis are different paths. As for the rectal cancer below the peritoneal reflection, conventional lymphadenectomy should be performed [29]. But Grinnell in the United States reported that positive rate of the lateral lymph node is only 1.9 %. In addition, the author thinks that lateral lymph node metastasis should belong to distant metastasis; dissection has no clinical significance. Therefore, lateral pelvic lymphadenectomy is not recommended [30]. Why the study results between eastern and western scholars are so different? Yano et al. recently studied and compared many years of literature of both parties to the dispute and think that difference in the results of both parties is likely caused by different rectal cancer staging concept between east and west. If staging standard of rectal cancer is unified, lateral lymph node metastasis of low rectal cancer perhaps may result in similar positive rate in Japan and western countries [31].

As range of lateral lymphadenectomy is big, incidence rate of postoperative micturition and sexual dysfunction caused by intraoperative damage to the pelvic autonomic nerve also increases. For this reason, some scholars proposed extended radical resection of PANP, called as "functional extended radical resection." After performing this operation, 62.3 % and 57.1 % of the patients can maintain normal erectile and sexual functions, respectively, and postoperative 5-year survival rate is 61.2 % [32]. However, Wan Yuanlian et al. also reported that lateral dissection may reduce pelvic recurrence from 17.7 % by adoption of traditional radical resection to 5.6 %, but there is no significant improvement of 5-year survival rate. Further analysis was conducted on the cases that had lateral lymph node metastasis and received radical resection and lateral dissection. Recurrence still occurred in 80 % of the patients within 2 years after operation; distant metastasis occurred in 75 % of the patients, and 3- and 5-year survival rate after operation was only 16.7 % and 0, which indicates that as lateral metastasis breaks through the barrier of fascia propria, it is not only local pathological change in the pelvic cavity, but also belongs to a part of pathological change of the whole body. Lateral dissection can reduce local recurrence rate, but cannot significantly improve survival rate [33, 34].

From the above analysis, although rectal cancer lateral lymphadenectomy can reduce postoperative local recurrence rate, great dispute still exists on the significance of dissection. Lymphatic diversion path and rule of middle and low rectal cancer need further illustration. Whether or not biological behaviors of lateral lymph node metastasis belong to a part of systemic metastasis requires further study and demonstration, and whether or not conventional lateral lymphadenectomy should be conducted for rectal cancer below the peritoneal reflection needs validation through multicenter randomized clinical trial on a large size of samples.

1.3.4 Laparoscopic Radical Resection of Colorectal Cancer

In 1991, Jacobs M reported laparoscopic radical resection of colorectal cancer for the first time. Through nearly 20 years of development, laparoscopic radical resection of colorectal cancer has achieved great development. Laparoscopic radical resection of colorectal cancer should observe all basic principles for open operation. As range of surgical resection is big, operative gap is small, and field of vision is often disturbed by the small intestine, there is some difficulty to perform such operation. Along with the accumulation of experience and development of advanced devices, laparoscopic-assisted resection of colorectal cancer increasingly becomes mature, and its safety and effectiveness are also recognized by many scholars both at home and abroad.

US Clinical Outcomes of Surgical Therapy (COST) reviewed and analyzed clinical data of 372 cases that received laparoscopic-assisted resection of colorectal cancer before 1994. The results showed that cases of conversion to *open operation* accounted for 15.6 %, operative mortality was 2 %, and implantation incidence rate was 1.1 %. Cancer-related mortality relates to the stage of tumor. These data are almost equivalent to those of traditional open operation. So they think it is necessary to conduct randomized clinical trial to compare the two operation methods [35]. For this reason, in 1994, COST organized 66 surgeons from 48 hospitals to participate in the multicenter randomized clinical trial. A total of 872 patients were grouped. Median follow-up time is 4.4 years. The study showed that there is no significant difference in complications, postoperative 30-day mortality, incidence rate of rehospitalization and reoperation, recurrence rate, incision implantation rate, and 3-year survival rate between laparoscopic-assisted operation and open operation. Compared with open operation, laparoscopic-assisted operation has a shorter hospitalization time and less postoperative pain despite its longer operation time [36]. Exclusion criteria of this clinical trial include rectal cancer and transverse colon cancer, local progress period, or distant metastasis. However, tumor recurred in a total of 160 cases during follow-up period. Recurrence rate of the two groups is 16 % and 18 %, respectively. But the researcher did not make any explanation for such high recurrence rate.

The European Colon Cancer Laparoscopic or Open Research Study Group (COLOR) also started a multicenter randomized clinical trial in which 29 hospitals participated in 1997. The inclusion and exclusion criteria were almost the same as those in COST study. The results were almost close to those of COST, too. A total of 1248 patients were grouped in this study. Cases of conversion to open operation accounted for 17 %, operative mortality was less than 2 %, and median follow-up time is 4.4 years; there was no significant difference in 3-year disease-free survival rate of the two groups and overall survival rate. Based on this, the researcher thought that compared with open operation, laparoscopic-assisted operation is undoubtedly safe and effective. We should further increase sample size and improve study design, and find that whether laparoscopy is superior to open operation or not [37, 38].

After that, Hong Kong, China, UK MRC CLASSIC Group, and many other medical institutions in the world conducted some randomized clinical trial and discussed the advantages and disadvantages of laparoscopic radical resection of colon cancer. Study results obtained were also almost similar to those reported by COST or COLOR [39, 40]. According to these studies, Abraham analyzed 12 randomized clinical trials completed before 2002, involving a total of 2512 patients. The results showed that laparoscopic-assisted operation time increased by about 30 %, but postoperative complications and incision infection rate were lower than that of the open operation group, with quicker postoperative restoration and less pain. There was no significant difference in radical resection and operative mortality between the two groups [41]. Tjandra et al. analyzed 17 randomized clinical trials completed in 1991–2005. A total of 4013 patients were involved. The results were almost similar to those reported by Abraham NS [42].

To sum up the abovementioned study results, laparoscopic radical resection of colon cancer has a longer operation time but less bleeding, quicker postoperative restoration, less pain, lower incision infection rate, and shorter hospitalization time compared with traditional open operation. There is no significant difference in operative complications, mortality, recurrence rate, and long-term survival time between the two operation methods. However, most cases involved in these studies are colon cancer patients. Thus, laparoscopic radical resection of rectal cancer will complete TME standard operation within limited space and vision, does it have the same safety and effectiveness?

Study conducted by Leroy et al. indicates that the advantage of laparoscopic-assisted surgical resection of colon cancer can also be reflected in resection of rectal cancer. They reported 102 cases that received laparoscopic-assisted TME radical resection of rectal cancer from 1991 to 2000. Three percent of cases were converted to open operation, operative mortality is 2 %, 91.8 % received radical resection, average follow-up time is 3 years, there is no incision implantation metastasis, local recurrence rate is 6 %, and 5-year survival rate is 65 %. These data were similar to those of open operation or even better. They thought that laparoscopic radical resection of rectal cancer was safe, effective, and feasible [43]. In China, results of the clinical study conducted by Zheng Minhua, Zhou Zongguang, and others indicated that laparoscopic radical resection of low or even extra-low rectal cancer can reach the radical treatment rate of open operation and have some advantages in intraoperative bleeding, intestinal function restoration, off-bed activity time, incidence rate of postoperative complications, etc. There is no statistical difference in the length of intestinal segment resected, distance from tumor to low resection margin and lymphadenectomy range, local recurrence rate, distant metastasis rate, and accumulated 5-year survival rate compared with open operation [44, 45].

The Sixth Affiliated Hospital of Sun Yat-sen University made a statistical analysis on the data of laparoscopic radical resection of rectal cancer from March to July 2009. The results showed that if laparoscopic operation technology is skillfully mastered, laparoscopic radical resection of rectal cancer can shorten the operation time compared with open operation.

1.3.5 Hepatic Metastasis Treatment of Colorectal Cancer

Hepatic metastasis occurred in about 50 % of colorectal cancer during the whole course of disease [46], of which 15–25 % is synchronous hepatic metastasis and 20–25 % is asynchronous hepatic metastasis [47]. Among all hepatic metastasis patients, the liver of nearly 20 % of the patients is the only organ with metastasis. If not treated, the average survival time of these patients would not exceed 1 year [48]. Surgical treatment for hepatic metastasis has experienced a lot of controversy, firstly helpless, try, then objection and retry, and now widely accepted. And the important role of liver resection in hepatic metastasis of colorectal cancer was gradually established in recent 20 years. After colon cancer patients with hepatic metastasis received primary tumor resection and hepatic metastatic focus resection, 5-year survival rate can still reach 20–60 %, and even the 10-year survival rate reported was 26–42 % [49, 50]. Although it relates to subsequent adjuvant treatment and development of operating level, it is certain that hepatic resection plays an active role in extending survival time of colorectal cancer patients with hepatic metastasis.

In recent years, radio frequency ablation therapy for hepatic metastasis of colorectal cancer also achieved a good generalization, application, and development. Radio frequency ablation therapy is mainly used for the patients with hepatic metastasis where resection cannot be conducted. In this case, the disease mostly belongs to extensive metastasis. After radio frequency ablation, recurrence rate is high, and local recurrence rate is even higher especially when length-diameter of metastatic focus exceeds 3 cm [51]. Therefore, adjuvant chemotherapy is mostly conducted after radio frequency ablation. Related clinical trial is ongoing.

In addition, the mainstream tendency for hepatic metastasis of colorectal cancer is to select either adjuvant systemic chemotherapy or hepatic artery catheter perfusion chemotherapy, chemoembolization, chemotherapy and radiotherapy in the focus, etc. Various therapies are applicable to different patients. Multidisciplinary treatment will be an important model to improve overall prognosis for hepatic metastasis of colorectal cancer. Related content will be described in detail in Chap. 2 of this book.

1.3.6 Adjuvant Chemoradiotherapy and Neoadjuvant Chemotherapy

1.3.6.1 Significance of Adjuvant Chemoradiotherapy

Surgical operation is the only approach to obtain radical treatment of colorectal cancer. But in the past 30 years, surgical treatment effect of colorectal cancer is unsatisfactory; 5-year survival rate is about 50–60 %. Trial of surgical models, such as increasing surgical resection range, did not significantly improve survival rate. On the contrary, it resulted in greater wound and more complications. Furthermore, as mentioned above, hepatic metastasis has occurred in 15–25 % of colorectal cancer in diagnosis. Such cases cannot be cured only relying on surgical operation. For this reason, more and more scholars are probing adjuvant treatment other than surgical operation. Their study mostly emphasizes chemotherapy and radiotherapy.

Since it was discovered that nitrogen mustard had antitumor effect in 1943, studies on adjuvant chemotherapy for colorectal cancer have experienced probe and argument for more than half a century. Only in recent (nearly 30) years has the great development been obtained. These studies develop gradually along with the emergence of new chemotherapy drugs. In general, the present situation of chemotherapy for colorectal cancer is that 5-FU-based short-course (6 months) combination chemotherapy model has been established. Combination and optimization of chemotherapy regimen are still in exploration [52].

At present, 5-FU/CF is the standard adjuvant chemotherapy scheme. They will form a covalent compound with thymidylate synthase to realize the antitumor effect. To discuss the role of chemotherapy in adjuvant treatment of colorectal cancer, the National Surgical Adjuvant Breast and Bowel Project (NSABP) of the United States conducted systematic study in 1977–1990, including C-01, C-02, C-03, and C-04. A total of 3820 patients were grouped, of which the curative effect of the 5-FU/CF scheme (CF 500 mg/m^2, dripping for 2 h, 5-FU 500 mg/m^2, injecting it when half of CF is dripped; the above operation was conducted once a week, six times as a course of treatment; after each course of treatment is completed, stop it for 2 weeks and then enter the next course, a total of eight courses of treatment), MOF scheme, and 5-FU/CF/LEV scheme was compared in the C-03 and C-04 study, respectively. The study results showed that compared with the latter two schemes, the 5-FU/CF scheme has better tumor-free survival rate and overall survival rate [53, 54]. Therefore, NSABP experts thought that the abovementioned 5-FU/CF scheme is an adjuvant chemotherapy scheme acceptable by Stage II and III colon cancer patients [55].

As a standard chemotherapy drug, 5-FU/CF has been accepted by most scholars. However, the abovementioned schemes will take a long period, and consumption of CF is great. For this reason, many research organizations jointly conducted a multicenter randomized clinical trial with the code of INT-0089 in 1988. A total of 3759 patients were grouped. Follow-up time exceeded 5 years. The results indicate that LEV is not a necessary component part of adjuvant treatment of colon cancer. By adoption of the 5-FU/CF scheme, it is unnecessary to add LEV. In the event of low dosage of CF (CF 20 mg/(m^2·d), administrated for 5 days each week, 4–5 weeks as a course of treatment, a total of six courses of treatment), there is no significant difference in tumor-free survival rate and overall survival rate compared with CF dosage of the aforesaid C-03 or C-04. Therefore, INT-0089 study thinks that 5-FU/CF with 6-month adjuvant treatment is the most standard treatment scheme at present. It does not come singly, but in pairs. Results of another randomized clinical trial with the code of NCCTG 894,651, where 890 patients were grouped, are almost consistent with those of INT-0089 [56].

Along with the development of study on chemotherapy drugs, new chemotherapy drugs or dosage forms keep emerging. Focus of both pharmacology and clinical medical science is on whether or not synergetic effect exists among different 5-FU/CF-based chemotherapy schemes. For example, clinical application of the drugs such as oxaliplatin, irinotecan, CPT-11, Xeloda, etc. has demonstrated the adjuvant curative effect for metastatic colorectal cancer. In addition, it is discovered in study that oxaliplatin or irinotecan has significant synergetic effect with 5-FU. Effect of combination chemotherapy is better [57]. Targeting chemotherapy drugs bevacizumab, Avastin, and cetuximab, C225, have been approved for use in metastatic colorectal cancer in the United States and Europe. The present study indicates that combination chemotherapy scheme of Avastin or C225 may improve the median survival time of metastatic colorectal cancer patients from 12 to 24 months. Its clinical curative effect is encouraging. Related study progress will be described in detail hereinafter.

1.3.6.2 Significance of the Neoadjuvant Chemoradiotherapy

Because of the biological characteristics of colorectal cancer and concealed clinical manifestations, hepatic metastasis has occurred in 15–25 % of the patients in definite diagnosis of colorectal cancer, of which most patients cannot receive surgical resection. Recurrence occurs in nearly 60 % of patients after just resection of the focus of hepatic metastasis. In addition, because of the particularity of lymphatic diversion of rectal cancer and the close relation with pelvic organs, many patients have been in locally advanced period in diagnosis. So long as surgical resection is performed, most consequence is low radical treatment effect and high local recurrence rate. Adam et al. reported 701 cases of hepatic metastasis of colorectal cancer that cannot receive surgical resection in 2001. After neoadjuvant chemotherapy scheme by oxaliplatin combined with 5-FU/CF, the grade of 95 cases (13.5 %) was reduced to resectable grade, without any operative mortality, and the postoperative 5-year survival rate reached 35 %, almost consistent with the survival rate of resectable hepatic metastasis of colorectal cancer [58]. This study result greatly encourages the study enthusiasm of clinical medical scientists and leads to a revolutionary thinking for decision-making on clinical treatment of colorectal cancer: The neoadjuvant chemotherapy is probably the best choice of chemotherapy.

The study indicates that preoperative radiotherapy may reduce tumor volume, improve radical treatment rate of the operation, decrease local recurrence rate, and increase survival rate. As for locally advanced rectal cancer, it can lower tumor grade and raise anal preservation chance [59]. Stage III randomized clinical trial CAO/ARO/AIO-94 was conducted in Germany, where a total of 823 patients were grouped. 5-FU/CF served as the standard chemotherapy scheme. The results show that compared with traditional postoperative chemoradiotherapy, preoperative neoadjuvant chemoradiotherapy has better local tumor control effect, lower toxic and side effect, and higher survival rate, and anal preservation rate is improved [60]. Recently Rodel et al. conducted a multicenter Stage II randomized clinical trial, and indicates adoption of preoperative neoadjuvant adiochemortherapy with XELOX as standard chemotherapy regimen, in at least more than half of the patients, tumor can be regressed by 50%, and incidence rate of serious diarrhea side reaction is only 16 % [61]. Whether 5-FU/CF-based or XELOX-based neoadjuvant chemotherapy scheme is better requires further validation through clinical trials. Some clinical trials are ongoing to test the superiority of the neoadjuvant combination chemoradiotherapy scheme. For example, PETACC-6 is a Stage III randomized clinical trial that involves 1090 patients. The purpose is to compare the advantages and disadvantages of the neoadjuvant radiotherapy and postoperative radiotherapy-combined XELOX scheme or single Xeloda-based chemotherapy scheme. The results are still under follow-up and analysis.

Camma et al. analyzed 14 randomized clinical trials completed from 1970 to 1999, with a total of 6426 patients involved, of which 3081 patients only received surgical treatment. The analysis results indicate that compared with only operation, local recurrence rate of the patients that received neoadjuvant radiotherapy before operation is low, tumor-related mortality is low, and 5-year survival rate is high. But it is not associated with the incidence rate of distant metastasis [59]. Combining the aforesaid CAO/ARO/AIO-94 study results, neoadjuvant chemoradiotherapy can not only lower tumor grade and reduce local recurrence rate, but also has better effect than postoperative adjuvant chemoradiotherapy.

1.3.6.3 Chemotherapy for Stage II Colorectal Cancer

Dispute on whether or not Stage II colorectal cancer should receive chemotherapy always exists. At present some scholars think that colorectal cancer with recurrence and high-risk factors should receive adjuvant chemotherapy; otherwise, it is unnecessary. These high-risk factors include poor tumor differentiation, invasion into veins, obstruction or perforation, and number of lymph nodes analyzed <12, T4 [62].

Four clinical trials conducted by NSABP (C-01, C-02, C-03, C-04) involved a total of 3820 patients, of which there are 1565 Stage II cases and 2255 Stage III cases. Although the study results indicate that adjuvant treatment can improve patients' 5-year survival rate and tumor-free survival rate, the analysis on tumor staging and hierarchy discovered that adjuvant treatment resulted in a reduction of overall mortality of Stage II colon cancer by 30 %, while total mortality of Stage III colon cancer was only reduced by 18 %, and reduction of mortality of Stage II cases is not associated with the abovementioned "high-risk factors" of patients. Therefore, NSABP experts recommended all Stage II colon cancer patients to receive adjuvant chemotherapy [63]. But results of International Multicentre Pooled Analysis of Colon Cancer Trials (IMPACT) and INT-0089 are opposite. IMPACT summarized five randomized clinical trials that involved 1016 cases of Stage II and 1487 cases of Stage III colon cancer patients [64]. INT-0089 study involved a total of 3759 cases of colon cancer patients, with 20 % of high-risk Stage II and 80 % of Stage III patients [54]. The results of both studies indicated that adjuvant chemotherapy may benefit Stage III colon cancer patients, but it did not benefit Stage II patients. Schrag et al. analyzed clinical curative effect for global 3151T3 colon cancer cases without obstruction or perforation. Overall survival rate of the patients that received chemotherapy is 78 %, and that of patients that did not receive chemotherapy is 75 %. This result is similar to that of IMPACT and INT-0089. At the same time, it was found that adjuvant chemotherapy can improve the overall survival rate of Stage II colon cancer patients by 2–5 % at most, and chemotherapy mortality is 0.5–1 % [65].

The above mentioned study results indicated that survival rate of Stage II colon cancer patients that received adjuvant chemotherapy can be improved by about 5 %, but it also has 1 % of chemotherapy mortality risk, and side reaction of chemotherapy is unavoidable. Therefore, US National Comprehensive Cancer Network (NCCN) and American Society of Clinical Oncology (ASCO) do not recommend conventional chemotherapy for Stage II colon cancer patients. Through analysis on related clinical trials, some scholars still suggest adjuvant chemotherapy for Stage II colon cancer with high-risk recurrence factors, such as poor tumor differentiation, invasion into veins, obstruction or perforation, number of lymph nodes <12, T4, etc. But this viewpoint has not been validated. It needs further study, observation, and analysis through large-scale, multicenter clinical trials.

1.3.7 Related Study on Targeted Drugs

Along with in-depth fundamental research, some key molecules related to occurrence and progress of diseases are discovered. Targeted drugs for these highly specifical molecules are also applied in treatment of colorectal cancer. Targeting chemotherapy drugs bevacizumab, Avastin, and cetuximab, C225, have been approved for use in metastatic colorectal cancer in the United States and Europe and also been approved for clinical use in China. The former can combine and neutralize vascular endothelial growth factor (VEGF); the latter has high affinity to endothelial growth factor receptor (EGFR). Hurwitz et al. reported 813 cases of metastatic colorectal cancer in 2004, which randomly received IFL+Avastin (402 cases) or IFL+placebo (411 cases) treatment. The results showed that median survival time of the two groups was 20.3 months and 15.6 months, respectively, and effective rate was 44.8 % and 34.8 %, respectively [66]. Cunningham et al. reported BOND trial results in 2004. Patients on which CPT-11 chemotherapy has no effect randomly received C225+CPT-11 (218 cases) or only C225 treatment (111 cases). Effectiveness of the two groups was 22.9 % and 10.8 %, respectively, and median survival time was 8.6 months and 6.9 months, respectively [67]. It indicates that C225 may reverse the drug resistance of CPT-11. Curative effect of C225 is not correlated with EGFR expression level that is immunohistochemically determined, but correlated with seriousness of skin rash. The more serious the rash is, the better the prognosis will be. More and more studies indicated that combined Avastin or C225 chemotherapy scheme may improve the median survival time of metastatic colorectal cancer from 12 to 24 months. The clinical curative effect showed is really encouraging. Probe of optimization of combination chemotherapy scheme is ongoing [68, 69]. At the same time, in-depth study of the application of targeting drugs is also ongoing. For example, there is evidence to prove that only colorectal cancer of wild type KRAS gene has reaction to C225 chemotherapy, while it is ineffective in the case of mutation type [70]. Many studies are probing molecular marker that monitors chemotherapy reaction for better selection or adjustment of chemotherapy scheme [71].

1.4 Expectation

Prevention is better than treatment. The onset of colorectal cancer is concealed. There is no specificity of clinical manifestations. As for the patients with clinical symptoms, it should be highly vigilant and conduct systematic screening. The population with high-risk factors of colorectal cancer should get more attention and follow up. Along with the improvement of people's living standard, the incidence of colorectal cancer will further increase. Prevention and control work situation is becoming more and more serious.

Surgical operation-based multidisciplinary treatment is the best model for the treatment of the colorectal cancer at present. The neoadjuvant chemoradiotherapy may significantly improve overall prognosis of patients, and clinical curative effect of the targeting drugs is even encouraging. Standardized, scientific, and systematic treatment has significantly improved the clinical curative effect for colorectal cancer.

However, 5-year survival rate of colorectal cancer under this surgical operation-based multidisciplinary treatment is still around 50–60 %. The reason lies in the low proportion of early-stage patients and lack of revolutionary treatment results. Therefore, how to establish a mature colorectal screening mechanism and improve early diagnosis rate of colorectal cancer is our important topic in the future. In addition, no ideal curative effect makes colorectal cancer-related fundamental study attract more and more attention. Studies of many scholars are aimed at trying to find treatment target points of specificity from the pathogenetic mechanism so as to improve overall prognosis of colorectal cancer.

Adjuvant chemoradiotherapy and neoadjuvant chemoradiotherapy benefit Stage III colorectal cancer patients a lot. The neoadjuvant chemotherapy can reduce tumor volume, lower tumor grade, and decrease postoperative recurrence, which is more and more widely applied and generalized. But safety and effectiveness of adjuvant chemoradiotherapy for Stage II patients need further demonstration through multicenter randomized clinical trial on a large size of samples.

The 5-FU/CF-based chemotherapy scheme has been established. Along with the emergence of more and more new drugs, especially targeted drugs, more clinical studies are required to optimize and combine traditional and new drugs so as to produce a synergetic effect.

In general, overall treatment effect for colorectal cancer is gradually rising, but still not so satisfactory. To establish an effective survey and screening mechanism is a hard work. Selection of the treatment policy and treatment models involved needs further optimization. Related clinical operating procedures need further demonstration through clinical trials.

References

1. Sung JJ, Lau JY, Young GP, et al. Asia Pacific consensus recommendations for colorectal cancer screening. Gut. 2008;57:1166–6.
2. Lin C, Yang B, Donald M, et al. Cancer trends in Asian Pacific Rim Region. Tumor. 2004;24:422–6.
3. You WC, Jin F, Devesa S, et al. Rapid increase in colorectal cancer rates in urban Shanghai, 1972–97, in relation to dietary changes. J Cancer Epidemiol Prev. 2002;7:143–6.
4. Pfister DG, Benson AB, Somerfield MR. Clinical practice. Surveillance strategies after curative treatment of colorectal cancer. N Engl J Med. 2004;350:2375–2.
5. Hawk ET, Levin B. Colorectal cancer prevention. J Clin Oncol. 2005;23:378–1.
6. Shu Z, Hai Y, Gong Y, et al. Optimization of sequential screening scheme for colorectal cancer. Chinese Tumor. 1994;3:15–6.
7. Shinya H, Wolff WI. Morphology, anatomic distribution and cancer potential of colonic polyps. Ann Surg. 1979;190:679–3.
8. Al-Sukhni W, Aronson M, Gallinger S. Hereditary colorectal cancer syndromes: familial adenomatous polyposis and lynch syndrome. Surg Clin North Am. 2008;88:819–4.
9. Rex DK, Cutler CS, Lemmel GT, et al. Colonoscopic miss rates of adenomas determined by back-to-back colonoscopies. Gastroenterology. 1997;112:24–8.
10. Mak T, Lalloo F, Evans DG, Hill J. Molecular stool screening for colorectal cancer. Br J Surg. 2004;91:790.
11. Cotton PB, Durkalski VL, Pineau BC, et al. Computed tomographic colonography (virtual colonoscopy): a multicenter comparison with standard colonoscopy for detection of colorectal neoplasia. JAMA. 2004;291:1713–9.
12. Jianping W, Zuli Y, Yuanzhi T, et al. Effects of pelvic autonomic nerve preservation on male patients with rectal cancer. Chin J Pract Surg. 2003;23:44–6.
13. Jianping W, Huang M, Xinming S, et al. The assessment of curative effect after total mesorectal excision with autonomic nerve preservation for rectal cancer. Chin J Surg. 2005;43:1500–2.
14. Jianping W, Jun Z, Xinming S, et al. Analysis on pelvic autonomic nerve preservation in 120 female patients of rectal carcinoma undergoing radical resection. Chin J Gen Surg. 2005;20:619–21.
15. Jianping W, Guanfu C, Meijin H, et al. Influence of surgeon-related factors on postoperative sexual function in patients with rectal cancer. Chin J Pract Surg. 2005;25:688–9.
16. Ce Z, Zihai D, Guoxin L, et al. Anatomical observations of pelvic autonomic nerves concerning with total mesorectal excision. Chin J Clin Anat. 2006;24:60–4.
17. Willett CG, Compton CC, Shellito PC, Efird JT. Selection factors for local excision or abdominoperineal resection of early stage rectal cancer. Cancer. 1994;73:2716–20.
18. Greenberg JA, Shibata D, Herndon JE, et al. Local excision of distal rectal cancer: an update of cancer and leukemia group B 8984. Dis Colon Rectum. 2008;51:1185–4.
19. Paty PB, Nash GM, Baron P, et al. Long-term results of local excision for rectal cancer. Ann Surg. 2002;236:522–30.
20. McCall JL. Total mesorectal excision: evaluating the evidence. Aust N Z J Surg. 1997;67:599–2.
21. Kockerling F, Reymond MA, Altendorf-Hofmann A, et al. Influence of surgery on metachronous distant metastases and survival in rectal cancer. J Clin Oncol. 1998;16:324–9.
22. Heald RJ, Smedh RK, Kald A, et al. Abdominoperineal excision of the rectum – an endangered operation. Norman Nigro Lectureship. Dis Colon Rectum. 1997;40:747–1.
23. Carlsen E, Schlichting E, Guldvog I, et al. Effect of the introduction of total mesorectal excision for the treatment of rectal cancer. Br J Surg. 1998;85:526–9.
24. Law WL, Chu KW. Anterior resection for rectal cancer with mesorectal excision: a prospective evaluation of 622 patients. Ann Surg. 2004;240:260–8.
25. Martling AL, Holm T, Rutqvist LE, et al. Effect of a surgical training programme on outcome of rectal cancer in the County of Stockholm. Stockholm Colorectal Cancer Study Group, Basingstoke Bowel Cancer Research Project. Lancet. 2000;356:93–6.
26. Martling A, Cedermark B, Johansson H, et al. The surgeon as a prognostic factor after the introduction of total mesorectal excision in the treatment of rectal cancer. Br J Surg. 2002;89:1008–3.

27. Martling A, Holm T, Rutqvist LE, et al. Impact of a surgical training programme on rectal cancer outcomes in Stockholm. Br J Surg. 2005;92:225–9.
28. Takahashi T, Ueno M, Azekura K, Ohta H. Lateral node dissection and total mesorectal excision for rectal cancer. Dis Colon Rectum. 2000;43:59–8.
29. Xinshu D, Zhigao L, Binbin C, et al. Clinical significance of lateral lymphadenectomy in lower rectal cancer therapy. Chin J Bases Clin Gen Surg. 2003;10:103–4.
30. Grinnell RS. Lymphatic block with atypical and retrograde lymphatic metastasis and spread in carcinoma of the colon and rectum. Ann Surg. 1966;163:272–80.
31. Yano H, Moran BJ. The incidence of lateral pelvic side-wall nodal involvement in low rectal cancer may be similar in Japan and the West. Br J Surg. 2008;95:33–9.
32. Xinshu D, Haitao X, Zhigao L, et al. Effect of lateral lymph nodes dissection and autonomic nerve preservation in anterior resection for rectal cancer: 124 cases review. Chin J Surg. 2007;45:1164–6.
33. Wan Y, Pan Y, Yucun L, et al. Patterns of lymph node metastasis and extent of lymph node dissection for middle or lower rectal cancer: analysis of 462. Chin J Surg. 2001;39:425–8.
34. Wan Y, Pan Y, Yucun L, et al. The characteristics of lateral node metastasis in middle/lower rectal cancer and its influence on the prognosis. Chin J Gastrointest Surg. 2004;7:104–6.
35. Fleshman JW, Nelson H, Peters WR, et al. Early results of laparoscopic surgery for colorectal cancer. Retrospective analysis of 372 patients treated by Clinical Outcomes of Surgical Therapy (COST) Study Group. Dis Colon Rectum. 1996;39:53–8.
36. Nelson H, Sargent D, Wieand H, et al. A comparison of laparoscopically assisted and open colectomy for colon cancer. N Engl J Med. 2004;350:2050–9.
37. Veldkamp R, Kuhry E, Hop WC, et al. Laparoscopic surgery versus open surgery for colon cancer: short-term outcomes of a randomised trial. Lancet Oncol. 2005;6:477–4.
38. Buunen M, Veldkamp R, Hop WC, et al. Survival after laparoscopic surgery versus open surgery for colon cancer: long-term outcome of a randomised clinical trial. Lancet Oncol. 2009;10:44–2.
39. Weeks JC, Nelson H, Gelber S, et al. Short-term quality-of-life outcomes following laparoscopic-assisted colectomy vs open colectomy for colon cancer: a randomized trial. JAMA. 2002;287:321–8.
40. Jayne DG, Guillou PJ, Thorpe H, et al. Randomized trial of laparoscopic-assisted resection of colorectal carcinoma: 3-year results of the UK MRC CLASICC Trial Group. J Clin Oncol. 2007;25:3061–8.
41. Abraham NS, Young JM, Solomon MJ. Meta-analysis of short-term outcomes after laparoscopic resection for colorectal cancer. Br J Surg. 2004;91:1111–4.
42. Guillou P, Quirke P, Thorpe H, et al. Short-term endpoints of conventional versus laparoscopic-assisted surgery in patients with colorectal cancer (MRC CLASICC trial): multicentre, randomised controlled trial. Lancet. 2005;365:1718–6.
43. Leroy J, Jamali F, Forbes L, et al. Laparoscopic total mesorectal excision (TME) for rectal cancer surgery: long-term outcomes. Surg Endosc. 2004;18:281–9.
44. Minhua Z, Yanyan H, Aiguo L, et al. Clinical comparison of laparoscopic and open total mesorectal excision for lower rectal cancer. Chin J Gastrointest Surg. 2004;7:177–80.
45. Mei H, Zongguang Z, Wenzhang L, et al. Laparoscopic versus open total mesorectal excision with anal sphincter preservation for low rectal cancer: a randomized trial on short-term outcomes. Chin J Gastrointest Surg. 2003;6:368–71.
46. Lochan R, White SA, Manas DM. Liver resection for colorectal liver metastasis. Surg Oncol. 2007;16:33–5.
47. Altendorf-Hofmann A, Scheele J. A critical review of the major indicators of prognosis after resection of hepatic metastases from colorectal carcinoma. Surg Oncol Clin N Am. 2003;12:165–2.
48. Bengtsson G, Carlsson G, Hafstrom L, et al. Natural history of patients with untreated liver metastases from colorectal cancer. Am J Surg. 1981;141:586–9.
49. Minagawa M, Makuuchi M, Torzilli G, et al. Extension of the frontiers of surgical indications in the treatment of liver metastases from colorectal cancer: long-term results. Ann Surg. 2000;231:487–9.
50. Nagakura S, Shirai Y, Yokoyama N, et al. Major hepatic resection reduces the probability of intrahepatic recurrences following resection of colorectal carcinoma liver metastases. Hepatogastroenterology. 2003;50:779–3.
51. Solbiati L, Livraghi T, Goldberg SN, et al. Percutaneous radio-frequency ablation of hepatic metastases from colorectal cancer: long-term results in 117 patients. Radiology. 2001;221:159–6.
52. Desen W. Adjuvant chemotherapy and neoadjuvant chemotherapy for colorectal cancer. In: Desen W, editor. Colorectal cancer. Beijing, China: Peking University Medical Press; p. 203–20.
53. Wolmark N, Rockette H, Fisher B, et al. The benefit of leucovorin-modulated fluorouracil as postoperative adjuvant therapy for primary colon cancer: results from National Surgical Adjuvant Breast and Bowel Project protocol C-03. J Clin Oncol. 1993;11:1879–7.
54. Haller D, Catalano P, Macdonald J, et al. Fluorouracil (FU), leucovorin and levamisole adjuvant therapy for colon cancer: five year report of INT-0089. Proc Am Soc Clin Oncol. 1998;17:256a.
55. Wolmark N, Colangelo L, Wieand S. National surgical adjuvant breast and bowel project trials in colon cancer. Semin Oncol. 2001;28:9–3.
56. O'Connell MJ. North Central Cancer Treatment Group – Mayo Clinic trials in colon cancer. Semin Oncol. 2001;28:4–8.
57. Kelly H, Goldberg RM. Systemic therapy for metastatic colorectal cancer: current options, current evidence. J Clin Oncol. 2005;23:4553–60.

58. Adam R, Avisar E, Ariche A, et al. Five-year survival following hepatic resection after neoadjuvant therapy for nonresectable colorectal. Ann Surg Oncol. 2001;8:347–3.
59. Camma C, Giunta M, Fiorica F, et al. Preoperative radiotherapy for resectable rectal cancer: a meta-analysis. JAMA. 2000;284:1008–5.
60. Sauer R, Becker H, Hohenberger W, et al. Preoperative versus postoperative chemoradiotherapy for rectal cancer. N Engl J Med. 2004;351:1731–40.
61. Rodel C, Liersch T, Hermann RM, et al. Multicenter phase II trial of chemoradiation with oxaliplatin for rectal cancer. J Clin Oncol. 2007;25: 110–7.
62. Van CE, Dicato M, Wils J, et al. Adjuvant treatment of colorectal cancer (current expert opinion derived from the Third International Conference: perspectives in Colorectal Cancer, Dublin, 2001). Eur J Cancer. 2002;38:1429–6.
63. Baddi L, Benson 3rd A. Adjuvant therapy in stage II colon cancer: current approaches. Oncologist. 2005;10:325–1.
64. Efficacy of adjuvant fluorouracil and folinic acid in colon cancer. International Multicentre Pooled Analysis of Colon Cancer Trials (IMPACT) investigators. Lancet. 1995;345:939–4.
65. Schrag D, Rifas-Shiman S, Saltz L, et al. Adjuvant chemotherapy use for Medicare beneficiaries with stage II colon cancer. J Clin Oncol. 2002;20:3999–5.
66. Hurwitz H, Fehrenbacher L, Novotny W, et al. Bevacizumab plus irinotecan, fluorouracil, and leucovorin for metastatic colorectal cancer. N Engl J Med. 2004;350:2335–2.
67. Cunningham D, Humblet Y, Siena S, et al. Cetuximab monotherapy and cetuximab plus irinotecan in irinotecan-refractory metastatic colorectal cancer. N Engl J Med. 2004;351:337–5.
68. Tol J, Koopman M, Cats A, et al. Chemotherapy, bevacizumab, and cetuximab in metastatic colorectal cancer. N Engl J Med. 2009;360:563–2.
69. Hecht JR, Mitchell E, Chidiac T, et al. A randomized phase IIIB trial of chemotherapy, bevacizumab, and panitumumab compared with chemotherapy and bevacizumab alone for metastatic colorectal cancer. J Clin Oncol. 2009;27:672–80.
70. Lievre A, Bachet JB, Le CD, et al. KRAS mutation status is predictive of response to cetuximab therapy in colorectal cancer. Cancer Res. 2006;66:3992–5.
71. Ogino S, Meyerhardt JA, Cantor M, et al. Molecular alterations in tumors and response to combination chemotherapy with gefitinib for advanced colorectal cancer. Clin Cancer Res. 2005;11:6650–6.

2 Diagnosis and Treatment of Liver Metastases

Antoine Brouquet and Bernard Nordlinger

2.1 Introduction

The most frequent cause of death in patients with colorectal cancer is due to liver metastases. Approximately 50% of patients develop liver metastases at some point in the course of their disease, translating into approximately 500,000 patients worldwide [1]. Without any treatment, the median survival of patients with colorectal cancer liver metastases rarely exceeds 1 year, ranging from 3.8 to 21 months. The volume of liver involvement, the presence of extrahepatic disease, the metastatic lymph nodes in the mesentery, the carcinoembryonic antigen (CEA) level, and the age of the patient all influenced the survival rate [2].

If only a minority of patients with liver metastases is amenable to surgery, surgical resection remains the only treatment that can, to date, ensure long-term survival and cure in some patients [3]. Even if the presence of liver or lung metastases from colorectal cancer is associated with a poor prognosis, it does not always preclude curative treatment.

Recent progress including new chemotherapeutic regimens, ablative techniques, and interventional radiology may permit to increase the number of patients that can be treated with a curative intent. Unfortunately, recurrences are still observed in most patients after resection of liver metastases. To reduce this risk, new therapeutic modalities are based on combined strategy of treatment.

A. Brouquet • B. Nordlinger (✉)
Department of Digestive and Oncologic Surgery, Ambroise Paré Hospital Boulogne, Boulogne Cedex, France
e-mail: bernard.nordlinger@apr.aphp.fr

2.2 Diagnosis and Preoperative Assessment of Colorectal Liver Metastases

Clinical symptoms of colorectal liver metastases are usually late occurrences. In most cases, colorectal liver metastases are found during routine radiographic screening leading to the diagnosis of colorectal cancer or during the follow-up after resection of a colorectal primary tumor.

Because hepatic resection is the sole treatment associated with prolonged survival on patient with colorectal liver metastases, the pretherapeutic work-up in patients with colorectal liver metastases should determine whether lesions can be safely and completely removed and whether patients' conditions allow liver surgery. This work-up should precise the extent of the hepatic and extrahepatic disease, liver function, and comorbidities of the patient that could contraindicate the surgery.

Physical general status of patients has to be assessed before planning surgery. In particular, the question is to determine whether the patient can tolerate general anesthesia, clamping maneuvers required by liver surgery. American Society of

X. Qin et al. (eds.), *Multidisciplinary Management of Liver Metastases in Colorectal Cancer*, DOI 10.1007/978-94-017-7755-1_2

Anesthesiologists (ASA) score is a good tool to predict postoperative morbidity and mortality after liver resection and allows selection of patient who can safely undergo liver resection [4].

Preoperative imaging work-up of liver metastases should precise the respectability of the lesions and is currently based on ultrasound, multiphase helical computed tomography (CT) scan, and magnetic resonance imaging (MRI). These investigations should help to precise the number, the location, and the relationship to major liver vessels, and the distance from the anterior and posterior liver surface of the lesions. Liver metastases should be considered as resectable when all hepatic disease can be safely removed or locally treated leaving sufficient future liver remnant with adequate vascular inflow, venous outflow, and biliary drainage. Number, size, location of primary tumor, and CEA level should not be used as criteria to contraindicate liver resection.

Positron emission tomography–computed tomography (PET-CT) is valuable to rule out an extrahepatic spread of the disease since liver resection should not be performed in case of non-resectable extrahepatic disease [5, 6]. In case of unresectable liver metastases, treatment is initially based on chemotherapy, and imaging work-up is performed every 3 months to evaluate the tumor response and to determine whether a local treatment of the lesions can be considered. In addition, colonoscopy or CT colonography should be performed to exclude a local recurrence or metachronous colorectal neoplasia.

Liver function can be assessed using the Child-Pugh classification, blood liver function tests, and in some cases, the indocyanine green (ICG) retention tests. The volume of the non-tumorous parenchyma that will be left in place after hepatic resection should be evaluated by computed tomography (CT) scan volumetry.

2.3 Surgery for Colorectal Liver Metastases

2.3.1 Intraoperative Assessment

Surgery should start with a careful exploration of the abdominal cavity to rule out an extrahepatic spread of the disease or an unexpected bilobar involvement of the liver which could contraindicate the resection. This exploration includes palpation of the liver and intraoperative ultrasound (IOUS). IOUS is particularly useful to better precise the relationship of the lesions with vascular pedicles and can help to select the type of resection. IOUS can also guide radiofrequency ablation (RFA) of deep lesions in the future liver remnant.

2.3.2 Principles of Liver Resection for Colorectal Liver Metastases

Liver resection should be considered only in a curative intent. To date, there is no data to recommend debulking surgery for colorectal liver metastases. The size of surgical margin for the resection of colorectal liver metastases remains debated. Free surgical margin is an independent prognostic factor survival, and consequently, R0 resection is recommended [7–11].

The extent of liver resection depends on the number, the size, and the location of the lesions. If remnant liver parenchyma is normal, up to six of the eight anatomical segments, i.e., up to 75 % of the liver parenchyma, can be safely resected with low risk postoperative liver insufficiency. However, the majority of patient candidates for a liver resection have received a preoperative chemotherapy that could induce liver damage [12–17].

Liver resections are usually classified in anatomical (i.e., removing one or several segments) or atypical ("wedge") resections. Oncological results of these two types of resection are similar in the setting of colorectal liver metastases [17]. Resections removing three or more continuous segments are defined as major hepatic resections. Superficial small metastases can be resected with wedge resections. Larger lesions often require major resections.

2.3.3 Increasing the Resectability

Although liver resection is the sole treatment associated with prolonged survival in patients with colorectal liver metastases, only 10–15 % of patients have resectable liver metastases at the time of diagnosis [18]. During the past decades, refinements and improvements of surgical skills have led to extend the frontiers of resectability in patients with colorectal liver metastases [19].

2.3.3.1 Radiofrequency Ablation

In some cases, curative liver resection can be contraindicated because lesions are bilobar, and the extent of the planned liver resection is too large that could induce postoperative liver failure. Treatment of the lesions located in the future liver remnant can be achieved using tools for local destruction. Cryotherapy of liver metastases has been firstly used in this indication [20], but in situ recurrence rate was elevated. To date, radiofrequency ablation (RFA) is preferred [21].

RFA can be performed either percutaneously or intraoperatively. Different types of needle electrode can be used to treat liver metastases. The area of necrosis induced by RFA should be larger than the size of the tumor, by 1 cm, similar to the surgical margin obtained after surgical resection. Tumors of less than 3 cm located in the future remnant liver are currently the better indication of RFA. Indeed, in case tumor of 3 cm or more, oncologic results remain uncertain with the increased risk of in situ local recurrence [22].

2.3.3.2 Preoperative Portal Vein Embolization

If the future remnant liver after liver resection is too small to provide sufficient postoperative liver function, preoperative selective portal vein embolization has been proposed to induce ipsilateral atrophy and contralateral hypertrophy of the future remnant liver, thus preventing postoperative liver failure [23]. Following embolization, a liver resection judged primarily impossible, due to insufficient volume of remnant liver, is feasible in 60 % of cases, with mortality and morbidity rates comparable to those observed following liver resections without embolization. In case of bilobar lesions, induced liver regeneration or hypertrophy can be associated with an accelerated increase in the size of metastases located in the non-embolized liver [24]. Whether preoperative chemotherapy should be stopped after the embolization to avoid to decrease the hypertrophy of the liver or continued to control the disease during the time interval between the embolization and the hepatectomy is still debated [25–27].

2.3.3.3 Two-Stage Hepatectomy

Multiple bilobar liver metastases are often considered as unresectable. In selected cases, bilobar liver metastases can be resected in two stages. The first stage includes the resection or local destruction of lesions located in the future remnant liver which is in most cases the left liver. The second hepatectomy is generally a right or an extended right hepatectomy. During the first procedure, a right portal vein ligation can be performed if the volume of the left lobe is judged to be insufficient. Although this strategy can only be proposed in selected patients with unresectable liver metastases, oncologic outcome can be close to those observed in patients' resectable liver metastases [28].

2.3.3.4 Repeat Liver Resections for Recurrent Metastases

Recurrence limited to the liver following previous hepatic resection occurs in 25–50 % of cases and may be amenable to repeat resection [29]. Postoperative mortality and morbidity do not differ from those reported after a first resection, and the mean survival approaches 2 years. Hepatic recurrences should therefore be resected whenever technically feasible.

2.3.3.5 Preoperative Chemotherapy

In case of resectable liver metastases, preoperative chemotherapy can be administered to decrease the risk of recurrence, to test the chemosensitivity of the tumor, to guide the choice for postoperative treatment, and to facilitate the resection. One randomized trial [30] has recently showed that perioperative chemotherapy decreases the risk of recurrence after liver resection for resectable colorectal liver metastases (see Chap. 13).

In case of unresectable liver metastases, chemotherapy is initially the sole treatment that can be proposed. During the past decade, the introduction of new cytotoxic agents (camptothecin and oxaliplatin) and targeted therapies (bevacizumab and cetuximab) has led to increase the response rate and survival of patients with advanced colorectal cancer [31–36]. In patients with unresectable liver metastases, in case of tumor shrinkage during chemotherapy, curative liver resection may be considered. Several retrospective studies have showed that oncologic outcome of patients operated of initially unresectable liver metastases downstaged by chemotherapy may be good even in case of initial large hepatic involvement. Recurrence rate is close to 80 % and remains elevated in these patients, and 5-year survival rate can range from 25 to 35 % [20, 37, 38].

2.3.4 Postoperative Outcome

2.3.4.1 Early Postoperative Outcome

In most recent studies, in-hospital mortality rates vary from 0 to 5 % and are strongly influenced by intraoperative blood loss, preoperative liver function, and extent of liver resection [4]. Reversible postoperative complications are observed in 25–40 % of patients. Morbidity after hepatic resection is usually due to transient liver failure, hemorrhage, sub-phrenic abscesses, or biliary fistula. The mean hospital stay after liver surgery ranges from 10 to 15 days in the absence of complications.

Recent studies suggest that administration of preoperative chemotherapy could increase the risk of liver resection for colorectal liver metastases. Morbidity rate may be slightly increased in patients who have received a preoperative chemotherapy [14–16]. The impact of preoperative chemotherapy on postoperative mortality after liver resection is debated, and to date, only one study has reported that chemotherapy could increase the mortality after liver resection. In this study, the mortality rate was increased in patients who had lesions of chemotherapy associated steatohepatitis [15].

2.3.4.2 Oncologic Results

Liver resection of colorectal metastases is associated with 3- and 5-year survival rates close to 40 % and 30 %, respectively. After resection, recurrences are observed in two-thirds of patients and involve the liver in 50 % of cases.

Several studies have assessed factors influencing survival. Risk factors of recurrence have been identified using multivariate analysis on two large series of more than 1,000 patients [7–9]: age, size of the largest metastasis, elevated CEA level, stage of the primary tumor and lymph node involvement, disease-free interval <12 months, number of liver nodules, and involved surgical margin. However, these studies did not take into account the potential impact of associated treatment and in particular the administration of chemotherapy.

Response to chemotherapy is a very strong prognosis factor of survival in patients operated of colorectal liver metastases [39–42].

2.4 Treatment Strategy for Colorectal Liver Metastases

Although liver resection allows prolonged survival in a subset of patients with colorectal liver metastases, recurrences are still observed. Recurrence rate after hepatectomy approaches two third. To decrease the risk to tumor relapse, combined strategy using chemotherapy before, after, or both in association with surgery has been proposed.

2.4.1 Results of Combined Therapeutic Strategies for Colorectal Liver Metastases

Adjuvant treatment has firstly been evaluated for the treatment of resected colorectal liver metastases. Efficacy of postoperative treatment using systemic chemotherapy or hepatic arterial infusion with 5-FU, folinic acid, or floxuridine has been tested after resection of liver metastases from colorectal cancer (CRC) in several randomized studies [43–47], but survival benefit has not yet been clearly demonstrated. These data have been confirmed in a recent meta-analysis that showed that adjuvant CT with a 5-FU-based regimen versus no postoperative chemotherapy tends to improve disease-free and overall survival after complete resection of CRC metastases, but the observed improvement in survival was not statistically significant [48].

More recently, the administration of a perioperative oxaliplatin-based chemotherapy for the treatment of colorectal liver metastases has been evaluated in a randomized trial. Administration of perioperative chemotherapy (six cycles before and six cycles after surgery) was associated with a slight increase of reversible complication rate after liver resection when compared to surgery alone. This study showed that perioperative chemotherapy was associated with a decrease of recurrence rate after liver resection [30]. To date, administration of perioperative chemotherapy should be the standard of care for resectable colorectal liver metastases (see Chap. 13).

2.4.2 Synchronous Liver Metastases

Treatment strategy of patients with synchronous liver metastases depends on the resectability of liver metastases, the location of the primary tumor, and the eventual symptoms or complications due to the presence of the primary tumor.

2.4.2.1 Resectable Liver Metastases

In case of resectable liver metastases, treatment strategy depends on the extent of the hepatic disease and the location of the primary tumor. In patients with colon cancer, resection of primary tumor is usually performed first. After resection of primary tumor, preoperative chemotherapy can be administered before the resection of liver metastases to reduce the risk of recurrence. If hepatic disease is localized, combined surgery may be discussed after a preoperative chemotherapy. In patients with rectal cancer, the treatment strategy depends on whether treatment of primary tumor required a preoperative chemoradiotherapy.

2.4.2.2 Unresectable Liver Metastases

In case of unresectable liver metastases, chemotherapy is the treatment of choice (Benoist *Br J Surg*). The resection of the primary tumor before the start of chemotherapy can be discussed according to the risk of local complication (bleeding or obstruction). In case of major response to chemotherapy and downstaging of liver disease, resection of the residual disease may be considered. In this situation, liver resection can be performed after, in the same operating time, or after the resection of the primary tumor [49–52].

2.5 Conclusion

To date, a subgroup of patient with colorectal liver metastases can be cured by liver resection. For this reason, early detection of colorectal liver metastases in patients treated for colorectal cancer is needed and justified.

Liver resection allows prolonged survival in a subset of patients with resectable lesions. This is an efficient and safe treatment so far. Unfortunately, only a minority of patients (10–15 %) with colorectal liver metastases have a resectable disease at the time of the diagnosis and more than half of operated patients will develop recurrences during the follow-up.

Objectives in the future for the treatment of colorectal liver metastases should be to increase the resectability rate and to decrease the recurrence rate after curative liver resection. Multimodality treatment including combined strategy could lead to improve oncologic results of surgery for colorectal liver metastases.

References

1. Jemal A, Siegel R, Ward E, Hao Y, Xu J, Thun MJ. Cancer statistics. CA Cancer J Clin. 2009;59:225–49.
2. Stangl R, Altendorf-Hofmann A, Charnley RM, Scheele J. Factors influencing the natural history of colorectal liver metastases. Lancet. 1994;343:1405–10.
3. Scheele J. Hepatectomy for liver metastases. Br J Surg. 1993;80:274–6.
4. Belghiti J, Hiramatsu K, Benoist S, Massault P, Sauvanet A, Farges O. Seven hundred forty-seven hepatectomies in the 1990s: an update to evaluate the actual risk of liver resection. J Am Coll Surg. 2000;191:38–46.
5. Bipat S, van Leeuwen MS, Comans EF, et al. Colorectal liver metastases: CT, MR imaging, and PET for diagnosis – meta-analysis. Radiology. 2005;237:123–31.
6. Truant S, Huglo D, Hebbar M, Ernst O, Steinling M, Pruvot FR. Prospective evaluation of the impact of [18F]fluoro-2-deoxy-D-glucose positron emission

tomography of resectable colorectal liver metastases. Br J Surg. 2005;92:362–9.
7. Fong Y, Fortner J, Sun RL, Brennan MF, Blumgart LH. Clinical score for predicting recurrence after hepatic resection for metastatic colorectal cancer: analysis of 1001 consecutive cases. Ann Surg. 1999;230:309–18.
8. Nordlinger B, Jaeck D, Guiguet M, Vaillant JC, Balladur P, Schaal JC. Surgical resection of hepatic metastases. Multicentric retrospective study by the French Association of Surgery. In: Nordlinger B, Jaeck D, editors. Treatment of hepatic metastases of colorectal cancer. Paris: Springer; 1992. p. 129–46.
9. Nordlinger B, Guiguet M, Vaillant J-C, et al. Surgical resection of colorectal carcinoma metastases to the liver. A prognostic scoring system to improve case selection, based on 1568 patients. Cancer. 1996;77: 1254–62.
10. Pawlik TM, Scoggins CR, Zorzi D, Abdalla EK, Andres A, Eng C, Curley SA, Loyer EM, Muratore A, Mentha G, Capussotti L, Vauthey JN. Effect of surgical margin status on survival and site of recurrence after hepatic resection for colorectal metastases. Ann Surg. 2005;241:715–22.
11. Bodingbauer M, Tamandl D, Schmid K, Plank C, Schima W, Gruenberger T. Size of surgical margin does not influence recurrence rates after curative liver resection for colorectal cancer liver metastases. Br J Surg. 2007;94:1133–8.
12. Rubbia-Brandt L, Audard V, Sartoretti P, et al. Severe hepatic sinusoidal obstruction associated with oxaliplatin-based chemotherapy in patients with metastatic colorectal cancer. Ann Oncol. 2004;15:460–6.
13. Fernandez FG, Ritter J, Goodwin JW, Linehan DC, Hawkins WG, Strasberg SM. Effect of steatohepatitis associated with irinotecan or oxaliplatin pretreatment on resectability of hepatic colorectal metastases. J Am Coll Surg. 2005;200:845–53.
14. Karoui M, Penna C, Amin-Hashem M, et al. Influence of preoperative chemotherapy on the risk of major hepatectomy for colorectal liver metastases. Ann Surg. 2006;243:1–7.
15. Vauthey JN, Pawlik TM, Ribero D, et al. Chemotherapy regimen predicts steatohepatitis and an increase in 90-day mortality after surgery for hepatic colorectal metastases. J Clin Oncol. 2006;24:2065–72.
16. Brouquet A, Benoist S, Julie C, Penna C, Beauchet A, Rougier P, Nordlinger B. Risk factors for chemotherapy-associated liver injuries: a multivariate analysis of a group of 146 patients with colorectal metastases. Surgery. 2009;145:362–71.
17. Finch RJ, Malik HZ, Hamady ZZ, Al-Mukhtar A, Adair R, Prasad KR, Lodge JP, Toogood GJ. Effect of type of resection on outcome of hepatic resection for colorectal metastases. Br J Surg. 2007;94:1242–8.
18. Scheele J, Stang R, Altendorf-Hofmann A, et al. Resection of colorectal metastases. World J Surg. 1995;191:59–71.
19. Chun YS, Vauthey JN. Extending the frontiers of resectability in advanced colorectal cancer. Eur J Surg Oncol. 2007;33:S52–8.
20. Rivoire M, De Cian F, Meeus P, Négrier S, Sebban H, Kaemmerlen P. Combination of neoadjuvant chemotherapy with cryotherapy and surgical resection for the treatment of unresectable liver metastases from colorectal carcinoma. Cancer. 2002;95: 2283–92.
21. Abdalla EK, Vauthey JN, Ellis LM, Ellis V, Pollock R, Broglio KR, Hess K, Curley SA. Recurrence and outcomes following hepatic resection, radiofrequency ablation, and combined resection/ablation for colorectal liver metastases. Ann Surg. 2004;239:818–25.
22. Berber E, Siperstein A. Local recurrence after laparoscopic radiofrequency ablation of liver tumors: an analysis of 1032 tumors. Ann Surg Oncol. 2008;15: 2757–64.
23. Azoulay D, Castaing D, Smail A, Adam R, Cailliez V, Laurent A, Lemoine A, Bismuth H. Resection of nonresectable liver metastases from colorectal cancer after percutaneous portal vein embolization. Ann Surg. 2000;231:480–6.
24. Elias D, De Baere T, Roche A, Mducreux, Leclere J, Lasser P. During liver regeneration following right portal embolization the growth rate of liver metastases is more rapid than that of the liver parenchyma. Br J Surg. 1999;86:784–8.
25. Goéré D, Farges O, Leporrier J, Sauvanet A, Vilgrain V, Belghiti J. Chemotherapy does not impair hypertrophy of the left liver after right portal vein obstruction. J Gastrointest Surg. 2006;10:365–70.
26. Beal IK, Anthony S, Papadopoulou A, Hutchins R, Fusai G, Begent R, Davies N, Tibballs J, Davidson B. Portal vein embolisation prior to hepatic resection for colorectal liver metastases and the effects of periprocedure chemotherapy. Br J Radiol. 2006;79:473–8.
27. Brouquet A, Belghiti J. Chemotherapy and its effect on liver hypertrophy: implications for portal vein embolization and resection. Semin Interv Radiol. 2008;25:162–6.
28. Jaeck D, Oussoultzoglou E, Rosso E, Greget M, Weber JC, Bachellier P. A two-stage hepatectomy procedure combined with portal vein embolization to achieve curative resection for initially unresectable multiple and bilobar colorectal liver metastases. Ann Surg. 2004;240:1037–49.
29. Nordlinger B, Vaillant JC, Guiguet M, Balladur P, Paris F, Bachellier P, Jaeck D. Survival benefit of repeat liver resections for recurrent colorectal metastases: 143 cases. Association Francaise de Chirurgie. J Clin Oncol. 1994;12:1491–6.
30. Nordlinger B, Sorbye H, Glimelius B, Poston GJ, Schlag PM, Rougier P, Bechstein WO, Primrose JN, Walpole ET, Finch-Jones M, Jaeck D, Mirza D, Parks RW, Collette L, Praet M, Bethe U, Van Cutsem E, Scheithauer W, Gruenberger T. Perioperative chemotherapy with FOLFOX4 and surgery versus surgery alone for resectable liver metastases from colorectal cancer (EORTC Intergroup trial 40983): a randomised controlled trial. Lancet. 2008;371:1007–16.
31. de Gramont A, Figer A, Seymour M, Homerin M, Hmissi A, Cassidy J, Boni C, Cortes-Funes H,

Cervantes A, Freyer G, Papamichael D, Le Bail N, et al. Leucovorin and fluorouracil with or without oxaliplatin as first-line treatment in advanced colorectal cancer. J Clin Oncol. 2000;18:2938–47.
32. Douillard JY, Cunningham D, Roth AD, Navarro M, James RD, Karasek P, Jandik P, Iveson T, Carmichael J, Alakl M, Gruia G, Awad L, et al. Irinotecan combined with fluorouracil compared with fluorouracil alone as first-line treatment for metastatic colorectal cancer: a multicentre randomized trial. Lancet. 2000;355:1041–7.
33. Falcone A, Ricci S, Brunetti I, Pfanner E, Allegrini G, Barbara C, Crinò L, Benedetti G, Evangelista W, Fanchini L, Cortesi E, Picone V, et al. Phase III trial of infusional fluorouracil, leucovorin, oxaliplatin, and irinotecan (FOLFOXIRI) compared with infusional fluorouracil, leucovorin, and irinotecan (FOLFIRI) as first-line treatment for metastatic colorectal cancer: the Gruppo Oncologico Nord Ovest. J Clin Oncol. 2007;25:1670–6.
34. Cunningham D, Humblet Y, Siena S, Khayat D, Bleiberg H, Santoro A, Bets D, Mueser M, Harstrick A, Verslype C, Chau I, Van Cutsem E. Cetuximab monotherapy and cetuximab plus irinotecan in irinotecan-refractory metastatic colorectal cancer. N Engl J Med. 2004;351:337–45.
35. Hurwitz H, Fehrenbacher L, Novotny W, Cartwright T, Hainsworth J, Heim W, Berlin J, Baron A, Griffing S, Holmgren E, Ferrara N, Fyfe G, et al. Bevacizumab plus irinotecan, fluorouracil, and leucovorin for metastatic colorectal cancer. N Engl J Med. 2004;350:2335–42.
36. Van Cutsem E, Köhne CH, Hitre E, Zaluski J, Chang Chien CR, Makhson A, D'Haens G, Pintér T, Lim R, Bodoky G, Roh JK, et al. Cetuximab and chemotherapy as initial treatment for metastatic colorectal cancer. N Engl J Med. 2009;360:1408–17.
37. Meric F, Patt YZ, Curley SA, Chase J, Roh MS, Vauthey JN, Ellis LM. Surgery after downstaging of unresectable hepatic tumors with intra-arterial chemotherapy. Ann Surg Oncol. 2000;7:490–5.
38. Adam R, Delvart V, Pascal G, Valeanu A, Castaing D, Azoulay D, Giacchetti S, Paule B, Kunstlinger F, Ghémard O, Levi F, Bismuth H. Rescue surgery for unresectable colorectal liver metastases downstaged by chemotherapy: a model to predict long-term survival. Ann Surg. 2004;240:644–57.
39. Adam R, Pascal G, Castaing D, Azoulay D, Delvart V, Paule B, Levi F, Bismuth H. Tumor progression while on chemotherapy: a contraindication to liver resection for multiple colorectal metastases? Ann Surg. 2004;240:1052–61.
40. Rubbia-Brandt L, Giostra E, Brezault C, Roth AD, Andres A, Audard V, Sartoretti P, Dousset B, Majno PE, Soubrane O, Chaussade S, Mentha G, Terris B. Importance of histological tumor response assessment in predicting the outcome in patients with colorectal liver metastases treated with neo-adjuvant chemotherapy followed by liver surgery. Ann Oncol. 2007;18:299–304.
41. Allen PJ, Kemeny N, Jarnagin W, DeMatteo R, Blumgart L, Fong Y. Importance of response to neoadjuvant chemotherapy in patients undergoing resection of synchronous colorectal liver metastases. J Gastrointest Surg. 2003;7:109–15.
42. Blazer 3rd DG, Kishi Y, Maru DM, Kopetz S, Chun YS, Overman MJ, Fogelman D, Eng C, Chang DZ, Wang H, Zorzi D, Ribero D, Ellis LM, Glover KY, Wolff RA, Curley SA, Abdalla EK, Vauthey JN. Pathologic response to preoperative chemotherapy: a new outcome end point after resection of hepatic colorectal metastases. J Clin Oncol. 2008;26:5344–51.
43. Lorenz M, Muller HH, Schramm H, et al. Randomized trial of surgery versus surgery followed by adjuvant hepatic arterial infusion with 5-fluorouracil and folinic acid for liver metastases of colorectal cancer. German Cooperative on Liver Metastases. Ann Surg. 1998;228:756–62.
44. Kemeny N, Huang Y, Cohen AM, et al. Hepatic arterial infusion of chemotherapy after resection of hepatic metastases from colorectal cancer. N Engl J Med. 1999;341:2039–48.
45. Kemeny MM, Adak S, Gray B, et al. Combined-modality treatment for resectable metastatic colorectal carcinoma to the liver: surgical resection of hepatic metastases in combination with continuous infusion of chemotherapy-an intergroup study. J Clin Oncol. 2002;20:1499–505.
46. Portier G, Elias D, Bouche O, et al. Multicenter randomized trial of adjuvant fluorouracil and folinic acid compared with surgery alone after resection of colorectal liver metastases: FFCD ACHBTH AURC 9002 trial. J Clin Oncol. 2006;24:4976–82.
47. Langer B, Bleiberg H, Labianca R. Fluorouracil (FU) plus l-leucovorin (l-LV) versus observation after potentially curative resection of liver or lung metastases from colorectal cancer (CRC): results of the ENG (EORTC/NCIC CTG/GIVIO) randomized trial. J Clin Oncol. 2002;20:149a (abstr 592).
48. Mitry E, Fields A, Bleiberg H, et al. Adjuvant chemotherapy after potentially curative resection of metastases from colorectal cancer. A meta-analysis of two randomized trials. J Clin Oncol. 2006;24(18S):3524.
49. Benoist S, Pautrat K, Mitry E, Rougier P, Penna C, Nordlinger B. Treatment strategy for patients with colorectal cancer and synchronous irresectable liver metastases. Br J Surg. 2005;92:1155–60.
50. Mentha G, Majno PE, Andres A, Rubbia-Brandt L, Morel P, Roth AD. Neoadjuvant chemotherapy and resection of advanced synchronous liver metastases before treatment of the colorectal primary. Br J Surg. 2006;93:872–8.
51. Bretagnol F, Hatwell C, Farges O, Alves A, Belghiti J, Panis Y. Benefit of laparoscopy for rectal resection in patients operated simultaneously for synchronous liver metastases: preliminary experience. Surgery. 2008;144:436–41.
52. Martin 2nd RC, Augenstein V, Reuter NP, Scoggins CR, McMasters KM. Simultaneous versus staged resection for synchronous colorectal cancer liver metastases. J Am Coll Surg. 2009;208:842–50.

3 Molecular Mechanism of Hepatic Metastasis of Colorectal Cancer

Shu Zheng

3.1 Overview of the Study on Hepatic Metastasis of Colorectal Cancer

In the event of distant metastasis of colorectal cancer, the liver is the main metastatic site, accounting for about 38–60 % [1]. Early-stage hepatic metastasis of colorectal cancer has few clinical manifestations. Only 20 % of patients are suitable for surgical treatment [2], and 5-year survival rate of the patients with hepatic metastasis of colorectal cancer is nearly zero if they do not receive any treatment. Hepatic metastasis is one of the main reasons for the death of colorectal cancer patients. It is a problem that should be solved to probe the mechanism of hepatic metastasis of colorectal cancer and find molecular markers for early diagnosis and treatment targets.

Tumor metastasis is a complex biological phenomenon. It is one of the biological characteristics of malignant tumors, which can be realized from the following four stages:

1. Metastatic process includes three steps, i.e., detachment of tumor cells from the primary focus, transportation, and growth, including:
   (a) Local infiltration: adhesion force between tumor cells will decrease; extracellular matrix of various enzymes secreted by tumor cells promotes metastasis.
   (b) Detachment of tumor cell: under the action of enzymes, tumor cells pass through blood vessel endothelium and basement membrane and enter blood circulation.
   (c) Tumor cells survive in circulation. Cell subgroups with high metastatic potential adhere to blood vessel endothelium and effuse out of vessel wall to form a metastatic focus.
   (d) Tumor cell adheres to endothelial cell or subendothelial basement membrane and capillary bed.
   (e) Tumor cells proliferate and grow in a new microenvironment.
2. Nodes and network. Numerous and complicated links of transduction, regulation, inhibition, or activation exist between tumor-related genes. Numerous genes and proteins play their roles in different pathways. Metastasis of colorectal cancer is also a complex process regulated by many genes and involving many pathways. A small part of genes plays a role as driver [3]. Only from the perspective of pathways or even the whole network, more systematic studies can discover their important roles in this process.

S. Zheng
Cancer Institute, The Second Affiliated Hospital, Zhejiang University School of Medicine, Hangzhou, China
e-mail: zhengshu@zju.edu.cn

X. Qin et al. (eds.), *Multidisciplinary Management of Liver Metastases in Colorectal Cancer*, DOI 10.1007/978-94-017-7755-1_3

3. Epithelial-mesenchymal transition. "Epithelial-mesenchymal transition" (EMT) [4, 5] refers to the process in which epithelial cell loses its original epithelial characteristics and polar arrangement, etc., and transits to mesenchymal phenotype. During the course of tumor metastasis, tumor cell exhibits some characteristics of mesenchymal cell, such as adhesion characteristic, enhancement of protein hydrolysis and activity, etc., which enables tumor cell to metastasize and form metastatic focus at distant site. On the contrary, "mesenchymal-epithelial transition" (MET) enables tumor cell to inhabit the site.
4. Primary tumor cell decides metastasis. Gene phenotype of tumor cell decides its metastatic characteristics. The quantity of metastasis-related gene expression directly influences the occurrence of hepatic metastasis [6].

3.2 Factors Influencing Hepatic Metastasis of Colorectal Cancer

The formation of metastatic focus of colorectal cancer is closely associated with biological characteristics of tumor cells, immunity status of human body, and microenvironment of organs. Only when the condition in each aspect is satisfied can tumor cells form metastatic focus in a certain organ.

3.2.1 Host Immunity and Tumor Metastasis

After occurrence of tumor, human body may play an antitumor role through immune response mechanism [7]. The antitumor immune mechanism of human body includes cellular immunity and humoral immunity. They work with each other to jointly kill and wound tumor cells. Cellular immunity is the main antitumor immunity mode. Humoral immunity has a synergetic effect in some cases generally.

3.2.2 Metastatic Capability of Tumor Cells

Animal experiment study found that there are 2×106 cells that will enter blood circulation every day for a 1 mm^3 size cancer, while not more than 1 % can survive within 24 h, and not more than 0.1 % of tumor cells that enter circulation can eventually survive and form metastasis [8]. Tumor metastasis is the result of selective proliferation of cell subgroups with metastatic potential.

Tumor stem cell theory makes a new explanation for this. A small group of cells with stem cell characteristic exists in tumor tissue, called as tumor stem cells. A single cell can develop into a tumor, with self-renewal and multilineage differentiation capabilities of stem cells. Most other tumor cells only have relative proliferation capability. Tumor stem cells are initiating cells to form tumor, which maintain the growth of tumor and probably the source of tumor metastasis and recurrence [9].

3.2.3 Local Microenvironment of Organs

The occurrence of metastasis not only depends on the characteristics of tumor cells but also on host reaction. Microenvironment affects the stability of tumor cells and has a highly selective inhibitory effect on final survival and growth of metastatic tumor cells [10]. In 1889, Paget put forward "seed and soil" theory. Growth of metastatic focus is affected by mutual action between certain tumor cells and the environment of certain organs. Only when seed and soil match each other can metastasis be successfully formed [11].

Recently some people also put forward that before reaching target organ, tumor cells would mobilize marrow cells to reach the target organ in advance or release some factors to change the microenvironment of the target organ so that it is suitable for the growth of tumor cells. Kaplan et al. [12] discovered that in the mouse that received the injection of positive marrow cells of VEGF receptor, tumor metastasis is more easy to occur. The possible mechanisms are as follows: positive marrow cells of VEGF receptor reach the metastatic focus earlier than tumor cells and improve the microenvironment so that they become suitable for the growth of tumor cells; primary tumor may produce some chemical active substances. Under the influence of such substances, the marrow will enhance the metastatic capability of the tumor cells that have existed in the marrow.

3.3 Hepatic Metastasis of Colorectal Cancer-Related Molecular Events

Infiltrated growth and metastasis of colorectal cancer relies on the changes in special phenotypes that it has gradually obtained. Such changes are caused by multiple molecular events. Here we will make a brief description for the related important molecular events:

3.3.1 Cell Adhesion

Cell adhesion event plays a very important role in tumor metastatic process. On one hand, change in the expression of some adhesion molecules of tumor cells may weaken the adhesion between the cells so that tumor cells are detached from the adjacent cells; on the other hand, some adhesion molecules of tumor cell expression enable the tumor cells that have entered the blood to be adhered to blood vessel endothelial cells or certain cells of the metastatic target organ, causing hematogenous metastasis and accelerating the formation of metastatic focus [13]. Metastatic process of tumor cells above all is the alternate process of adhesion and detachment. In this process, many adhesion molecules play their roles.

3.3.1.1 Cadherin-Catenin System

Cadherin is a kind of transmembrane glycoprotein responsible for adhesion between calcium-dependent cells. It is involved in mutual action between subfamily-specific cells. It is involved in the selective cell adhesion at different development stages of tissue. Cytoplasmic function field of cadherin is connected with catenin. Deactivation of cadherin leads to the damage to cell-cell adhesion. Its overexpression will cause closer cell-cell contact. E-cadherin (ECAD) with continuous expression and functional activity plays a role of maintaining cell integration in the epithelium. In colon cancer, expression of E-cadherin and α-catenin is downregulated. In about 80 % of primary colon cancer, α- and β-catenin expression decreases. Significant decrease in α-catenin expression is associated with poor differentiation, high metastatic potential, and bad prognosis [14–17].

3.3.1.2 Carcinoembryonic Antigen (CEA)

CEA is an important marker of expression in dedifferentiation process of colorectal cancer, which is one of the most valuable tumor markers. It is most widely applied in early-stage detection of hepatic metastasis of colorectal cancer. CEA receptor on liver Kupffer cell induces Kupffer cell to secrete cell factors (IL-1α, IL-1β, IL-6, TNFα) to induce expression of adhesion molecules of endothelial cells of hepatic antrum, which increases tumor adhesion and retention in the liver. Apply reverse transcription polymetase chain reaction (RT-PCR) to detect expression of CEA mRNA in peripheral blood and marrow so as to judge if there is tumor cell in peripheral blood of colorectal cancer patient or not [18].

3.3.1.3 CD44

CD44 is a kind of transmembrane hyaluronic acid receptor, which mediates the adhesion to endothelial cell. High expression of its aberrants CD44v6 and CD44v8-10 is deemed as closely associated with hepatic metastasis of colorectal cancer. Interception of this combination of adhesion molecule with related ligand perhaps can block the occurrence of hepatic metastasis of colorectal cancer. CD44 aberrant splicing may influence the conglomeration and distribution of cytoskeletal protein of tumor cell so as to influence tumor cell migration and movement capability. Joint effect in several aspects results in the formation of tumor metastasis [19]. Aberrant tumor cell expression of CD44 may escape the reorganization and avoid clearance by host immunity system in metastatic process.

3.3.1.4 Integrin

Integrin can integrate intracellular skeleton and extracellular matrix to form an entirety. At the same time, integrin also participates adhesion between cells. Results of the immunohistochemical experiment conducted by Akamura et al. [20] indicate that tissue integrin α VLA3 staining of 58 % (11/19) of colorectal cancer with hepatic metastasis is positive, significantly higher than that of the tissue without metastasis (0 %). The expression level of integrin α3β1 in the tissue of hepatic metastasis of colorectal cancer is also significantly higher than that of primary tissue. In addition, integrin is very important in invasion as it combines with MMP2 and uPAR.

3.3.2 Movement and Invasion

In the movement and invasion of colon cancer cells, hepatic growth factor (HGF) is a major influencing factor produced by the liver. Overexpression of the receptor c-met of HGF plays an important role in the progress of colorectal cancer, inducing tumor cell migration. In recent years, much evidence indicates that HGF is associated with the formation of hepatic metastasis of colorectal cancer [21]. c-met level in hepatic metastatic focus is relatively high. Overexpression of c-met only occurs in 50 % of primary tumor, while c-met level of about 70 % of hepatic metastatic foci is higher than that of the primary tumor of the same patient. All these results indicate that overexpression of c-met plays an important role in screening tumor cells with migration and formation of distant metastasis.

Transforming growth factor (TGF) is a normal colon epithelial cell growth inhibitor and is also associated with the enhancement of movement and migration of colon tumor cells. The study indicates that expression of TGF in metastatic tumor is higher than that in primary tumor [22], and TGF-β1 can inhibit tumor metastasis at the early stage of formation of tumor. Downregulation of its expression level may promote tumor growth. Perhaps it can reduce adhesion between tumor cells and participate in basement membrane degradation and tumor angiogenesis, etc. But at late stage, it may promote tumor expansion.

3.3.3 Degradation of Extracellular Matrix

During the course of invasion and metastasis, tumor cells must damage intercellular matrix and basement membrane (BM) extracellular matrix (ECM). ECM and BM are composed of collagen, laminin, protein polysaccharides, and other molecules produced by epithelial cells, matrix cells, and even tumor cells. Proteins that may participate in this process mainly include matrix-degrading metalloproteinases (MMPs), serine proteinase, elastase, aspartase, and cysteine protease, etc. [23].

3.3.3.1 Matrix-Degrading Metalloproteinases (MMP)

Both tumor and connective tissue cells can secrete MMPs, which is divided into four subfamilies, i.e., collagenases, gelatinases, stromelysins, and metalloelastases. MMP1 and MMP13 in MMP family promote the damage to peripheral mesenchymas of the cancer and cancer proliferation and infiltration. MMP2, MMP3, MMP7, and MMP9 may damage type IV collagenase that constitutes basement membrane and promote cancer cells to enter blood vessel [24]. At the same time, there exist three kinds of MMP-specific inhibitors, called as tissue inhibitor of metalloproteinases (TIMPs). Balance between MMPs and TMPs influences tumor invasion and phenotype [25].

3.3.3.2 Plasminogen/Fibrinase System

Plasminogen activator (PA) and plasminogen activator inhibitor (PAI) system are other important proteinase systems related to tumor metastasis. It was originally discovered in blood circulation. PA may be divided into urokinase-type plasminogen activator (uPA) and tissue-type plasminogen activator (tPA). They belong to serine proteinase family and can transform plasminogen to fibrinase so as to play a synergetic role in the degradation of ECM and activation of proteinases and promote tumor invasion and metastasis [14].

3.3.4 Formation of Tumor Vessel

Since Folkman discovered the phenomenon that tumor grows relying on the formation of blood vessel, many factors that positively and negatively regulate the formation of blood vessel have been discovered, such as vascular endothelial growth factor (VEGF), basic fibroblast growth factor (BFGF), transforming growth factor (TGF), interleukin 8 (IL-8), matrix metalloproteinase (MMP), blood platelet-activating factor, and so on. Tumor survival and metastasis rely on the comprehensive results of positive and negative regulating factors, which tend to result in tumor angiogenesis.

VEGF is a mitogenetic factor of special endothelial cell. It plays its part mainly through three receptors on the endothelial cell, i.e., flk, flt1, and flt4. VEGF may be secreted by tumor cell. The high expression level of VEGF was improved not only by the influence of stimulation signal,such as hypoxia, but also cell regulation, such as IL-1, IL-6, IL-8, TGF, platelet-derived growth factor (PDGF). Block of the activity of VEGF with antibody that resists VEGF receptor or with specific tyrosine kinase inhibitor that blocks the action of VEGF receptor can reduce quantity, size, and vessel density of hepatic metastatic foci of mice colon cancer model [26].

Sialyl-Lewis x (sLex) antigen, as the ligand of E-selectin receptor on the surface of hepatic blood vessel endothelial cell, plays an important role in hepatic metastasis of colorectal cancer. Tumor cell highly expressing sLex antigen is detached from the primary focus, enters the blood vessel, adheres to hepatic blood vessel endothelium, and grows to form a hepatic metastatic tumor. High expression sLex antigen cell is more easy to infiltrate basement membrane and adheres to activated human blood vessel endothelial cell to form hepatic metastasis. This is because that sLex antigen on the surface of tumor cell, serving as the ligand of E-selectin on the surface of capillary vessel endothelial cell, mediates adhesion of tumor cell to blood vessel endothelial cells of the target organ and promotes the directional chemotactic movement of tumor cell so that metastasis is produced. Many studies also verify that expression of sLex antigen in metastatic focus of colorectal cancer is stronger than that in primary focus [27, 28].

3.4 Colorectal Tumor Metastasis-Related Gene Study

The Cancer Research Institute of Zhejiang University conducted the following work in the aspect of genetic study related to the hepatic metastasis of colorectal tumor:

1. Based on Affymetrix GeneChip system, screened out osteopontin and maspin genes with differential expression in hepatic metastasis tissue from more than 12,000 known genes and EST
2. Studied the biological role of SNC19/ST14 genes obtained in suppression subtractive hybridization library of colorectal cancer and related normal mucosa in hepatic metastasis of colorectal cancer
3. Conducted integrated analysis by combining gene expression profile and cytoband, searched for related genes in hepatic metastasis of colorectal cancer, and discovered SPARCL1
4. Literally reviewed the possible action mechanism of PRL-3 hepatic metastasis of colorectal cancer in occurrence and development process

3.4.1 Osteopontin (OPN)

Based on the detection of 21 pairs of colorectal cancer, normal intestinal mucosa, lymph node, and hepatic metastatic tissue specimens by using Affymetrix GeneChip system, the Cancer Research Institute of Zhejiang University screened out the high expression gene, OPN, in hepatic metastatic tissue from more than 12,000 known genes and EST [29]. Based on the screening results of gene chip, expression difference in OPN mRNA was detected in normal intestinal mucosa, colorectal cancer tissue, and hepatic metastatic tissue of colorectal cancer. It was found that OPN mRNA expression level is highest in hepatic metastatic tissue of colorectal cancer,second place in primary tissue of colorectal cancer,and lowest in normal large intestinal mucosa. It demonstrated the significant correlation between OPN and hepatic metastasis of colorectal cancer. By detecting histological positioning of OPN mRNA using in situ hybridization technology, it was found that expression in colorectal cancer cell was positive and in normal hepatic metastatic tissue was negative. When detecting histological positioning of OPN protein by applying immunohistochemistry technology, it was found that expression in colorectal cancer cell and in normal hepatic metastatic tissue was also positive (Fig. 3.1).

By combining the related functional detection results of colorectal cancer cells after OPN transfection, a hypothesis is proposed that OPN influences occurrence and development of hepatic metastasis of colorectal cancer: for the colorectal cancer cells with high expression of OPN, homotypic adhesion capability between cells is reduced so that tumor cells are easy to detach from primary focus and complete the first step of metastasis; GJIC function between cancer cells is inhibited and intercellular communication is weakened; OPN also can enhance heterotypic adhesion between colorectal cancer cell and blood vessel endothelial cell, and expression of metastasis-related gene CD44 is strengthened, and expression of E-cadherin is inhibited, which urges tumor cell to adhere to extracellular matrix. During the course of reflux through portal vein, OPN provides possibility for colorectal cancer cell to invade peripheral vessel and to easily remain in the liver. The combined ligand-receptor action between OPN and its chemotactic receptor CD44 and another receptor integrin makes colorectal cancer easy to form metastatic focus in the liver, which demonstrates that OPN is one of the important genes involved that can influence occurrence and development of hepatic metastasis of colorectal cancer.

Through the experimental study on expression of OPN and metastasis-related mechanism, and combining their related literature, we deduce the possible action mechanism of OPN that promotes hepatic metastasis of colorectal cancer. OPN is secreted from colorectal cancer cell, which accounts for decreased expression of adhesion molecules such as E-cadherin, reduced homotypic adhesion and adhesion force between cancer cells, inhibited GJIC function, and enhanced invasive movement capability of cells. Thus cancer cells can be detached from the

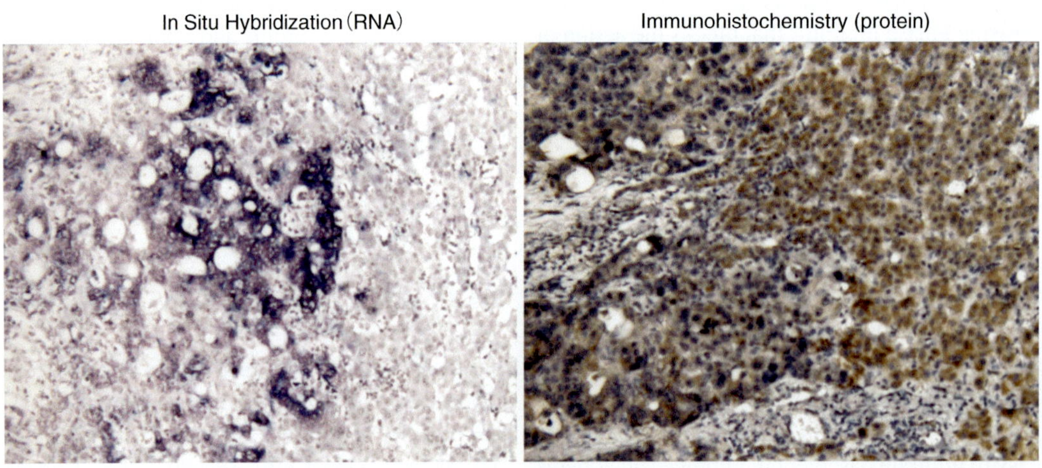

Fig. 3.1 Expression of OPN in colorectal cancer and hepatic metastatic tissue

primary focus to enter peripheral circulation so as to initiate metastasis of colorectal cancer. At the same time, due to the expression of OPN, expression of another metastasis-related factor CD44 also increases, and heterotypic adhesion action between colorectal cancer cell and ECM and blood vessel endothelial cell is enhanced. In addition, chemotactic receptor CD44 of OPN and another receptor integrin exist in the liver. Ligand-receptor action between them makes colorectal cancer easy to form metastatic focus in the liver.

3.4.2 Secreted Protein, Acidic and Rich in Cysteine-Like 1 (SPARCL1)

Based on the results of Affymetrix GeneChip system and by adoption of mathematical analysis method singular value decomposition (SVD), the Tumor Research Institute of Zhejiang University conducted an integrated analysis on cytobands and genes expression profile data, of which cytoband 4q22 with the most significant difference was further analyzed, and discovered the main contributing gene osteopontin (OPN) of high expression and the main contributing gene secreted protein, acidic and rich in cysteine-like 1 (SPARCL1) of low expression.

Both SPARCL1 and osteopontin belong to adhesion molecule that mediates cell matrix mutual action. SPARCL1 was discovered in the study on non-small cell lung cancer conducted by Schraml et al. for the first time in 1994, named as MAST9 [30]. SPARCL1 protein belongs to secreted protein, acidic and rich in cysteine (SPARC) family, with 62 % of homologous nature as secreted protein, acidic and rich in cysteine (SPARC) sequence. Both of them have cysteine-rich follistatin-like (FS) structure field structural domain and extracellular calcium binding (EC) structural domain. But N end of SPARCL1 is far longer than that of SPARC, as shown in Fig. 3.2. It is also named as SPARC-like 1 because its structure is highly homologous as SPARC. In recent

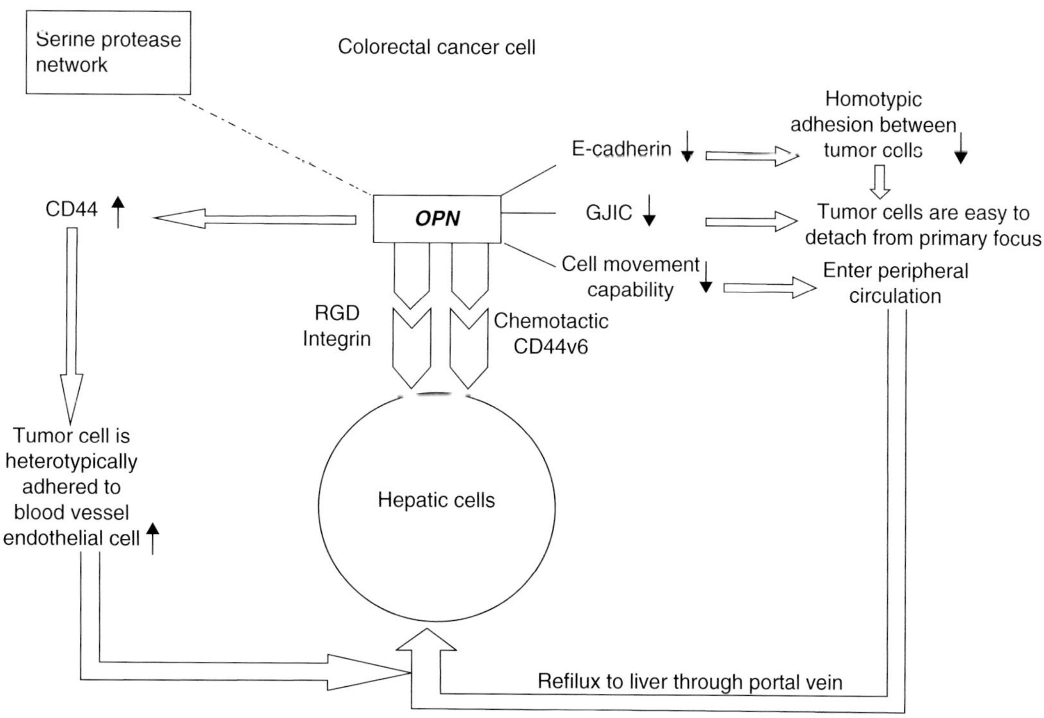

Fig. 3.2 Schematic diagram of action mechanism of OPN in hepatic metastasis of colorectal cancer. *RGD* arg-gly-asp (arginine-glycine-aspartic acid), *GJIC* gap junction intercellular communication (cell gap junction)

years, the study discovered that downregulation of the expression of SPARCL1 in CD133+/CD34+ cell indicates the possible regulation related to malignant tumors and other diseases [31].

Immunohistochemical detection discovered that expression of SPARCL1 in cytoplasm and cell membrane of non-metastatic colorectal cancer is significantly higher than that in primary focus tissue of hepatic metastatic colorectal cancer, but its expression in hepatic metastatic focus is significantly lower than the paired primary focus tissue of colorectal cancer. Through real-time quantitative PCR validation, the difference in the abovementioned SPARCL1 is also significant in mRNA level.

Western blot and RT-PCR method verified that there is no expression of SPARCL1 protein and mRNA in the three kinds of colorectal cancer cell lines, i.e., RKO, SW480, and SW620. In in vitro experiment, by adoption of MTT method and through cell scratch test, it was discovered that SPARCL1 recombinant protein did not significantly change the proliferation capability of the three kinds of colorectal cancer cells, but migration capability of RKO cells was weakened significantly. Such inhibitory action was not observed in SW480 and SW620.

The present studies on SPARCL1 are summed up as follows: (1) Expression level of SPARCL1 is high in non-metastatic colorectal cancer tissue while low in hepatic metastatic focus, which indicates that SPARCL1 perhaps is an early event in the process of hepatic metastasis of colorectal cancer and may serve as the marker for early prediction of hepatic metastasis of colorectal cancer. (2) In in vitro experiment, it was observed that SPARCL1 recombinant protein mainly has the ability of inhibiting the migration of colorectal cancer cells. SPARCL1 may become a candidate target in hepatic metastatic treatment.

3.4.3 Mammary Serine Protease Inhibitor (Maspin)

Maspin was obtained through suppression subtractive hybridization and differential display between the normal mammary epithelial cells and breast cancer cells by Zhou et al. in 1994. Encoded protein maspin has relatively high homology with other members of serine proteinase inhibitor superfamily, of which homology with equine and human neutral, monocyte elastase inhibitor is 43 % and 39 % respectively. Expression of maspin has been found in mammary epithelial cells, mammary myoepithelial cells, and prostatic epithelial cells.

By applying mRNA differential display analysis technology, the Cancer Research Institute of Zhejiang University screened out ten pairs of paired specimens of cancer tissue of solid tumor (two pairs of cardia cancer, esophageal cancer, gastric cancer, colorectal cancer, and ovarian cancer, respectively) and normal tissue through 32 primers from ten pairs of clinical tumor tissue samples. One hundred twenty-seven differential display fragments were obtained. A human solid tumor-related gene EST pool was preliminarily established. Among these differential display fragments, we found that expression of maspin increased in four pairs of specimens of gastric cancer, cardia cancer, and colorectal cancer. In the study applying gene chip of more than 12,000 genes and EST, we also found that expression of maspin significantly increased in 16 pairs of colorectal cancer through the detection for 21 pairs of specimens of colorectal cancer and normal mucosa tissue.

Through the experimental study relating to the expression of maspin in colorectal cancer and metastasis, it was found that:

1. When importing exogenous antisense maspin (AsCOLO205) into COLO205 colorectal cancer cell line, it was discovered that CD44 was positively related to maspin and negatively related to CD62, while there is no significant change in CD54.
2. When applying gene chip and bioinformatical analysis on the change in expression of AsCOLO205, change was discovered in adhesion-related genes, such as cadherin genes; movement-related genes, such as actin-gene; and cell information transmission-related genes, such as cell linker protein gene.
3. When applying laser confocal technology to detect functional change in cell linker protein of

AsCOLO205, it was discovered that expression level of gap junction protein of AsCOLO205 increased, and the function was somewhat restored, but its function is still poor compared with normal fibroblast.

4. Antisense maspin transfected COLO205 cell line of colorectal cancer. Morphological changes such as aggregation and proliferation of colorectal cancer cells and enhancement of adhesion occurred.

Therefore, we infer that possible action mechanism of maspin in colorectal cancer metastasis is as follows: At the early stage of metastasis of colorectal cancer, expression of maspin will increase; adhesion function of colorectal cancer cells is reduced through downregulation of the expression of some adhesion molecules, such as CD44 and cadherin, which is favorable for detaching cancer cells from primary tumor so as to initiate metastasis. Upregulation of P-selectin makes cancer cells easy to become oncogenic at the transportation stage so as to improve survival capability of cancer cells. At the late stage of colorectal cancer metastasis, i.e., the stage where secondary tumor is formed, downregulation of the expression of maspin enhances the adhesion capability of colorectal cancer cells so that oncogenesis of cancer cell increases, which is favorable for forming secondary tumor in target organ; growth of cancer cell is also accelerated, which is favorable for growth of colorectal cancer. Intercellular communication of cancer cells is restored to a certain degree, which is favorable for cancer cells to quickly obtain the characteristics of a certain tumor. Perhaps this is one of the reasons for the difference in phenotype between secondary tumor and primary one in most cases.

3.4.4 ST14 Gene

ST14 gene was discovered by the study group of Prof. Zheng Shu of the Cancer Research Institute of Zhejiang University for the first time. The encoded ST14 protein belongs to type II serine proteinase. It is deemed as one of the embers of protein hydrolase family that involves tumor-invasive metastasis [32]. Besides self-activation, possessing activity of collagenase, and degradation of extracellular matrix, this protein can identify and activate such proteins as proteinase-activated receptor 2 (PAR2), precursor of hepatocyte growth factor/scatter factor (HGF/SF), and precursor of urokinase-type plasminogen activation factor [33, 34]. These proteins are closely associated with the growth and metastasis of tumor [35].

The Cancer Research Institute of Zhejiang University applied GeneChip (microarray) technology to detect the change in gene expression profile before and after colorectal cancer cell line RKO transfected ST14 gene and discovered that high expression of ST14 gene may cause upregulation of the metastasis-related integrin β1 (ITGB1),

Table 3.1 Differential expression genes after RKO cell line transfected ST14

Top 10 upregulation probe sets			Top 10 downregulation probe sets		
	Probe set ID	Gene symbol		Probe set ID	Gene symbol
1	1553538_s_at	N/A[a]	1	1554237_at	SDCCAG8
2	1553551_s_at	MTND2	2	1555623_at	N/A[a]
3	1553575_at	N/A[a]	3	1555801_s_at	ZNF533
4	1555461_at	N/A[a]	4	1558048_x_at	N/A[a]
5	1555653_at	MTND5	5	1558105_a_at	N/A[a]
6	1555731_a_at	AP1S3	6	1561775_at	N/A[a]
7	1558250_s_at	N/A[a]	7	1564220_a_at	N/A[a]
8	1558678_s_at	MALAT1	8	1569110_x_at	PDCD6
9	1560514_at	LOC285205	9	200600_at	MSN
10	1561042_at	ITGB1	10	200916_at	TAGLN2

[a]*N/A* not available

matrix metalloproteinase 1 (MMP1), MALAT1, AP1S3 genes, and oxidative phosphorylation pathway (as shown in Table 3.1).

According to the present study results, encoded protein of ST14 may participate in signal transduction, jointly influence matrix degradation and epithelium migration, and enhance tumor infiltration and metastasis through direct degradation of extracellular matrix and activation of other membrane proteins or matrix source proteins in certain condition, such as growth factor, protein hydrolase, G protein-linked receptor on cell surface, etc. It can be summed up as ST14-centered network relation, where ECM, scHGF/SF, and Pro-UPA are its stroma, F-action, and HAI-1 are binding proteins (as shown in Figs. 3.3, 3.4, and 3.5).

3.4.5 Phosphatase of Generating Liver 3 (PRL-3)

PRL-3 is a kind of protein tyrosine phosphatase. It is a key enzyme in multiple signal transduction pathways and plays an important regulation role in cell growth, differentiation, and cell cycle. Loss or abnormality of its expression will lead to abnormal tyrosine phosphatization. In recent years many studies indicate that PRL-3 can promote tumor cell migration and metastatic activity. It is closely associated with tumor metastasis.

In 2001, Vogelstein et al. [36] screened differential genes of metastatic focus of colorectal cancer, primary focus and normal intestinal mucosa by adoption of serial analysis of gene expression (SAGE) and quantitative PCR method. It was discovered that there is little or no expression of PRL-3 in primary focus of colorectal cancer and normal mucosa, while the expression is high in metastatic focus, which indicates that PRL-3 is closely associated with hepatic metastasis of colorectal cancer. PRL-3 may become a new target of hepatic metastatic treatment. After that, studies related to PRL-3 and colorectal cancer metastasis gradually increase. Many studies indicate that expression of PRL-3 in primary focus is significantly related to hepatic metastasis, but not significantly related to lymph node metastasis (as shown in Table 3.2).

Tumor invasion and metastatic capability is associated with angiogenesis promotion capability of tumor cells. The study discovered expression of PRL-3 rises in tumor vessel [40]. Furthermore, expression of PRL-3 in tumor metastatic focus is mainly concentrated on tumor vessel [41]. CHO cells of PRL-3 expression intravenously injected into nude mouse tail can promote the formation of pulmonic tumor in the nude mouse [42]. PRL-3 in colorectal cancer cells with intravenous infiltration and distant metastasis significantly rises compared with that without intravenous infiltration [37]. In in vitro experiment, DLD-1 cell of PRL-3 expression

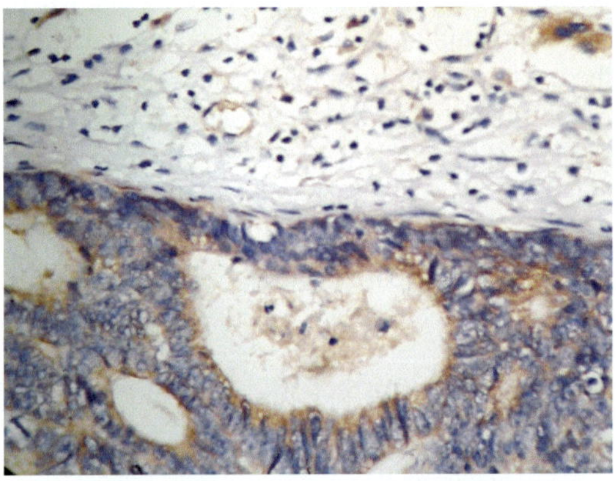

Fig. 3.4 Expression of SPARCL1 in colorectal cancer tissue

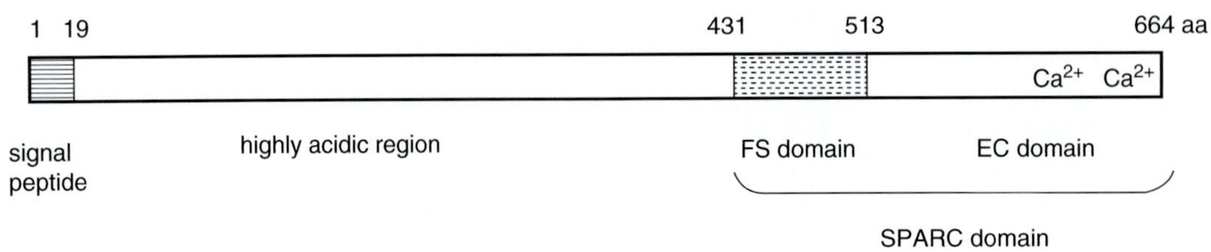

Fig. 3.3 Schematic diagram of structural domain of SPARCL1 protein

may aggregate human umbilical vein endothelial cells and promote angiogenesis through umbilical vein endothelial cells [43].

PRL-3 may promote the enhancement of colorectal cancer cell migration and invasion capability. The in-depth study on related molecular mechanism discovered that PRL-3 is associated with multiple signal transduction pathways. Cecile Rouleau et al. [44] transfected colon cancer cell line DLD-1 to make the expression of PRL-3 high. It was discovered that invasion capability was improved. Hirotaka Kato et al. [37] transfected PRL-3-specific miRNA in DLD-1 cell line to downregulate the expression of PRL-3 and discovered that tumor cell activity was reduced and aggregation in liver decreased. But proliferation of tumor cells did not change.

Wang et al. [45] discovered that in the DLD-1 colon cancer cell line with continuous high expression of PRL-3, serine/threonine protein kinase Akt was phosphatized and activated, and stroma of Akt was phosphatized and deactivated. These events rely on phosphoinositide-3 kinase (PI3K) and can be blocked by specificity inhibitor LY294002 of PI3K, which indicates that PRL-3 is associated with PI3K-related signal transduction pathways. In cell line DLD-1, expression of PRL-3 may reduce epithelial cell marker protein, such as E-cadherin (ECAD), γ-catenin, and integrin β3 and increase the expression of mesenchymal cell

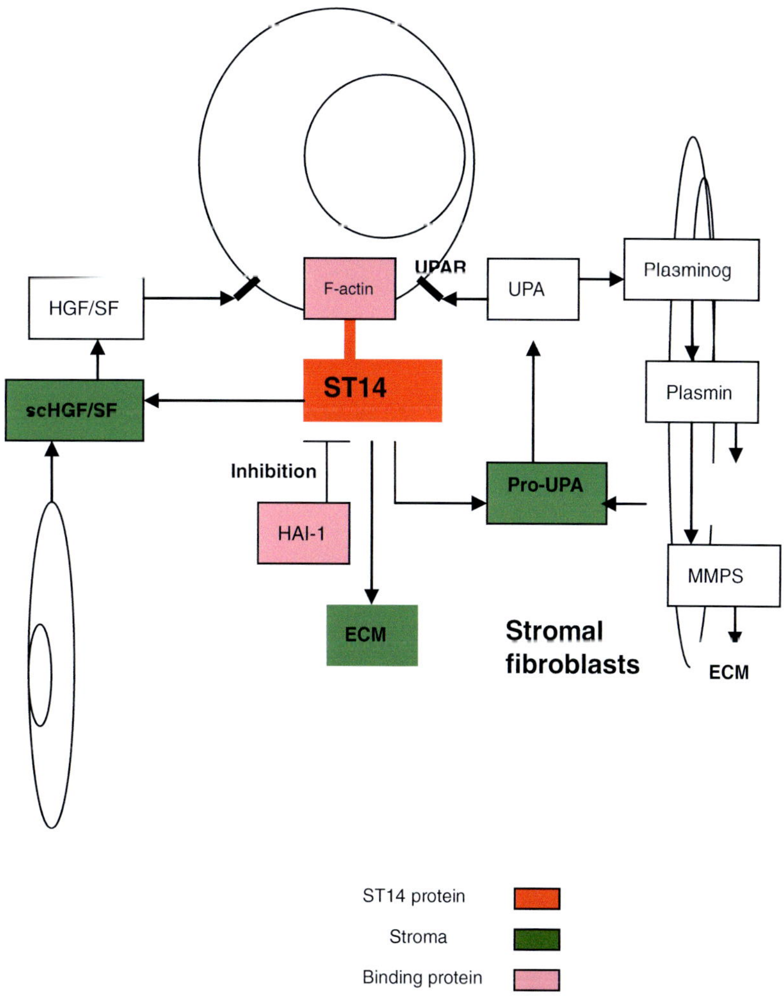

Fig. 3.5 ST14 gene regulatory network

Table 3.2 Expression of PRL-3 in colorectal cancer and metastatic focus

Sample (colorectal cancer)	Method	Positive standard	PRL-3 in primary focus	PRL-3 in metastatic focus	Correlation of PRL in primary focus and metastasis	Reference
177 cases of colorectal cancer 23 cases of hepatic metastasis 6 cases of pulmonic metastasis 59 cases of lymphatic metastasis 4 cases of peritoneal metastasis	In situ hybridization	≥10 % tumor cell expression signal	44.6 %	91.3 % in the liver 100 % in the lung 47 % in metastatic lymph node 50 % in peritoneal metastatic focus	Related to hepatic metastasis Related to pulmonic metastasis	[37]
88 cases of colorectal cancer 12 cases of hepatic metastasis 41 cases of lymphatic metastasis 28 cases of normal colonic mucosa	Immunohistochemistry	≧5 % cell staining	23.9 % 7.1 % (normal intestinal mucosa)	66.7 % in the liver 53 % in metastatic lymph node	Related to hepatic metastasis	[38]
49 cases of colorectal cancer 14 cases of lymphatic metastasis	Immunohistochemistry	Positive: 20–60 % cell staining Strong positive: ≧60 % cell staining	Positive: 16.3 % Strong positive: 0	Strong positive: 100 % metastatic lymph node	Among 14 patients with positive PRL-3 in lymph node, positive PRL-3 only occurs in primary focus of two cases; therefore PRL is not significantly associated with lymphatic metastasis	[39]

marker protein, such as Snail and fibronectin, which indicates that PRL-3 can mediate EMT so as to promote tumor metastasis. Fiordalisi et al. [46] discovered that in the colorectal cancer cell line SW480, PRL-3 can improve RhoA and RhoC activity. The use of Rho-associated protein kinase (ROCK) (a kind of kinase that activates Rho in upstream) inhibitor can block the migration and invasion capability of PRL-3-dependent cell migration and invasion capability, which indicates that PRL-3 promotes cell migration and invasion by its action in the upstream of Rho.

3.5 Prospect

More and more metastasis-related genes and proteins are discovered and studied, and metastasis-related pathways and networks are depicted continuously. New metastasis-related concepts and theories are too numerous to be counted. Along with the development of high-throughput technology, such as biological chip, sequencing technology, etc., more molecular events related to hepatic metastasis of colorectal cancer will be discovered, and the whole metastasis-related molecular network will be eventually depicted.

Although understanding about molecular mechanism of metastasis keeps increasing, there is still no good method for early diagnosis of hepatic metastasis of colorectal cancer. Progress regarding hepatic metastatic treatment is not noticeable. The discovery of new genes and development of hepatic cell theories provide a new breakthrough point and new direction for our further study on metastasis and also bring hope for diagnosis and treatment of hepatic metastasis of colorectal cancer. When fundamental studies keep development, an important issue that we face is how to conduct translational study and how to convert the existing study results to a tool to serve clinical work. On the way to conquer tumor, cancer researchers will shoulder heavy responsibilities.

References

1. Kemeny N, Seiter K. Colon and rectal carcinoma. In: Handbook of chemotherapy in clinical oncology. SCI ed. 1993:589–94.
2. Stangl R, Altendorf-Hofmann A, Charnley RM, et al. Factors influencing the natural history of colorectal liver metastases. Lancet. 1994;343(8910):1405–10.
3. Greenman C, et al. Patterns of somatic mutation in human cancer genomes. Nature. 2007;446(7132): 145–6.
4. Barrallo-Gimeno A, Nieto MA. The Snail genes as inducers of cell movement and survival: implications in development and cancer. Development. 2005;132: 3151–61.
5. Moody SE, et al. The transcriptional repressor Snail promotes mammary tumor recurrence. Cancer Cell. 2005;8:197–209.
6. De Vita VT, Hellman S, Rosenberg S. Principles of oncology. 5th ed. Philadelphia: Lippincott Raven Publisher; 1997. p. 135 [M].
7. Lanier LI. Activating and inhibitory NK cell receptor. Adv Exp Med Biol. 1998;18(2):452.
8. Fidler IJ. Metastasis: quantitative analysis of distribution and fate of tumor emboli labeled with 125I-5-iodo-2′-deoxyuridine. J Natl Cancer Inst. 1970;45:773.
9. Reya T, Morrison SJ, Clafke MF, et al. Stem cells, cancer, and cancer stem cells. Nature. 2001;414(6859): 105–511.
10. Fidler IJ. Modulation of the organ microenvironment for treatment of cancer metastasis. J Natl Cancer Inst. 1995;87:1588–92.
11. Paget S. The distribution of secondary growths in can cer of the breast. Lancet. 1889;1:571.
12. Kaplan RN, et al. VEGFR1-positive haematopoietic bone marrow progenitors initiate the pre-metastatic niche. Nature. 2005;438(7069):750–1.
13. Liotta LA. Cancer cell invasion and metastasis. Sci Am. 1992;266(2):54–9, 62–3.
14. Jorg H, et al. Cell surface molecules and their prognostic values in assessing colorectal carcinomas. Ann Surg. 2000;231:11.
15. Mohri Y. Prognostic significance of E-cadherin expression in human colorectal cancer tissue. Surg Today. 1997;27:606–12.
16. Ilyas M, Novelli M, Wilkinson K, et al. Tumour recurrence is associated with Jass grouping but not with differences in E-cadherin expression in moderately differentiated Dukes' B colorectal cancers. J Clin Pathol. 1997;50:218–22.
17. Skoudy A, Gomez S, Fabre M, et al. p120-catenin expression in human colorectal cancer. Int J Cancer. 1996;68:14–20.
18. Castells A, Boix L, Bessa X, et al. Detection of colonic cells in peripheral blood of colorectal cancer patients by means of reverse transcriptase polymerase chain reaction. Br J Cancer. 1998;78(10):1368.
19. Gothy DC, Fawcett S, Walsh D, et al. Alternatively spliced variants of cell adhesion molecule CD44 and tumor progression in colorectal cancer. Br J Cancer. 1996;74(3):342.
20. Takamura H, Endo Y, Ninomiya I, et al. Comparison of the pattern of integrin expression between primary tumors and liver metastasis of gastric and colorectal cancers. Nippon Rinsho. 1995;53(7):1678–82.

21. Fujita S, Sugano K. Expression of c-met proto-oncogene in primary colorectal cancer and liver metastases. Jpn J Clin Oncol. 1997;27:378–83.
22. Picon A, Gold LI, Wang J, et al. A subset of metastatic human colon cancers expresses elevated levels of transforming growth factor beta1. Cancer Epidemiol Biomarkers Prev. 1998;7:497–504.
23. Kawano, Osawa T, Ito I, et al. Expression of gelatinase A, tissue inhibitor of metalloproteinases-2, matrilysin, and trypsin(ogen) in lung neoplasms: an immunohistochemical study. Hum Pathol. 1997;28(5):613–22.
24. Yasumitsu H, Shofuda K, Nishihashi A, et al. Assignment of human membrane-type matrix metalloproteinase-2 (MT2-MMP) gene to 16q12 by FISH and PCR-based human/rodent cell hybrid mapping panel analysis. DNA Res. 1997;4(1):77–9.
25. Ichikawa Y, Ishikawa T, Tanaka K, et al. Extracellular matrix degradation enzymes: important factors in liver metastasis of colorectal cancer and good targets for anticancer metastatic therapy. Nippon Geka Gakkai Zasshi. 2001;102(5):376–80.
26. Takahashi Y, Bucana CD, Liu W, et al. Platelet-derived endothelial cell growth factor in human colon cancer angiogenesis: role of infiltrating cells. J Natl Cancer Inst. 1996;88:1146–51.
27. Nobuya Y, Yong-Suk C, Kiyoshi M, et al. Increased expression of sialyl Lewis a and sialyl x in liver metastasis of human colorectal carcinoma. Invasion Metastasis. 1995;15:95–102.
28. Shoji N, Masao K, Shingi I, et al. Increased expression of sialyl lewis x antigen correlates with poor survival in patients with colorectal carcinoma: clinicopathological and immuno-histochemical study. Cancer Res. 1993;53(15):3632–7.
29. Ding Ling, Zheng Shu, Cao Jiang. Relation between the expression of mRNA of Osteopontin and protein in large intestinal cancer and hepatic metastasis. Natl Med J China. 2002. 82(14):970–73.
30. Schraml P, et al. cDNA subtraction library construction using a magnet-assisted subtraction technique (MAST). Trends Genet. 1993;9(3):70–1.
31. Okamoto OK, et al. Common molecular pathways involved in human CD133+/CD34+ progenitor cell expansion and cancer. Cancer Cell Int. 2007;7:11.
32. Ge Weiting, Zheng Shu, Sun Lifeng, Shi Ying, Hhu Hanguang, Ding Kefeng. Expression and purification of ST14, a tumor metastasis-associated protein, and its activity assay. J Biochem Mol Biol. 2004. 20(5): 685–89.
33. Lin CY, Wang JK, Torri J, Dou L, Sang QA, Dickson RB. Characterization of a novel, membrane-bound, 80-kDa matrix-degrading protease from human breast cancer cells. Monoclonal antibody production, isolation, and localization. J Biol Chem. 1997;272(14): 9147–52.
34. Lin CY, Anders J, Johnson M, Sang QA, Dickson RB. Molecular cloning of cDNA for matriptase, a matrix-degrading serine protease with trypsin-like activity. J Biol Chem. 1999;274(26):18231–6.
35. Takeuchi T, Shuman MA, Craik CS. Reverse biochemistry: use of macromolecular protease inhibitors to dissect complex biological processes and identify a membrane-type serine protease in epithelial cancer and normal tissue. Proc Natl Acad Sci U S A. 1999;96(20):11054–61.
36. Saha S, VogelsteinSaha B, et al. A phosphatase associated with metastasis of colorectal cancer. Science. 2001;294:1343–6.
37. Kato H, Semba S, Miskad UA, Seo Y, Kasuga M, Yokozaki H. High expression of PRL-3 promotes cancer cell motility and liver metastasis in human colorectal cancer: a predictive molecular marker of metachronous liver and lung metastases. Clin Cancer Res. 2004;10:7318–28.
38. Peng L, Ning J, Meng L, Shou C. The association of the expression level of protein tyrosine phosphatase PRL-3 protein with liver metastasis and prognosis of patients with colorectal cancer. J Cancer Res Clin Oncol. 2004;130:521–6.
39. Wang Y, Li ZF, He J, Li YL, Zhu GB, Zhang LH. Expression of the human phosphatases of regenerating liver (PRLs) in colonic adenocarcinoma and its correlation with lymph node metastasis. Int J Colorectal Dis. 2007;22:1179–84.
40. St Croix B, Rago C, Velculescu V, Traverso G, Romans KE, Montgomery E, et al. Genes expressed in human tumor endothelium. Science. 2000;289: 1197–202.
41. Bardelli A, Saha S, Sager JA, Romans KE, Xin B, Markowitz SD, et al. PRL-3 expression in metastatic cancers. Clin Cancer Res. 2003;9:5607–15.
42. Guo K, Li J, Tang JP, Koh V, Gan BQ, Zeng Q. Catalytic domain of PRL-3 plays an essential role in tumor metastasis: formation of PRL-3 tumors inside the blood vessels. Cancer Biol Ther. 2004;3:945–51.
43. Guo K, Li J, Wang H, Osato M, Tang JP, Quah SY, et al. PRL-3 initiates tumor angiogenesis by recruiting endothelial cells in vitro and in vivo. Cancer Res. 2006;66:9625–35.
44. Rouleau C, Roy A, St Martin T, Dufault MR, Boutin P, Liu D, et al. Protein tyrosine phosphatase PRL-3 in malignant cells and endothelial cells: expression and function. Mol Cancer Ther. 2006;5:219–29.
45. Wang H, Quah SY, Dong JM, et al. PRL-3 down-regulates PTEN expression and signals through PI3K to promote epithelial-mesenchymal transition. Cancer Res. 2007;67:2922–6.
46. Fiordalisi JJ, Keller, et al. PRL tyrosine phosphatases regulate rho family GTPases to promote invasion and motility. Cancer Res. 2006;66:3153–61.

4 Metastatic Liver Cancer and Microenvironment

Jia Fan and Qiang Gao

The metastasis to adjacent locations and distance is one of the most important biological characteristics that distinguish malignant tumors from benign tumors. In 1976, Bross and Blumenson proposed the famous "metastatic cascade theory" [1], i.e., the complicated, dynamic, and continuous biological process of invasion and metastasis can be basically divided into the following relatively independent steps:

1. The proliferation of cancerous cells and angiogenesis in primary foci.
2. The detachment, directional movement, and degradation matrix of tumor cells.
3. Penetration into vascular circulation and migration.
4. Cancerous cells move to the target organs, adhere to the vascular endothelial cells of the target organs, and adhere to the basement membrane.
5. Disassociate out of the vessels and reach secondary sites, have adhesions with secondary sites, and form clones.
6. The proliferation and angiogenesis of cancerous cells form metastasis.

J. Fan (✉) • Q. Gao
Liver Cancer Institute, Zhongshan Hospital, Fudan University, Shanghai, China
e-mail: fan.jia@zs-hospital.sh.cn

However, these steps do not occur in the random modes, but rather have certain targets. As early as in 1889, Paget proposed "seed and soil theory," which holds that the formation of tumor metastasis is due to that the tumor cells in the flourishing growth status serve as "seeds," and when they encounter such suitable substrate environments as organs or tissue, i.e., the soil, the tumor metastasis will occur. Forty years later, Ewing challenged this theory, proposing that the occurrence of metastasis resulted from the pure mechanical factors associated with anatomical vascular structures. On the basis of summarizing the clinical experiences, Dr. Sugarbaker concluded that common local metastasis should be attributed to anatomical or mechanical factors, for example, venous return or lymphatic flow into regional lymph nodes, but distant metastasis should be attributed to organ specificity [2]. Later, this view became widely accepted, and there was more and more clinical experiment support. The liver metastasis process of colorectal cancer is a typical example. The liver is the most common organ for the distant metastasis of colorectal cancer, and the metastasis process is the result of co-activation of anatomical and biological factors.

On the other hand, although tumors occur as a result of the accumulation of genetic changes and colonial selection, tumors are independent but working together with the promotion of tumor invasion and metastasis as the mutual goal,

X. Qin et al. (eds.), *Multidisciplinary Management of Liver Metastases in Colorectal Cancer*,
DOI 10.1007/978-94-017-7755-1_4

including tumor cells and host stromal cells (vascular endothelial cells, endothelial cells, peripheral vascular cells, fibroblasts, myofibroblasts, macrophages, lymphocytes, dendritic cells, and mast cells) as well as functional organs comprising extracellular components; these cells are embedded into the extracellular matrix (ECM) and mutually constitute tumor's microenvironment with the vasculature and its surrounding tissue fluid, and this is what we commonly call the tumor microenvironment in a narrow sense, and the external environment that tumor cells are in or the external environment that tumor tissues are in can also be understood as the tumor microenvironment. A tumor is like a society, in which tumor cells maintain a relation of mutual fighting and mutual utilization with the surrounding "normal" cells. The dynamic interaction between the tumor cells and microenvironment is indispensable in the process of tumor occurrence and development: microenvironment regulates the growth of tumor cells and determines its metastatic potential and metastasis target organ and affects curative effects [3]. There are even some opinions that chronic carcinogenic factors first lead to the mutation of tumor interstitium components, and the mutated interstitium further promotes the mutations of adjacent epithelium, genetic instability, and ultimate carcinogenesis [4].

Liver metastasis is one of the major causes of deaths from colorectal cancer. During the whole course of disease, simultaneous liver metastases are about 15–25 %, while metachronous liver metastases are 20 %. That is to say, about 50 % of the colorectal cancer will ultimately have liver metastasis. With the deepening of studies on tumor's biological behaviors and cancer molecular biology, people have gained deeper and deeper understanding on colorectal cancer; however, there are still a number of critical issues that have not been clarified. From the prospect of microenvironment, it is beneficial to deepening the understanding of the biological nature of malignant tumors. The occurrence of liver metastasis of colorectal cancer not only needs the coordination and promotion of the microenvironment in which the cancerous cells are in, and the microenvironment of the liver itself plays an indispensable important role. In view of this, this paper introduces the important role that tumor microenvironment and hepatic microenvironment play in the liver metastasis of colorectal cancer.

4.1 Tumor Microenvironment and Liver Metastasis of Intestinal Cancer

4.1.1 Cellular Components of Tumor Microenvironment

The non-tumor cells in tumor microenvironment mainly comprise of fibroblasts, fat cells, endothelial cells, peritubular cells, and some cells in blood, such as lymphocytes, mononuclear/macrophages, granulocytes, natural killer cells, etc. Although they are not malignant in nature, the special local environment they are in and the mutual effects between them and the tumor cells bestow them abnormal phenotypes different from the relevant phenotypes in normal tissue and unique functions. In view that the non-tumor cells in the microenvironment have consistency between different tumor types, this paper shall also make a brief introduction on the important discoveries and their characteristics in other types of tumor-related microenvironments.

4.1.1.1 Fibroblasts

Compared with the fibroblasts in normal tissue, tumor-associated fibroblasts (TAF) in tumor microenvironment are in continued active state, not only not to be restored to the normal nonactivated state but also not to have apoptosis or be eliminated. (1) The activation of local fibroblast, (2) the epithelial–mesenchymal transition (EMT) of cancerous cells or microenvironment epithelial cells, and (3) the differentiation and activation of bone marrow-derived precursor cells [5] are generally thought as the sources of TAF. TAF are mostly distributed in the tumor invasion front, endothelial cells in the tumor–stromal interface, or tumor interstitium near the tumor vessels and wrap the ovaries. It is found through mouse tumor model that the activated fibroblasts of overexpression of hepatocyte growth factor (HGF) or TGF-β can induce carcinogenesis in such a multitude of tissues and organs as stomach and intestinal cancer. The research of human breast cancer tissue also found that stromal cells feature chromosomal rearrangements, while malignant epithelial cells do not, indicating abnormalities in matrix may be before tumor epithelial and stimulate the occurrence of tumors. TAF plays an important role in the invasion and metastasis of tumors through various kinds of growth factors, chemokines, angiogenic factors, and matrix degradation enzymes of matrix-degrading enzymes [5]. Experimental results of in vitro co-culture also indicate that TAF has the effects of stimulating the growth, invasion, and metastasis of tumor cells, while the fibroblasts derived from normal tissues do not feature such effects, indicating TAF's unique phenotype and functions. TAF not only features interactions with tumor cells and endothelial cells but also has complicated regulatory networks with microenvironment immune cells. For example, TAF can synthesize tenascin-C and tenascin-C and further play inhibiting roles on the local immunity of tumor tissue through or directly inhibiting the migration of immune cells of the contact barriers of immune cells and tumor cells [6].

4.1.1.2 Endothelial Cells

During the developmental process of tumors, tumor vessels play a very significant role, not only providing tumors with nutrients but also providing a path for the tumor metastasis. Since the endothelial cells of tumor vessels are in the tumor microenvironment for long terms, their phenotypes and functional characteristics have undergone obvious changes, including some changes in immunological characteristics, for example, the decrease of expression of adhesion molecules, the weakening of leukocyte adhesion and the trans-endothelial cell migration, the downregulation of major histocompatibility complex (MHC) molecule expression and antigen presentation dysfunction, the enhancement of the ability of anti-free radical damage, the synthesis of large amounts of extracellular matrix and combination of various kinds of growth factors, and the increase of the tumor cells and resistance to damages. Using the means of high-throughput gene chips, the comparison of the variations of genetic expressions of the vascular endothelial cells in normal tissues and in relevant tumors has found many molecules and their signaling pathways involving movements, invasion and metastasis, and angiogenesis, among which some genes and their products can serve the indicators for the tumor's capacities of invasion and metastasis and prognosis [7]. Research has indicated that there are striking differences in the sensitivities to drugs and adoptive immunotherapy (such as lymphokine-activated killer (LAK)) before and after the formation of tumor vessels: some tumors which were sensitive to drugs and adoptive to immunotherapy are usually insensitive or tolerant after the formation of blood vessels, which indicates the important role of endothelial cells of tumor vessels in tumor progression and therapy. Endothelial cells of tumor vessels are the first barrier to the entry of immune cells and therapeutic drugs into the tumor tissue, and the specific functional characteristics of endothelial cells of tumor vessels may be associated with the escaping from immunity monitoring and elimination of tumor cells. And there exist interactions between the tumor cells endothelial cells: on the one hand, tumor cells express relevant Notch ligands through the mitogen-activated protein kinases (MAPK) signaling pathway, thus further activating the Notch signaling pathway of endothelial cells and promoting the formations of tumor vessels [8]; on the other hand, the experiments of in vitro co-culture and in vivo nodule formation have all indicated that endothelial cells can also directly enhance the growth, movements, substrate degradation, and nodule formation of cancerous cell lung metastases [9].

4.1.1.3 Immune/Inflammatory Cells

Under the influence of chemotaxis factors, immune/inflammatory cells migrate from bone marrow or peripheral lymphoid tissues to the tumor microenvironment. More and more evidences have indicated that such innate immune cells as mononuclear/macrophages, granulocytes, mast cell, and B cell play important roles in the promotion of tumor occurrence and progress. The tumor-associated macrophages (TAM) are M2 type, and compared with M1 type macrophages under common inflammatory conditions, the antigen presentation effect and the activities of tumor-killing cells of M2 type TAM type are completely lost but play the roles of promoting tumor growth, invasions, and metastasis [10]. TAM not only promote the proliferations of tumor cells, angiogenesis, chemotaxis of immunosuppressive cells, and the inhibition of antitumor immunity responses by secreting various kinds of active factors (VEGF, HGF, IL-8, IL-10, TGF-β, CCL22, etc.) and enzymes (MMPs, etc.) but also enhance the elevation of the invasion and metastasis potentials through the direct interactions between the tumor cells themselves [11]. For example, the direction effects of the prostate's cancerous cells dismiss its growth dependence on sex hormone, make the invasion of the cancerous cells have a qualitative leap, downregulate the expression of surface adhesion molecules of hepatoma cells, and enhance their mobility [12]. The tumor-associated neutrophils (TAN) in the microenvironment also play a proactive and active role in the process of creating a local microenvironment that is beneficial to tumor growth, invasion, and angiogenesis through similar mechanisms: in addition to the participation of tumor progress with active secretion of PDGF, EGF, TGF-β, MMPs, etc., research has found that under the influence of the GM-CSF secreted by the tumor cells and the direct effects of intracellular contacts, large amount of TAN is synthesized, and oncostatin M (OSM) is released, and in turn the member of this IL-6 family of OSM enhances the detachment between the tumor cells, angiogenesis, and invasion and metastasis [13]. These phenomena indicate immune cells of tumor microenvironment; besides the mediation of the immunologic tolerance and immune escape through the traditional immunological means, they can also directly enhance the invasion and metastasis potentials of tumor cells through such non-immunological means as intracellular contacts and the combination of receptors and ligands and signaling pathways. The dendritic cells, which are renowned for their antigen presentation effects, in addition to the main existent modes of immature state or tolerant phenotype in the tumor microenvironment, have also been proven to directly enhance the growth proliferation and malignant transformation and invasion and metastasis of tumor cells through the signaling pathways of NF-kB and B cell-activating factor [14]. A smartly designed animal experiment has also proven B cells' tumor-promoting effects [15] – the positive HPV16 which was prepared through genetic transformation – and meanwhile it does not express the HPV16/RAG-1–/– of RAG-1; the knockout of RAG-1 gene leads to the complete loss of B and T cells, and compared with the HPV16 mouse model that has not knocked out the RAG-1, there is infiltration of innate immune cells in its precancerous lesions. This is not only substantially associated with the local low-level matrix-degrading enzymes and angiogenic factors, the weakening of epithelial cell proliferation, and the good differentiation of horn cells of the oncogene but also the malignancy rate which greatly decreases (6.4 %, control mice was 50 %); the infusion of B cells derived from mice on HPV16/RAG-1–/–mice restores the process of typical canceration–infiltration by large amount of innate immune cells, uncontrolled angiogenesis of tumors, epithelial hyperplasia, and dedifferentiation of keratinocytes and also elevates the malignancy rate. Clinically, the correlation between B cells and tumor progress and poor prognosis has also been proven [16].

As main members of specific immunity, in addition to the T cells featuring tumor-killing effects, T cells also include subgroups with various other functions. In the mouse tumor model, CD4+CD25+ regulatory T cells, Treg directly affects the progress of chemical induction of carcinogenesis [17]: adoptive transfusion of Treg speeds up the process of induction of carcinogenesis by MCA; after the elimination of the regulatory T cells by administering of anti-CD4 or CD25 antibodies, the original process of carcinogenesis was restored. Clinically, the evidence suggests that FOXP3+Treg is associated with the occurrence, development, and invasion: the analysis of the expression distribution status of tumor microenvironment Treg in the normal pancreas tissues, atypical hyperplasia, carcinoma in situ, and even patients with pancreatic cancer in the progressive stage has found that with the occurrence and progress of tumors, the quantities and proportions of Treg gradually increase, while the CD8+TIA+CTL with local infiltration gradually decreases or even disappears; Treg can be used as an independent index of poor prognosis of pancreatic cancer patients [18]. The research in liver cancer has also found that there exists a substantial correlation between the Treg in the microenvironment and the tumor vessel invasion and the high-invasive phenotype of incomplete envelope [19]. Recently, it has also been proven that the CD8+T cell subgroups in the tumor microenvironment can also enhance tumor progression [20]: in the mouse model of carcinogenesis induced by DMCA (double methlycholanthrene), the cell subgroups of TCRαβ+CD8+CD44+CD62-T in microenvironment have not only a defect of the tumor-killing effect mechanism of perforin but also large amounts of expressions of such inflammatory mediators as TNF-α, IFN-γ, and Cox2. The existence of these mediators greatly increases the occurrence rate of carcinogenesis and speed of carcinogenesis. It is worth mentioning that in addition to the view of most researches that tumor's local infiltration or the quantity of Treg in peripheral blood has a negative correlation with the prognosis, colorectal cancer research also holds that in para-carcinoma, its quantity is associated with prognosis and has a positive correlation with prognosis in cancer [21].

Recently, two studies based on such high-throughput approaches as gene chips, PCR chips, and tissue chips have found, for colorectal cancer, that the comprehensive immunological factors of tumor localities, including the four aspects of categories, density, distribution, and functional states, are even a stage superior than TNM (tumor, Lymph nodes, metastasis), and up till now, they are the most accurate independent prognostic index; the author infers that the T cells in the tumor microenvironment can alter the invasion and metastasis of cancerous cells by directly affecting the cancerous cells or indirectly affecting the tumor interstitium [22, 23]; for liver cancer, the expression spectrum of specific immune/inflammatory genes in paracarcinoma liver tissue can predict the vascular invasion and prognosis of tumors, although the author also holds that immunological factors can affect tumor's invasion and metastasis potentials, yet he is more inclined to the view that the invasion and metastasis potential of the cancerous cells themselves and the individual specific genetic factors affect the expression orientation of immune/inflammatory factors in paracarcinoma liver tissue and make them prone to metastasize [24], further demonstrating the crucial and even decisive influence of immune microenvironment on tumor progression.

It is worth mentioning that in addition to direct impacts on the tumor cells, there also exist mutual utilization and mutual cooperation between the microenvironment and the non-tumor cells, and one kind of non-tumor cells also indirectly impacts the tumor cells via another kind of non-tumor cells. For example, the mast cells of microenvironment themselves can directly enhance the angiogenesis and invasion and metastasis of tumors; in addition, mast cells are not only one of the important mechanisms for the regulatory T cells to play immunosuppression, and the mast cells that are clustered in peritumoral fibrous tissue can also inhibit the growth proliferation of tumor cells through such active substances as heparin that are released by them [25]. Thus, it indicates the complexity of the association between the functional diversities of microenvironment non-tumor cells and the tumor microenvironment.

4.1.2 Extracellular Component

4.1.2.1 Extracellular Matrix Degradation Enzymes of Matrix-Degrading Enzymes

Extracellular matrix (ECM) is mainly composed of such four components as collagen, elastin, glycoproteins, and proteoglycans. Normal ECM structure is of great importance to maintaining the polarity of cells, intracellular connections, and the prevention of malignant transformation. ECM reconstruction is the typical characteristic of changes in tumor interstitium, and it includes the changes of nature and quantity of ECM component expression and the abnormalities of ECM protease levels. Many ECM components have two way effects. Fibronectin (FN), type IV collagen, thrombospondin (TSP-1), etc. can both promote and inhibit the formation of tumor vessels, mainly depending on their assembly methods and the structural integrity. Type XVIII endostatin and type IV collagen degradation products tumstatin inhibit the proliferation and migration effects of endothelial cells on VEGF by inducing their apoptosis so as to play their effects as endogenous angiogenesis inhibitor. Certain integrins play a critical role in the tumor's resistance to drug mediated by cellular adhesion.

In the early stage of tumor growth, extracellular matrix and basement membrane play barrier effects on the infiltration of early-stage tumor cells, and they are the physiological barriers that must be overcome in tumor metastasis. For colorectal cancer, growth and metastasis first need to invade the local tissue, and only after they have invaded into the muscularis mucosa and submucosal layer can they gain the chances of entering the blood or lymphatic vessels. Even after the initial invasion, the tumor cells retained on the liver still need to invade into the liver tissue before they can form metastasis. If tumor cells are to form metastasis, they need to penetrate through the basement membrane (BM) and extracellular matrix (ECM). During this process, tumor cells and interstitial cells will secrete some enzymes so as to destroy these barriers, and among them, the most studied and most important must be matrix metalloproteinases (MMPs). In the tumor invasion and metastasis, MMPs [26] degrade the extracellular matrix, are involved in the formation of neovascularity, regulate cell adhesion, can activate the potential activities of ECM structural proteins, and play an important role in the chemotaxis of inflammatory cells and stimulation of tumor migration. Integrin plays important roles in cell invasion and regulates the migration of regulatory cells in ECM; it can also regulate the MMPs' expression and activate proteins with potential activities. Other enzymes, enzyme inhibitors, cytokines, and growth factors in the tumor microenvironment and their receptors and adhesion molecules are all the substrates of MMPs. MMPs regulate the local microenvironment by activating and degrading these substrates; for example, through the shearing of different locations of IL-1β, they decide whether their directions are activated or deactivated. MMPs initiate EMT and induce the genetic instability of the tumor cells. An angiostatin, which is an MMPs' degradation product, is a powerful inhibitor of endogenous angiogenesis.

What correspond to MMPs are tissue inhibitors of metalloproteinase (TIMP), which is a natural inhibitor of MMPs. The imbalance between TIMP and MMPs has been proven to be closely associated with a multitude of pathological state, especially tumor's invasion and metastasis. Regarding interstitial cells of tumor microenvironment, TIMP can also directly play anti-apoptosis functions through the PI3K and JNK signaling means. In addition, the contrast imbalance of other enzymes and their inhibitors in the microenvironment, for example, uPA and PAI, also plays a role that cannot be ignored in the degradation of substrates and the release of relevant signals of the accumulation of proinflammatory cells, angiogenesis and tumor invasion, and metastasis. uPA levels and the expression of uPA receptors on the cell surface are associated with the invasion and metastasis of intestinal cancer.

4.1.2.2 Cytokines and Growth Factors

Cytokines and growth factors released by tumor cells and microenvironment interstitial cells are unanimously acknowledged to have biological behaviors on tumor cells and mainly include TGF-β, stromal cell-derived factor 1 (SDF-1)/CXCL12, VEGF, HIF-1α, and secreted protein acidic and rich in cysteine (SPARC).

Under normal circumstances, TGF-β is renowned for its functions of inhibiting growth, promoting apoptosis, and suppressing immunity, and it plays an important role in maintaining the tissue homeostasis. Tumor cells not only lose the inhibition effects on the growth of TGF-β, manifested in strong proliferation response, but also it can secrete high levels of TGF-β.

TGF-β is the most effective inhibiting molecule that mediates tumor immune escape; it is responsible for the invasion and metastasis capacities of tumor cells; for example, it stimulates the expression of integrin α3β1 in noninvasive hepatoma cells and transform them to invasive liver cancer [27], the EMT that induces cancerous cells and enhances its invasion and metastasis; it affects the microenvironment interstitial cells, such as the ECM and cytokines, that stimulate the secretion of TAF, enhancing the migration of progenitor cells and angiogenesis, indirectly accelerating the tumor progress.

The constitutive expression SDF-1 of mesenchymal cells and interstitial cells, i.e., CXCL12, is a member of the chemokine family, and its ligand CXCR4 has high expression in large amount of tumor cells, and meanwhile tumor cells can also have autocrine of SDF-1. Like other chemokines and their ligands (see the following), SDF-1/CXCR4 axis plays a critical role in the growth and proliferations and invasion and metastasis of tumor cells and angiogenesis and in the process of directional transfer of target organs [28].

As a transcription factor, HIF-1α can regulate the gene expressions in downstream after it is activated, and these protein products mostly involve angiogenesis, energy metabolism, cell proliferations, and survival vasomotor response. Research has found that the expression of HIF-1α has significant correlation with the tumor's benign and malignant natures and characteristics of tumor invasion and metastasis. The functions of microenvironment HIF-lα in tumor's occurrence and development mainly include promoting the formations of neovascularity, creating conditions for the invasion and metastasis of tumor cells, and promoting the production of a multitude of glycolytic enzymes, and the elevation of glycolysis can make the tumor cells more adaptable to the adverse environment of ischemia and hypoxia in the surrounding.

4.1.2.3 Chemokine

In tumor microenvironment, chemokine affects the growth and metastasis of tumors in the following aspects: regulating the migration of inflammatory/immune cells to tumor tissue. The infiltration of CD8+CTL by CCL2 and CCL5 into the tumor microenvironment plays a critical role; in the tumor model prepared with the tumor cell lines with CCL2 and CCL3 expressions, it is found that in the transplanted tumors, the lymphocyte infiltration has increased, the tumor growth has been slowed, and metastasis foci have decreased, indicating such transformed tumor cells can enhance the host's antitumor immunity [29]. However, in the mouse tumor model prepared with transfected Ras tumor cells, tumor cells demonstrate high Ras-dependent expression of CXCL8 and CXCL8 chemotaxis of large amounts of inflammatory cells, which leads to local severe chronic inflammation response and the formation of tumor vessels [30], affects the body's eliminating capacity of tumor cells, and regulates the angiogenesis of tumor tissues: CXC chemokines containing ELR motif (Glu-Leu-Arg), such as IL-8, can enhance the tumors' angiogenesis, but CXC chemokines not containing ELR can resist tumors' angiogenesis. In addition, partial chemokines of CC type also have the effects of enhancing angiogenesis. Therefore, the balance of microenvironment chemokines is one of the important mechanisms of tumors' angiogenesis; it stimulates the tumors to produce growth factors in the forms of autocrine or paracrine: chemokines mostly stimulate tumor cells and interstitial cells in the form of autocrine and make tumor cells survive and grow. Melanoma cells not only can express CXCR2 but can also secrete large amount of corresponding ligands CXCL1, and such autocrine can lead to the speedup of proliferation of tumor cells. Chemokines can also stimulate the growth of tumor cells in the form of paracrine. When the tumor cells express CXCL12, they can produce TNF-α, thus enhancing the proliferation of tumor cells and affecting the invasion and metastasis potentials of tumor cells. The combination of chemokine receptors and ligands can induce the movement of tumor cells and make them transfer to target organs, and the corresponding ligands that exist in the target organs in large quantity not only lead to the transfer of organ specificity of tumor target organs but also can strengthen their movements, invasion, and substrate degradation. For example, in the CCR1 expression of hepatoma cells, those with higher metastatic potential have stronger expressions, and the downregulation of CCR1 significantly decreases the metastatic capacity of hepatoma cell lines with high metastatic potential, such chemokines; as CCR1's main ligands, RANTES and MIP-1α are mainly expressed and distributed in the portal area of paracarcinoma liver tissue and lobular central vein area. The liver cells are almost not expressed, indicating the important role of the interaction of CCR1 and its ligands in the process of selective invasion of the portal vein of liver cancer and the value of CCR1 for judging liver cancer invasion [31].

4.1.3 Vascular Structure of Microenvironment

In order to maintain the necessary nutrition metabolism, tumors must depend on certain vascular structures, and neovascularities are also the necessary conditions for tumor cells' invasion and metastasis. Tumor cells themselves, as well as the fibroblasts, inflammatory cells, and bone marrow-derived precursor cells in the microenvironment, secrete large amounts of angiogenic factors and activate the angiogenic switch; among them, in over 20 kinds of polypeptide vascular growth factors that have been discovered so far, the most important one and the one that plays the central regulatory role is VEGF. Sprouting and growing on the basis of the existing vascular structures and having chemotaxis on endothelial progenitor cells to generate new vessels and vasculogenic mimicry (VM) (the pathway structures with tumor cells as linings) are the main formation modes of tumor vessels. Among them, the "vasculogenic mimicry (VM)" is only seen in highly invasive tumors, and it is rarely seen in low-invasion tumors or benign tumors. VM's existence not only greatly enriches the blood flow of tumor tissue, but also since the tumor cells directly construe the vascular walls and are free of the linings of endothelial cells, the tumor cells release protease to degrade the basement membrane within the vessels and come into direct contact with blood circulation, thus making VM more conducive to the growth and invasion and metastasis of tumors. This was further proved in clinical tumor research, and there were primary liver cancer with VM that has poor differentiation, high invasion and metastasis potentials, and poor prognosis [32]. Compared with the vascular structures of normal tissues and organs, the vascularity in tumor microenvironment is uneven and has a relatively lower average density and long dispersion distance. Other characteristics include having abnormal and twisting morphologies, irregularities of lumen and structure of the wall, and branch disorders and often ending in dead ends; it has no normal arteriole–capillary–veinlet structure, and in replacement it has arteriovenous fistula and plasma channels free of red blood cells. The vasculature possesses extremely high permeability, which can lead to high interstitial pressure of the microenvironment, worsen hypoxia, and further promote the formation of VEGF. Angiogenesis is the indication of malignant tumors' progress, and in clinical practice, angiogenesis parameters have been regarded as independent indicators in the judgment of tumor prognosis.

The total loss of functional lymphatic vessels inside the tumors is another important characteristic of microenvironment, but on the other hand, more and more researches indicate that lymphatic metastasis is the active behavior of tumor inducing the generation of lymphatic vessels. Due to the unique anatomy of the lymphatic vessels (the lack of closely connected single-layer lymphatic endothelial cells, incompletion of basement membrane and thin vessel walls) as well as the hydrodynamics characteristics (slow flow rate and shear force), compared with hematogenous spread, lymphatic spread is a more effective means of tumor metastasis. In view of the nonfunctional lymphatic vessels inside tumors, some scholars think that without the newly formed lymphatic vessels inside the tumors, only the lymphatic vessels on the tumors' edges are sufficient in order for lymphatic metastasis to occur. Histological studies have also found that peritumoral lymphatic vessels are not only larger in quantity and lumen, but they are also significantly associated with the lymph node metastasis in the tumor area [33]. VEGF-C/D are the two most important factors for the formation of tumor lymphatic vessels, and they also directly promote the chemotaxis and invasion of tumor cells on lymphatic vessels. Antagonistic VEGF-C/D therapy can inhibit tumors' lymphatic metastasis. The expression of VEGF-C/D or lymph vascular invasion (LVI) and lymphatic microvessel density (LMVD) in such tumor tissues as human breast cancer, stomach cancer, colorectal cancer, and lung cancer has been used as the molecular markers and the predictors of tumors' lymphatic metastasis and has become the prognostic markers that independently indicate tumor-free survival rates and total survival rates [34, 35].

4.1.4 Abnormal Metabolic State of Microenvironment

Under the co-activation of tumor cells and vascular structures, tumor microenvironment has formed three symbolic characteristics: low oxygen partial pressure/hypoxia, high interstitial fluid pressure (IFP) and acid extracellular fluid. They are the most important external factors that lead to the genetic instability of tumor cells. In the different locations of the same tumor, or at different times of the same location, and at the different individual tumors of the same pathological grades and developmental phases, these characteristics are not necessarily the same; therefore, they are also the important causes of tumor heterogeneity.

4.1.4.1 Hypoxic State

Due to the unique structural characteristics of blood vessels of tumor microenvironment, for example, lumens are irregular and can easily collapse, thus leading to intratumoral chronic hypoperfusion temporary acute hypoxia, inducing the apoptosis or necrosis of tumor cells. However, there are still some tumor cells that are tolerant to hypoxia, can survive after escaping the selective pressure of apoptosis and necrosis, and manifest more malignant biological characteristics: the increase of invasion and metastasis capacity, decrease of sensitivity to chemoradiotherapy and having stronger capacity of angiogenesis. Hypoxia results in the reduction and activity decrease of DNA mismatch repair enzyme and the mutations of tumor-prone points; the gene amplification induced by hypoxia increased the tumor cells' genetic instability, and the release of a large amount of active molecules (HIF-1α,VEGF, IL-8, HGF, etc.) induced by hypoxia and inflammatory reactions is a major mechanism for hypoxia to function [36]. It can be seen that hypoxia, a representative microenvironment characteristic that runs through the process of tumor growth, not only bestows tumor cell potentials of constant growth, malignant progression, and invasion and metastasis, and the hypoxia-induced neovascularities maintain the tumor growth but also lay a necessary foundation for tumor metastasis. Hypoxic microenvironment can also lead to a change in the dendritic cells' (DC) migration activity by influencing the expression balance of MMP-9/TIMP-1; thus it can lead to functional abnormalities, produce local immune suppression, and enable the tumor cells, especially the tumor cells in hypoxic areas, to immunologically escape, thus forming local infiltration and distant metastasis. Finally, the evolutionary selection caused by hypoxia makes tumor cells more invasive and metastatic.

4.1.4.2 Abnormal pH Values

The pH of tumor cells in malignant tumors is higher than that outside the cells but is lower than the pH within the relatively normal cells; the pH outside tumor cells is 6.5–7.0, and the pH outside the relevant normal cells is 7.1–7.6. Such an intracellular and extracellular pH grade and acidic extracellular environment have different effects on antitumor drugs: it is easy for drugs of weak acid to infiltrate into the cells to function, but it is hard for alkaline drugs to permeate into the cells, thus leading to restricted curative effects. In normal mammals, malignant cells characteristically display mutated metabolic models and rely on anaerobic metabolism of sugar as lactic acid increases, even with sufficient oxygen; the low efficiency of anaerobic metabolic pathways is supplemented by the flow increase of sugar, and the latter indicates that in human tumor, the glycolytic phenotype is nearly a common phenomenon. Some researchers have studied the role of glycolytic phenotype in the enhancement of tumor infiltration using the tumor-host mathematical model [37]. The glycolytic phenotype successfully adapts to environmental selection parameters, and it gives tumor cells the infiltration capacity; glycolytic phenotype allows cells to migrate from the microenvironment of precancerous lesions to adjacent normal tissues. These cells compete with the surrounding normal cells, while the normal cells are not adapted to the microenvironment with rich relevant substrates as compared with cell groups in tumor. Consequently, the unlimited proliferation of tumor leads to the formation of glycolytic phenotype, and meanwhile the precancerous lesion converts into infiltrative tumor.

4.1.4.3 Elevation of Interstitial Pressure

The permeability of solid tumor vasculature is commonly higher than that of normal tissue. The high permeability of the vasculature results in leakage of blood, which enters interstitial space. In addition, the reconstruction of tumor microenvironment ECM, contraction induction mediated by TAF, and a lack of functional lymphatic vessels leads to abnormally high interstitial space pressure. The elevation of peripheral blood osmolality leads to the decrease of osmotic pressure of the entry of drive drug molecules into the tumor tissue. Meanwhile, the accumulation of body fluids in the interstitial space will make the tumors swell swiftly. Clinical studies on intestinal cancer patients indicate that the abnormalities of vasculature permeability, the subsequent high interstitial fluid pressure, and the coexistent immunologic tolerance are the main causes of metastasis. In addition, the tumor cells carried in the tumor effusion fluid and the protein molecules formed by various kinds of vascular and lymphatic vessels are means that cause the diffusion of tumor cells. More understanding of molecules' mechanism on the regulation of tumor permeability provides assistance to the strategy of better treatment of tumors from the field of molecular medicine.

4.1.5 Microenvironment's Apparent Genetic Regulation on Tumor Cells

In the cross dialogue between the microenvironment's immune cells and tumor cells, the critical regulators of both parties' phenotypes and functional changes are the relevant signaling pathways of signal transducer and activator of transcription 3 (STAT3) [38]. In most tumor cells, STAT3 is in sustained active state, and under the effects of cytokines and growth factors that exist in large amounts in tumor microenvironment, such as IL-10, VEGF, and TGF-β, it further activates the signaling pathways in the tumor cells and promotes the expressions of many apoptosis-inhibiting genes and angiogenesis genes. More importantly, under the effects of the products expressed under the regulation of STAT3 signaling pathways and the factors that already exist in microenvironment, the STAT3 signaling pathways in the microenvironment's immune cells are activated, resulting in the induction, activation, amplification, and functioning of regulatory T cells; inhibition of the differentiation, maturing, and activation of myeloid dendritic cells; and the reduction of the tumor-killing activities of NK and macrophages [39]. Meanwhile, the STAT3 signaling pathways in the microenvironment's endothelial cells are also activated and coupled with the release of angiogenesis substances in large amount and greatly elevate the generation capacity of tumor vessels [40].

MAPK and Notch signaling pathways play an important role in tumor cell enhancement of endothelial cells' process of neovascularity [8]. Under the induction of activated MAPK signaling pathways, cancerous cells express Jagged1, Jagged1 in large amount as Notch's ligands, thus activating the Notch signaling pathways in the adjacent endothelial cells, leading to the proliferation of endothelial cells and angiogenesis; it is further discovered that the Jagged1 as the Notch's ligands is more closely associated with microvessel density and tumor progression.

The Nodal signal in the TGFβ superfamily is the critical signal for the induction of mesoderm production in early embryos and the maintenance of multilineage differentiation of embryonic stem cells. And the highly invasive subtypes of such a multitude of tumors as breast cancer, testicular cancer, and melanoma also express Nodal signaling pathways, the difference being the loss of the relevant inhibitor Lefty and the continued close relation between invasion and metastasis capacity [41]. Expose the human metastatic melanoma cells to the microenvironments of human embryonic stem cells, zebrafish embryos, to weaken its invasion and reduce the nodule formation capacity. And the inhibitor lefty of Nodal signals released in the embryonic microenvironment is considered one of the mechanisms of its effects [41] Lefty inhibits the Nodal-mediated SMAD phosphorylation and the relevant gene expression of the transcription factor forkhead box H1 (FOXH1) of its downstream, ultimately leading to the positive regression of cancerous cells.

4.1.6 Impacts of Tumor Cells on Microenvironment

There exist active conversations featuring two-way interactions between the tumor cells and the microenvironment they are in, ultimately forming vicious cycles that enhance tumor progression. Some scholars hold that tumor cells are the "leading roles" in its progression process, while the various kinds of nontransforming cells in the microenvironment and the relevant extracellular components are "supporting roles" and are selected constantly and modified by the "leading roles" beginning from the early stage of canceration. The soluble small molecules in the microenvironment play an extremely important role in the process of cross dialogues and mutual modifying of both parties: although the changes of the reactive stroma of prostate cancer can be used as the predictors of recurrence and metastasis, this kind of change originates from the shaping role released by TGF-β and interstitial cells released by cancerous cells [42]. In addition, the direct contact of tumor cells and interstitial cells and the exocrine vesicles of tumor cells are the other two important mechanisms for the change of the microenvironment by tumor cells. Although there is still no confirmed conclusion on whether the initial factors are the abnormalities of the epithelial cells themselves that lead to canceration or it is the abnormalities of the microenvironment that lead to the canceration of epithelial cells, some studies indicate that the selective pressure produced by the core suppressor genes that specifically inhibit the cell aging relevant signaling pathways in the cancerous cells (i.e., the growth of fibroblasts free of p53 mutation is limited) can induce the increase of a large number of p53 mutant fibroblasts in the microenvironment and further produces reactive interstitial environment conducive to the growth and invasion of cancerous cells [43]. This partially explains why TAF can enhance the tumor's invasion and metastasis as stated above, but normal tissue-derived fibroblasts are not the same; this also indicates tumor cells' active transformation of the microenvironment, as well as the necessity of such transformations to tumor progression.

In the processes of the formation of immune suppression network of tumor microenvironment, as well as their diffusion to regional lymph nodes, the spleen, and even the whole body, the tolerogenic substances produced by tumor cells play a critical role [44]. The VEGF, SDF-1, etc. produced by tumor cells stimulate chemotaxis of the immature myeloid cells in the circulation and induce these cells to be regionally differentiated into TAM and tolerogenic DC; tumor cells secrete soluble Fas, FasL, HLA-I, etc., to inhibit the killing capacity of locally infiltrated Nature Kill cell (NK) and CTL and promote their apoptosis; tumor-derived exocrine vesicles, consisting of large amounts of FasL, TRAIL, and soluble inhibitory molecules TGF-β, can also induce T-cell apoptosis and the differentiations of TAM and immature DC.

4.2 Hepatic Microenvironment and Liver Metastasis of Intestinal Cancer

The liver is the second most common target organ of tumor metastasis only next to lymph nodes. Based on the differences of the primary sites, liver metastasis can be seen in about 30–70 % of tumor patients. Among adults, the most common primary organs are melanoma, tumors of the gastrointestinal tract, breast cancer, lung cancer, neuroendocrine tumors, and sarcoma, while in children, the most common are neuroblastoma, Wilms' tumor, and leukemia. Most liver metastases are multifocal, and 77 % involve the left and right lobes of the liver, and only 10 % are single liver metastases. Although the effects of the genetics and phenotypes of metastatic tumor cells and the heterogeneity of the genetic and biological characteristics of the patients themselves on the occurrence and progress of liver metastasis have not been fully clarified, scholars unanimously hold that the structures and functional characteristics of hepatic microenvironment itself, such as the functional diversity of microcirculation structures, hepatic parenchymal cell, and mesenchyma cells, play an important role on liver metastasis.

On the whole, the liver filters the portal vein blood flow of internal organs, and blood circulation occupies 30 % of the cardiac output; the blood flow of hepatic microcirculation is slow and stagnant, and it is regulated by the Kupffer cells in blood sinusoid and astrocytes around sinusoid; the Kupffer cells that are prominent in sinusoid and endothelial cells provide rich adhesion mediation of cell surfaces, receptors, and highly effective endocytosis; large amounts of innate immune cells, such as macrophages, mast cells, dendritic cells, and NK cells, provide a specific tolerant microenvironment; parenchymal and stromal cells of the liver induce the formation of interstitial cells of metastatic tumor, inflammatory state, and angiogenesis depending on the necessity. This paper will elaborate this continuous process through four independent steps.

4.2.1 Capillary Phase That Enters Hepatoma Cells

After cancerous cells have entered the liver, they reach and are retained in the terminal branches of the portal veins, and also a few single cancerous cells stride over the sphincter of the preantral capillary to enter the proximal sinus, but there might still be a very few cancerous cells further entering the centrilobular vein along the liver sinusoid and finally reaching pulmonary circulation. Most hepatic cancerous cells will be eliminated by the following forces: the direct killing of NK cells, the reactive oxygen products released by Kupffer cells, the activation of passive anticancer immune response, and the obstruction of cancerous cells resulting in the release of free radicals in large quantity which are induced by ischemia–reperfusion injury. A small portion of cancerous cells survive by escaping killing via various kinds of active mechanisms. For example, CEA expressed by cancerous cells can induce the production of IL-10, thus inhibiting liver cells from releasing their NO, etc. inflammatory mediators; intestinal cancerous cells express MHC-I molecules so as to escape the cytotoxicity of NK cells; cancerous cells synthesize large amounts of glutathione so as to neutralize and offset the oxidative stress.

The cancerous cells that have subsequently survived, under the effects of inflammatory mediators and cytokines (TNF-α, IL-1, IL-18), are closely associated with the sinusoidal endothelial cells through the VCAM-1 on the endothelial cells. In experimental animals, the use of the neutralizing antibodies in VCAM can reduce liver metastasis by 75 %, from which we can see the core role of VCAM in this process [45]. In addition, the ICAM-1, P-selectin, and E-selectin expressed by endothelial cells play certain role in this step.

4.2.2 Formation of Micrometastasis Within the Hepatic Lobule

Cancerous cells further penetrate through sinusoidal endothelial cells and are colonized in the Disse gap or around the liver cells and have chemotaxis and attraction of sinus astrocytes, fibroblasts of portal area, and partial liver cells, gradually forming a subclinical, neovascularity-free micrometastasis. When the metastasis is formed in the surroundings of sinusoid, sinus astrocytes are the main source of its stroma and express the marker of activation α-SMA; when the metastasis is colonized in the periphery of hepatic lobule, fibroblasts of portal area are the source of mesenchyme; in addition, liver cells themselves can also become mesenchyme of metastasis through the transformation of epithelial matrix. These interstitial cells enhance the growth of micrometastasis and angiogenesis via the paracrine effects (VEGF, PDGF, HGF, TGF-β, and IL-8).

In-depth exploration of the functions of liver cells and interstitial cells and the heterogeneity of phenotypes in various regions of hepatic lobule or liver acinus is extremely important to the understanding of the selection formations of intrahepatic micrometastasis focus. There exist differences in the liver cell structures, metabolism, and enzyme activity in the different locations inside the liver acinus, which are known as the differences of structure and functional grades. Based on the relationship between the routing characteristics of hepatic microvascules and the regeneration of liver cells, Rappaport proposed that liver acinus is the smallest unit of microcirculation structures, i.e., the concept of Rappaport's liver acinus [46]. Liver acinus refers to the liver cell region that is formed with a terminal vessel (terminal portal branch and hepatic artery branch) that branches out from the interlobular artery and interlobular vein of the portal area as the axis and with the central veins at two ends as borders. A classical hepatic lobule contains six liver acinuses. The blood flow within the liver acinus unilaterally flows to the central vein from the axis. Based on the directions of blood flow, the liver acinuses are classified into three functional zones: the part near the axial vascular is Zone I, where liver cells get priority in obtaining the blood supply rich in oxygen and nutrients, and cellular metabolism is active, the volume of mitochondria is expanded, and phagocytic activity of cells and antivirus and regeneration capacities are relatively stronger. Liver cells have rich contents of succinic dehydrogenase, and the contents of cytochrome oxidase, enzymes, and transaminase are also relatively higher, and they are the major locations of protein and glycogen synthesis. The part near the central vein is Zone III, where liver cells have poorer nutrition and low resistance to harmful substances, and regenerative capacity is not strong; the part between Zone I and Zone III is Zone II, where the nutrition, metabolism, and regenerative capacity of liver cells are all between those of the previous two zones. Intrahepatic micrometastasis mostly occurs in the near portal area with rich oxygen supply and nutrients, i.e., Zone I, and it is closely associated with the adhesive molecules, phagocytic activities, and large amount of astrocytes and liver cells with active functions. In addition, colorectal cancer cells have high expression of CCR6, and the liver is the major source location of CCL20 in addition to lymph nodes (CCL20 is the sole ligand of CCR6); especially the mononuclear cells, macrophages, and dendritic cells of the portal area have high percentage of expression of CCL20 and CCR6/CCL20, playing an extremely important role in the directional metastasis of intestinal cancer in the hepatic portal area [47].

The difference from the main biological behaviors of large tumors is that micrometastasis is free of blood supply. Therefore, micrometastasis cells obtain oxygen and nutrition through permeation, which confines it from growing into a cancer nest of 2–3 mm. These cancerous cells maintain dormant on a long-term basis, and their cell dynamics and apoptosis are equal; therefore there is no pure growth. This balance is maintained until the cancerous cells are identified and eliminated by the immune monitoring system or obtain blood supply and grow.

4.2.3 Angiogenesis of Micrometastasis

The further development of micrometastasis into a general metastasis with clinical significance requires the formation of new blood vessels, which is an active process, including the degradation of extracellular matrix, proliferation and migration of endothelial cells, and the formation of new vessels, and among them, hypoxia and inflammatory mediators are the most important stimulants of angiogenesis. Since the discovery by Folkman of the phenomenon that tumor growth depends on angiogenesis, many factors that have positive and negative regulations of angiogenesis have been successively discovered. Tumor's survival and metastasis depend on the comprehensive results of positive and negative regulators, and the ultimate result tends to have the formation of tumor vessels. For colon cancer, among the multitude of relevant angiogenic factors, the vascular endothelial growth factor (VEGF) is by far the most important angiogenic factor and plays a main role on the initial degradation of extracellular matrix. There is a close relationship between the VEGF expressions of colon cancer patients at different stages of disease and vascular density and metastasis, and the expression of VEGF's receptor KDR on the vascular endothelial cells of tumor is also associated with vascular density and VEGF. On colon cancer patients with negative lymph nodes, vascular density is rather high, and the VEGF expresses relatively more unfavorable prognosis. A multitude of methods, such as the antibodies of anti-VEGF receptors or the tyrosine kinase inhibitor intercepting the VEGF receptor role, are adopted to block VEGF's activity which can reduce the quantity, sizes of hepatic metastasis of mice colon cancer model, and the vascular density of metastasis. In addition, sustained anti-VEGF therapy will lead to the death of tumor vessels and even tumor cells. Fibroblast growth factor (FGF) family is another group of powerful angiogenic cytokines, which enhance the removal of endothelial cells and the formation of small vessels, and there is coordination between VEGF and bFGF. What is more important in the metastasis of colon cancer is the platelet-derived endothelial cell growth factor (PD-ECGF).

The angiogenesis of liver metastasis of intestinal cancer is closely associated with three kinds of tumor growth patterns [48]: desmoplastic growth pattern, pushing growth pattern, and replacement growth pattern. Desmoplastic growth and pushing growth destroy substantial liver structure, with obvious angiogenesis, and replacement growth is maintained in the reticular fiber structure of the liver in the tumor-host interface, which guides the interstitial cells to grow along the residual reticular fiber structure of the liver, and these vessels in the interface not only have no expression of CD34 but also have no coverage of α-SMA+ interstitial cells, indicating smaller quantity of angiogenesis. However, the proportion of proliferation cancerous cells in the metastasis of replacement growth and the proportion of proliferated endothelial cells (but the quantity is the smallest of the three) are three to four times that of other growth patterns. The apoptosis proportion of cancerous cells in the pushing growth is the highest, and MVD is the lowest. The curative effects of the replacement growth in the anti-angiogenesis therapy are far lower than those of metastasis of other growth patterns.

4.2.4 The Final Formation Stage of Liver Metastasis

When the cancerous cells in metastasis have completed the above three steps, a liver metastasis of intestinal cancer of clinical significance is ultimately formed.

Regarding metastases, there exists a great heterogeneity between different individuals or within the same tumor: tumor interstitium and microvessel density and structure, hemodynamic differences between the blood supplies by the portal vein and hepatic arterial system, the heterogeneity of functions and phenotypes of tumor infiltration lymphocytes, and the differences in the growth and proliferation and gene expressions of cancerous cells themselves.

Based on the hepatic microenvironment, some scholars divide the whole process of intrahepatic metastasis of intestinal cancer into three phases (see Table 4.1) [49].

The contrasts between the surrounding liver tissue of metastasis and the normal liver distant from the metastasis have revealed that such genetic expressions as "extracellular matrix", "intercellular communication", "activation of astrocytes", and "cell growth" of paracarcinoma liver tissue are markedly upregulated, thus indicating the cancer-causing function of paracarcinoma hepatic microenvironment [50]. The spectrum of specific gene expression originated from paracarcinoma hepatic tissue or the interstitial cells in the metastasis can predict metastasis recurrence and patients' survivals after metastasis resection.

Table 4.1 The staging of liver metastasis based on hepatic microenvironment

	Stage I	Stage II	Stage III
Magnitude	<300 μm; undetectable	0.3–0.5 mm; a few are detectable	>5 mm; detectable
Clinical significance	Subclinical metastasis	Produce certain effects on focal liver	Produce systemic effects and may give rise to extrahepatic spread
Location and status	Confined within the hepatic lobule, free of angiogenesis, or only small amount of microvessel formations	It occupies the whole hepatic lobule and grows outward, with obvious angiogenesis	Clinically visible metastasis has been formed
Relation with liver cells[a]	Have not recruited vascular and interstitial components	Recruited liver cells and formed the mesenchyme and blood vessels of metastatic tumor	Affected by two aspects, the liver cells of normal liver beside the cancer and the liver cells infiltrated in the cancer
Effects on the liver	Only affect the liver cells in the colonized location	Jointly developing with the liver cells recruited into the cancerous focus	Affect normal hepatic tissue and structure, blood supply, and parenchymal molecular metabolism
Utilizable targets	Proinflammatory cytokines, immunosuppressive factor, stimulating factors of fibroblasts, oxidative stress-induced factors	Angiogenic factors, myelomonaytic growth factor (CMGF)	Tumor growth promotion factors, immunosuppressive factors

[a]Here " liver cells" include liver parenchymal cells and interstitial cells

4.3 Problems and Outlook

4.3.1 The Value of Microenvironment in Tumor Prevention and Cure

Tumor microenvironment plays an important role in tumor progression, tumor interstitium as anti-tumor target has obvious advantages, and if the interstitial cells are non-transformation cells, compared with tumor cells, their genome is relatively stable and they have a small chance of antigen loss and therapeutic tolerance; interstitial cells have little differences on different tumors, and therapy targeting at tumor interstitium can be used on various kinds of solid tumors on a wide spectrum.

The value of prevention is far greater than that of therapy. Various kinds of cells (macrophages, endothelial cells, fibroblasts, etc.) in the tumor microenvironment are all effective targets that can be prevented. First, the impacts on various kinds of anti-inflammatory treatments on TAM and TAN are quite obvious, for they are the main source of inflammatory mediators. Secondly, for the T lymphocytes of microenvironment, the mouse model has proven that the key molecules SMAD that selectively knock the TGF-β signaling pathways in T lymphocytes can lead to the defuse malignancy of the whole digestive tract; however, the mere selective knockout of the SMAD in the epithelial cells has no such effect [51]; at the early stage of the occurrence of human digestive tract tumor, it is also possible to detect the loss of TGF-β signaling pathways; drugs that can restore or strengthen the TGF-β signaling pathways mediated by SMAD can enhance the expression of downstream products (such as plasminogen activator inhibitor-1, TGFβR2) and inhibit the malignant transformation of canceration, indicating the prevention application value of the T lymphocytes of microenvironment [52]. In addition, various kinds of small molecule substances in the microenvironment, corresponding signaling pathway genes, and the formation of tumor vessels can all be taken as targets of prevention. Among them, the representative ones include the drugs that reconstruct the immune microenvironment with the relevant factors of antagonistic immune tolerance, such as small molecule substances of the major molecular mechanisms tolerant to microenvironment indoleamine 2, 3-dioxygenase (IDO), Arg, arginase I, inducible nitric oxide synthase (iNOS), and JAK-STAT signaling pathways. These drugs can activate the DC in patients, myeloid-derived suppressor cells (MDSCs), and CTL, recruit them in large amounts to the local microenvironment, and simultaneously block the cell-regulating functions of TAM and TAN [53].

The spontaneous treatment of microenvironment during the treatment of cancerous cells has become two undividable aspects of microenvironment treatment. After the plantation of cancerous cells with high invasion and metastasis potentials into the embryonic microenvironment, not only the cancerous cells manifest relatively better differentiation characteristics, even similar to the corresponding cells derived from normal sources, but also the capacity of nodule formation and invasion and metastasis is substantially reduced, indicating the shaping role of normal embryonic microenvironment on cancerous cells and its potential application value [41]. The balance between promoting and anti-angiogenic factors in the microenvironment makes the angiogenesis abnormal, and vessel structures tend to become normalized, thus correcting the abnormal metabolic state of microenvironment (pH values, gap pressure, and hypoxia) and restoring the sensitivity to chemoradiotherapy, etc. Research has indicated there exists an instantaneous "normalization window" in the angiogenesis therapy based on VEGFR2 antibodies, and the curative effects of combination therapies during this window are far greater than those of combination therapies of non-window period, indicating the importance of prolonging the vascular "normalization window" period and time selection in combination therapies [54]. The hindrance of tumor interstitium is considered as one of the reasons for the poor curative effects of antitumor immunity. Promoting the release of stromal antigens using such means as chemoradiotherapy, thus inducing the CTL reactions regarding the stromal antigen, or killing the interstitial cells with cross-presentation of tumor antigens, or stimulating the double immune responses from both antitumor and interstitial resistant cells, will be more conducive to the elimination of tumors and prevention of tumor recurrence [55].

4.3.2 Several Notable Aspects

Although tumor microenvironment is conducive to tumor progression, there still exists a certain balance relationship between the tumor suppressor factors and promoting factors in the microenvironment. Matrix degradation enzymes play an active role in the process of the formation and invasion and metastasis of blood vessels, but the endostatin, angiostatin, and tumstatin as the degradation products of MMPs are the main endogenous vascular resultants; therefore the experimental and clinical wide-spectrum MMPs have limited curative effects. Therefore, the development of specific inhibitors and the selections of specific patients and appropriate therapeutic targets (whether inhibiting the cellular functions or killing the cells) must be considered regarding the treatment of tumor microenvironment.

Selecting appropriate therapeutic targets and promoting the normalization of the abnormal tumor microenvironment are usually more effective. Excessive formation of tumor-inhibiting vessels can not only correct the abnormal angiogenesis but can also induce the tumors' resistance to angiogenesis and worsen the abnormalities of local vascular structure, thus worsening such metabolic disturbances as hypoxic microenvironment and uneven distribution of nutrients and the increase of the tumor cells' tolerance to chemoradiotherapy and capacity of invasion and metastasis. If it is dedicated to restoring the vascular structure of the tumor microenvironment and thus bringing about sufficient and evenly distributed oxygen and nutrient supply, it will not only give growing advantages to tumor cells with weaker tolerance to such adverse conditions as hypoxia and lower malignant biological characteristics, thus competitively inhibiting cancerous cells with relatively higher malignancies, but also is more beneficial for follow-up or simultaneous therapy focused on the tumor's invasion and metastasis, which is successively or simultaneously conducted, to play its role [56].

Although combination therapy is superior to monotherapy, if the design of combined application is inappropriate, on the contrary it will have exactly opposite effects. The dedication to immunologic tolerance of antagonistic microenvironment and reconstruction of the regulatory means conducive to antitumor immunity microenvironment, if rationally combining such traditional antitumor therapies as chemoradiotherapy, can play the synergistic and additive effects. Regarding radiotherapy, radiotherapy can promote the microenvironment's function of antigen-presenting cells and induce the T-cell infiltration, yet at present, for such reasons as the reduction of toxicity, clinically fractionated radiotherapies are more commonly adopted, so what kind of effects this will bring on the immune response induced by the first local irradiation and whether the radiotherapy interval or one-time large-intensity local irradiation must be considered in the combined reconstruction of local immune microenvironment.

In addition, the study of tumor microenvironment must have good models. In the embryonic microenvironment models utilizing zebrafish embryos and chicken embryos, it is found that normal embryonic microenvironment has reversal effect on the malignant characteristics of cancerous cells, the total control mechanism of embryonic stem cells, and highly malignant tumor cells and their potential application values. The development of the economical and efficient models applicable to different research objectives and maximally simulating the in vivo microenvironment will greatly enhance the development of tumor microenvironment study.

4.3.3 Hepatic Microenvironment and the Prevention of Liver Metastasis of Intestinal Cancer

Hepatic microenvironment plays an important role in the hepatic directional metastasis of intestinal cancer; the normal anatomical characteristic wherein blood flows into the liver from the intestines via the portal vein is unchangeable, and the spontaneously discovered intestinal cancer and liver metastasis are also irreversible. However, for those who are not subject to liver metastasis, we can alter the hepatic microenvironment so as to prevent the occurrence of liver metastasis of intestinal cancer, or halt the reactivation of the intestinal cancerous cells that have been colonized and in dormant state, or prevent the post metastasectomy relapse. The sinusoidal endothelial cells of hepatic microenvironment, astrocytes, immune and inflammatory cells, and hepatic parenchymal cells are all targets that can be tried. Specific chemokines and their receptors, such as CCR6 and CCL20 axis, as well as the newly discovered CCL2 [57], are also very good targets.

Currently, a new hypothesis, "pre-metastatic niche," holds that before the tumor cells arrive at the target organs, they will release several factors to activate hematopoietic progenitor cells (HPCs), and these cells will reach the target organs before the tumor cells, creating a microenvironment there that is suitable for the survival and proliferation of metastatic tumor cells so as to receive the arrival of tumor cells. The significance of this hypothesis for the liver metastasis of intestinal cancer may lie in the fact that the synergy of HPC and hepatic microenvironment promotes the occurrence of liver metastasis, and it also provides new challenges and opportunities to therapies targeting at hepatic microenvironment.

References

1. Bross IDJ, Blumenson LE. Metastatic sites that produce generalized cancer: identification and kinetics of generalizing sites. In: Fundamental aspects of metastasis. 1976. p. 359–75.
2. Sugarbaker EV. Patterns of metastasis in human malignancies. Cancer Biol Rev. 1981;2:235–78.
3. Wyckoff J, Wang W, Lin EY, et al. A paracrine loop between tumor cells and macrophages is required for tumor cell migration in mammary tumors. Cancer Res. 2004;64:7022–9.
4. Bindra RS, Glazer PM. Genetic instability and the tumor microenvironment: towards the concept of microenvironment-induced mutagenesis. Mutat Res. 2005;569:75–85.

5. Tse JC, Kalluri R. Mechanisms of metastasis: epithelial-to-mesenchymal transition and contribution of tumor microenvironment. J Cell Biochem. 2007;101:816–29.
6. Parekh K, Ramachandran S, Cooper J, et al. Tenascin-C, over expressed in lung cancer down regulates effector functions of tumor infiltrating lymphocytes. Lung Cancer. 2005;47:17–29.
7. Zhang T, Sun HC, Xu Y, et al. Overexpression of platelet-derived growth factor receptor alpha in endothelial cells of hepatocellular carcinoma associated with high metastatic potential. Clin Cancer Res. 2005;11:8557–63.
8. Zeng Q, Li S, Chepeha DB, et al. Crosstalk between tumor and endothelial cells promotes tumor angiogenesis by MAPK activation of Notch signaling. Cancer Cell. 2005;8:13–23.
9. Bagley RG, Weber W, Rouleau C, et al. Pericytes and endothelial precursor cells: cellular interactions and contributions to malignancy. Cancer Res. 2005;65: 9741–50.
10. Condeelis J, Pollard JW. Macrophages: obligate partners for tumor cell migration, invasion, and metastasis. Cell. 2006;124:263–6.
11. Sato E, Olson SH, Ahn J, et al. Intraepithelial CD8+ tumor-infiltrating lymphocytes and a high CD8+/regulatory T cell ratio are associated with favorable prognosis in ovarian cancer. Proc Natl Acad Sci U S A. 2005;102:18538–43.
12. Lu LF, Lind EF, Gondek DC, et al. Mast cells are essential intermediaries in regulatory T-cell tolerance. Nature. 2006;442:997–1002.
13. Queen MM, Ryan RE, Holzer RG, et al. Breast cancer cells stimulate neutrophils to produce oncostatin M: potential implications for tumor progression. Cancer Res. 2005;65:8896–904.
14. Kukreja A, Hutchinson A, Dhodapkar K, et al. Enhancement of clonogenicity of human multiple myeloma by dendritic cells. J Exp Med. 2006;203: 1859–65.
15. de Visser KE, Korets LV, Coussens LM. De novo carcinogenesis promoted by chronic inflammation is B lymphocyte dependent. Cancer Cell. 2005;7:411–23.
16. Dong HP, Elstrand MB, Holth A, et al. NK- and B-cell infiltration correlates with worse outcome in metastatic ovarian carcinoma. Am J Clin Pathol. 2006;125:451–8.
17. Nishikawa H, Kato T, Tawara I, et al. Accelerated chemically induced tumor development mediated by CD4+CD25+ regulatory T cells in wild-type hosts. Proc Natl Acad Sci U S A. 2005;102:9253–7.
18. Hiraoka N, Onozato K, Kosuge T, et al. Prevalence of FOXP3+ regulatory T cells increases during the progression of pancreatic ductal adenocarcinoma and its premalignant lesions. Clin Cancer Res. 2006;12: 5423–34.
19. Liu C, Gao S, Qu Z, et al. Tumor microenvironment: hypoxia and buffer capacity for immunotherapy. Med Hypotheses. 2007;69:590.
20. Roberts SJ, Ng BY, Filler RB, et al. Characterizing tumor-promoting T cells in chemically induced cutaneous carcinogenesis. Proc Natl Acad Sci U S A. 2007;104:6770–5.
21. Salama P, Phillips M, Grieu F, et al. Tumor-infiltrating FOXP3+ T regulatory cells show strong prognostic significance in colorectal cancer. J Clin Oncol. 2009;27:186–92.
22. Galon J, Costes A, Sanchez-Cabo F, et al. Type, density, and location of immune cells within human colorectal tumors predict clinical outcome. Science. 2006;313:1960–4.
23. Galon J, Fridman WH, Pages F. The adaptive immunologic microenvironment in colorectal cancer: a novel perspective. Cancer Res. 2007;67:1883–6.
24. Budhu A, Forgues M, Ye QH, et al. Prediction of venous metastases, recurrence, and prognosis in hepatocellular carcinoma based on a unique immune response signature of the liver microenvironment. Cancer Cell. 2006;10:99–111.
25. Samoszuk M, Kanakubo E, Chan JK. Degranulating mast cells in fibrotic regions of human tumors and evidence that mast cell heparin interferes with the growth of tumor cells through a mechanism involving fibroblasts. BMC Cancer. 2005;5:121.
26. Overall CM, Kleifeld O. Tumour microenvironment – opinion: validating matrix metalloproteinases as drug targets and anti-targets for cancer therapy. Nat Rev Cancer. 2006;6:227–39.
27. Giannelli G, Fransvea E, Marinosci F, et al. Transforming growth factor-beta1 triggers hepatocellular carcinoma invasiveness via alpha3beta1 integrin. Am J Pathol. 2002;161:183–93.
28. Burger JA, Kipps TJ. CXCR4: a key receptor in the crosstalk between tumor cells and their microenvironment. Blood. 2006;107:1761–7.
29. van Deventer HW, Serody JS, McKinnon KP, et al. Transfection of macrophage inflammatory protein 1 alpha into B16 F10 melanoma cells inhibits growth of pulmonary metastases but not subcutaneous tumors. J Immunol. 2002;169:1634–9.
30. Sparmann A, Bar-Sagi D. Ras-induced interleukin-8 expression plays a critical role in tumor growth and angiogenesis. Cancer Cell. 2004;6:447–58.
31. Wu X, Fan J, Wang X, et al. Downregulation of CCR1 inhibits human hepatocellular carcinoma cell invasion. Biochem Biophys Res Commun. 2007;355: 866–71.
32. Sun B, Zhang S, Zhang D, et al. Vasculogenic mimicry is associated with high tumor grade, invasion and metastasis, and short survival in patients with hepatocellular carcinoma. Oncol Rep. 2006;16: 693–8.
33. Franchi A, Gallo O, Massi D, et al. Tumor lymphangiogenesis in head and neck squamous cell carcinoma: a morphometric study with clinical correlations. Cancer. 2004;101:973–8.
34. Mylona E, Alexandrou P, Mpakali A, et al. Clinicopathological and prognostic significance of vascular endothelial growth factors (VEGF)-C and -D and VEGF receptor 3 in invasive breast carcinoma. Eur J Surg Oncol. 2007;33:294–300.

35. Schoppmann SF, Bayer G, Aumayr K, et al. Prognostic value of lymphangiogenesis and lymphovascular invasion in invasive breast cancer. Ann Surg. 2004; 240:306–12.
36. Chaudary N, Hill RP. Hypoxia and metastasis. Clin Cancer Res. 2007;13:1947–9.
37. Gatenby RA, Gawlinski ET. The glycolytic phenotype in carcinogenesis and tumor invasion: insights through mathematical models. Cancer Res. 2003;63: 3847–54.
38. Yu H, Kortylewski M, Pardoll D. Crosstalk between cancer and immune cells: role of STAT3 in the tumour microenvironment. Nat Rev Immunol. 2007;7:41–51.
39. Gamero AM, Young HA, Wiltrout RH. Inactivation of Stat3 in tumor cells: releasing a brake on immune responses against cancer? Cancer Cell. 2004;5: 111–2.
40. Yahata Y, Shirakata Y, Tokumaru S, et al. Nuclear translocation of phosphorylated STAT3 is essential for vascular endothelial growth factor-induced human dermal microvascular endothelial cell migration and tube formation. J Biol Chem. 2003;278:40026–31.
41. Topczewska JM, Postovit LM, Margaryan NV, et al. Embryonic and tumorigenic pathways converge via Nodal signaling: role in melanoma aggressiveness. Nat Med. 2006;12:925–32.
42. Ayala G, Tuxhorn JA, Wheeler TM, et al. Reactive stroma as a predictor of biochemical-free recurrence in prostate cancer. Clin Cancer Res. 2003;9: 4792–801.
43. Hill R, Song Y, Cardiff RD, et al. Selective evolution of stromal mesenchyme with p53 loss in response to epithelial tumorigenesis. Cell. 2005;123:1001–11.
44. Kim R, Emi M, Tanabe K, et al. Tumor-driven evolution of immunosuppressive networks during malignant progression. Cancer Res. 2006;66:5527–36.
45. Vidal-Vanaclocha F, Mendoza L, Telleria N, et al. Clinical and experimental approaches to the pathophysiology of interleukin-18 in cancer progression. Cancer Metastasis Rev. 2006;25:417–34.
46. Rappaport AM. The microcirculatory hepatic unit. Microvasc Res. 1973;6:212.
47. Ghadjar P, Coupland SE, Na I-K, et al. Chemokine receptor CCR6 expression level and liver metastases in colorectal cancer. J Clin Oncol. 2006;24:1910–6.
48. Vermeulen PB, Colpaert C, Salgado R, et al. Liver metastases from colorectal adenocarcinomas grow in three patterns with different angiogenesis and desmoplasia. J Pathol. 2001;195:336–42.
49. Vidal-Vanaclocha F. The prometastatic microenvironment of the liver. Cancer Microenviron. 2008;1:113–29.
50. Obul Reddy B, Martina G, Dennis K, et al. Global analysis of host tissue gene expression in the invasive front of colorectal liver metastases. Int J Cancer 2006;118:74–89.
51. Kim BG, Li C, Qiao W, et al. Smad4 signalling in T cells is required for suppression of gastrointestinal cancer. Nature. 2006;441:1015–9.
52. Suh N, Roberts AB, Birkey Reffey S, et al. Synthetic triterpenoids enhance transforming growth factor beta/Smad signaling. Cancer Res. 2003;63: 1371–6.
53. Muller AJ, Scherle PA. Targeting the mechanisms of tumoral immune tolerance with small-molecule inhibitors. Nat Rev Cancer. 2006;6:613–25.
54. Winkler F, Kozin SV, Tong RT, et al. Kinetics of vascular normalization by VEGFR2 blockade governs brain tumor response to radiation: role of oxygenation, angiopoietin-1, and matrix metalloproteinases. Cancer Cell. 2004;6:553–63.
55. Yu P, Rowley DA, Fu YX, et al. The role of stroma in immune recognition and destruction of well-established solid tumors. Curr Opin Immunol. 2006; 18:226–31.
56. Bello L, Lucini V, Costa F, et al. Combinatorial administration of molecules that simultaneously inhibit angiogenesis and invasion leads to increased therapeutic efficacy in mouse models of malignant glioma. Clin Cancer Res. 2004;10:4527–37.
57. Hu H, Sun L, Guo C, et al. Tumor cell-microenvironment interaction models coupled with clinical validation reveal CCL2 and SNCG as two predictors of colorectal cancer hepatic metastasis. Clin Cancer Res. 2009; 15:5485–93.

Screening and Identification of Molecular Marker for Metastatic Liver Cancer

5

Yinkun Liu, Chun Sun, and Binglin Chen

Metastatic liver cancer, also called as secondary liver cancer, refers to the tumor transferred from other parts of the body to the liver through portal vein, hepatic artery, or lymph. The metastatic liver cancer is generally from the lung, mammary gland, colon, pancreas, and stomach as well as leukemia and other hemocyte cancer. It is said that the stomach cancer, pancreatic cancer, and colon cancer could be transferred to the liver through the portal vein, while the breast cancer and lung cancer could be transferred to the liver through hepatic artery. Generally speaking, the metastatic liver cancer is free from HBV infection, hepatitis, and hepatocirrhosis. Here, AFP is normal, but CEA is raised. As per CT detection, various focal nodiules are found inside the liver. They may suffer from necrobiosis, cystic degeneration, bleeding, or calcification. Generally, the metastatic liver cancer is not merged with the portal vein cancer embolus, so that no well-defined symptoms are found at the early phase. In case the symptoms occur, the pathological changes are obvious. At the early phase, it mainly reflects the symptom of primary tumor. However, the symptom of metastatic liver cancer is not obvious. It is mostly found before the primary carcinoma operation, during the follow-up survey after the primary carcinoma operation or exploratory laparotomy. With the disease development, the symptom of metastatic liver cancer gradually appears with the enlargement of tumor. Also, for a minority of patients (mainly transferred from stomach and pancreas), the symptom of metastatic liver cancer is obvious. So, the symptom of metastatic liver cancer is found before the occurrence of primary carcinoma. However the symptom of protopathic tumor is not obvious.

As one of the common cancers in China, the primary liver cancer refers to the cancer swelling from liver cells or intrahepatic duct cells. According to the epidemic disease data for high-risk population, the sick rate hereof is the highest for the population at the age of 35–45, earlier than the age of previously defined high-risk population. When the primary liver cancer is found, 80 % thereof are at the middle or later period. Also, as the liver cancer is treated, the rate of recurrence and transform reaches 60 %. Therefore, the rate of death is very high. For the primary liver cancer patients, the positive rate of hepatitis B virus (HBV) in the serum reaches 90 %. Meanwhile, 90 % of the primary liver cancer is hepatocellular carcinoma and always goes along with the hepatocirrhosis and abnormality of liver function. The symptoms are unable to be found at the early phase of primary liver cancer. In terms of pathology, the primary liver cancer is generally divided into massive type, nodular

Y. Liu (✉) • C. Sun • B. Chen
Zhongshan Hospital, Fudan University, Shanghai, China
e-mail: liu.yinkun@zs-hospital.sh.cn

X. Qin et al. (eds.), *Multidisciplinary Management of Liver Metastases in Colorectal Cancer*,
DOI 10.1007/978-94-017-7755-1_5

type, and diffuse type. In terms of histology, it is divided into hepatocellular carcinoma, cholangiocarcinoma, and mixed cancer.

This chapter mainly covers the classification and definition of metastatic tumor molecular marker as well as the establishing and optimizing of related polymolecular diagnosis and prediction system. Also, systematic summary is made for the research on molecular marker of colon and rectal cancer and hepatic metastasis thereof.

5.1 Metastatic Tumor Molecular Marker

5.1.1 Definition of Tumor Molecular Marker

Tumor molecular marker (TM) is the substance produced from tumor tissue or reaction of the organism to tumor. For example, as examined, the molecular marker in the tumor-related microenvironment of inflammation or immunity could be adopted in the helper diagnosis of tumor, analysis of pathogenesis, treatment guidance, recurrence or transform monitoring, and prognosis. For tumor-related research and clinical practice, it is crucial to achieve the discovery, diagnosis, interposition, and treatment at the early phase. So, the tumor marker is provided with high use value in such aspects as general survey, diagnosis, and prognosis of tumor as well as the treatment evaluation and follow-up survey on the high-risk population. Actually, the primary liver cancer is similar to the secondary liver cancer or metastatic liver cancer in terms of the basic bionomics. In the target tissue, the focal nodes from the primary tumor position are similar in terms of pathology and clinical indices. However, no difference is found for the concept of tumor molecular marker.

5.1.1.1 Tumor Marker of Biochemistry

Tumor marker of biochemistry is mainly produced from the tumor cell and could secrete the substance in the conduction cell. So, the quantitative determination could be carried out via the zero-defect analytic method. Here, serum or urine, tissue fluid, and thoracic and abdominal fluid could be used as the specimen. The tumor marker is approximately divided into five types:

1. Protein-related tumor marker: α-fetoprotein (AFP), cancer embryo antigen (CEA), Bence-Jones protein (BJP), and monoclonal protein
2. Carbohydrate antigen-related tumor marker: antigen with CA such as CA 50, CA 125, CA 153, CA 199, and CA 242. Moreover, PSA and SCC could be adopted
3. Ganglioside-related tumor marker: sialic acid (SA)
4. Enzyme-related tumor marker: NSE, A2GT, AKP, LDH, ACP, and glutathione transferase
5. Steroids-related tumor marker: chorionic gonadotropin (HCG)

5.1.1.2 The Tumor Marker Could Be Divided as per the Source, Distribution, and Relationship with the Tumor

1. Primary tumor-related substance such as the enzymes quickly increased during cancerization
2. Ectopic tumor-related substance such as ectopic hormone and NSE
3. Placenta- and embryo tumor-related substance such as AFP and CEA
4. Viral tumor-related substance such as HTL-1 virus, thymus-derived cell leukemia, EB virus, Burkitt tumor, hepatitis B virus, and liver cancer
5. Oncogene, tumor suppressor genes, and the product thereof

5.1.1.3 Classification as per the Purpose of Application

1. Tumor molecular marker: it reflects the existence of disease, i.e., diagnosis indices; for the generalized concept, the tumor molecular marker could not only judge the tumor but also classify molecular marker of the tumor.
2. Molecular marker for tumor susceptivity: the potential occurrence of tumor could be detected, particularly, and the tumor patient could be found from the high-risk population, i.e., disease risk.
3. Molecular marker for tumor prediction: related to the clinical progress and result of

disease, so as to predict the occurrence of tumor, clinical outcome and development of tumor (prognosis), and recurrence and transform of tumor.

The clinical diagnosis of cancer generally relies on the iconography and several diagnosis markers. Such markers include various cancer cell antigens and carbohydrate antigens. However, both sensitivity and specificity thereof are not good enough. For instance, the sensitivity of alpha-fetoprotein (AFP) is only 39–64 %, and the specificity thereof is only 76–91 % in the diagnosis of hepatocellular carcinoma; the sensitivity of CEA is less than 70 % in the diagnosis of colon cancer; the sensitivity of CA 19-9 is less than 60 % in the diagnosis of gastrointestinal cancer. It is more important that the divergence still exists for definition of some markers' critical value. For example, as PSA is examined, the precision ratio of diagnosis is lower if the lower critical value (4 μg/L) is chosen, while only the patients at the late period are diagnosed if higher critical value (10 μg/L) is chosen, so as to lose the opportunity to treat at the early phase.

The single molecular marker-based disaggregated model for cancer diagnosis still lacks the convincing sensitivity and specificity. So, selection, identification, and assessment of new cancer-related tissue or serum molecular marker have become one of the important parts of tumor research [1, 2].

In recent years, with the further research on such preclinical medicine as immunology, molecular biology, and biochemistry as well as the development of detection technique and methodology, the tumor marker has gradually become the reliable index in the clinical diagnosis. The desirable tumor marker shall be provided with the following features: strong specificity and high sensitivity; also, the concentration examining is related to the size of tumor and phases, so that it could be used for curative effect monitoring and prognosis judgment. Though the current tumor markers are unable to reach 100 % sensitivity and 100 % specificity, the clinical application of tumor marker becomes more and more important thanks to the continuous improving of examination and evaluation procedures.

The cancer is a disease treated via multifactors and multiple paths. Thus, the disease signaling molecule shall be fully learned; also, the analysis of bioinformatics shall be made available. Today the establishing, verification and clinical application of multi-molecular diagnosis model have become the focal point in the research on tumor molecular marker.

5.1.2 Method of Screening the Tumor Molecular Marker

The development and progression of tumors is considered as a multistep procedure with involvement of multiple molecules. So, it is complicate to select and identify the tumor molecular marker. Here, it includes tumor cell line and tumor-bearing laboratory animal; comparative study on human tumor tissue, cancer-affected tissue, and normal tissue; comparative study on fluid from tumor patient and normal person (including blood, urine, transudate, and ascites); high flux reactor; and real-time research on meaningful tumor-related molecular or "group study" (genome, transcriptome, protein, or metabolism); thus, the molecular marker with differential expression could be screened out, and the probability of tumor molecular marker thereof could be further verified.

5.1.2.1 Genome and Transcriptome

Comparative Genome Hybridization (CGH)

There is genomic instability in a lot of tumors, among which the chromosomal instability (CIN) and microsatellite instability (MIN) are particularly concerned [3–5].

As a molecular cytogenetics-related technique developed since 1992, comparative genomic hybridization (CGH) could examine the changes of DNA copy number between two (or more) genomes and position these abnormalities on the special chromosome, so that it could be used in the research on the growth of various tumors classification of diagnosis and prognosis [6]. Here, the different types of fluorochrome are used to mark DNA of tumor tissues and normal cell or tissue via nick translation, so as to make the probe; also, hybridization is made with the intermediate chromosome of normal person, so that changes of DNA in the whole oncogene could be displayed on the chromosome through the difference between fluorescence intensity of tumor and that of normal tissue. In addition, the image analysis is used to conduct the quantitative investigation on the change of chromosome copy number. Therefore, there is no need to predict the affected positions and the preparation of cell at the middle period is avoided. So, it is suitable to the research on periphery blood, cultured cell, and tissue specimen as well as PCR increased specimen. However, owing to the low-level DNA augment and loss of small segment, the translocation of chromosome is undetected or non-detectable [7].

Array CGH could clone DNA or turn cDNAs into the array, so as to substitute the metaphase chromosome as the hybridization target. In this case, the resolution is increased; also, the tumor-related gene and precise positioning could be ascertained. The rule thereof is similar to CGH, i.e., DNA to be tested and contrast DNA with equal quantity but different fluorescent labels are hybridized with the array CGH from DNA clone or cDNAs after repetitive sequence of non-specific Cot-1 DNA. The change of copy number of DNA to be tested on the relevant series or gene could be reflected through the rate between two fluorescent singles of each target on the array [8–10].

Array CGH avoids the complex chromosome structure, so that the crossbred target series are only a short DNA segment with a minority of gene. In this case, the change of DNA copy number could be detected. However, the traditional CGH detection is impossible to detect the above changes. Meanwhile, the increased or unavailable scope could be exactly positioned on one or a couple of known genes on EST; both high sensitivity and accuracy are realized. In addition, the automation and routinization could be achieved simultaneously [11, 12]. For example, the US Vysis company offers genome research chip system: array 300 which covers 278 gene probes which are related to tumor, antepartum, and preimplantation, so that it could detect the change of 1/2/3 copy number, micro-deficiency, and non-euploidy of chromosome and unbalanced translocation. Thus, the new prospect is made available for the discovery of the related tumor molecular marker, clarifying of occurrence and development of tumor, genetic diagnosis, and individualized treatment.

Multicolor-Fluorescence In Situ Hybridization (mFISH)

FISH was created by Pinkel et al. [13] in 1986 on the basis of radioactive hybridization in situ. The fluorescently labeled nucleic acid probe is hybridized with the complementary nucleic acid inside the cell, so as to examine the conditions, quantity, and structure of the latter. As compared with the traditional radioactive hybridization probe and banding technique, FISH boasts higher specificity and resolution.

mFISH is based on the associated mark probe and proportional mark probe. With the associated mark technique, one probe could simultaneously adopt the half-antigen or fluorescein with different colors to mark, so that the capacity of mFISH is substantially increased. In principle, the associated mark could be available for the probe of 2n-1 (n is the number of hapten or fluorescein) [14]. If the fluorescein with different proportions is used to mark each probe, the capacity of FISH with associated mark will be further increased. Also, the quantitative analysis [15] could be carried out. The joint application of associated mark probe and proportional mark probe further optimizes the probe mark and testing result of mFISH.

In 1996, two study groups respectively used different methods to realize the simultaneous display of 22 pairs of euchromosome and two sex chromosomes through one hybridization. Speicher et al. [16] combined CCD with one group of filter lens to respectively mark the micro-cut probe through augment of DOP-PCR and five kinds of fluorochrome mixed from different proportions. The spectral filter series were used. Each type of spectral filter only permits certain specific wavelength to pass. So, the image of each marker chromosome position could be reflected through the change of different spectral filters. As treated via the computer software, one mFISH chromosome karyogram is made available, so that 24 kinds of the human chromosome were all provided with different fluorescence colors; even the long arm and short arm of single chromosome were respectively colored. Schrock et al. [17] adopted spectral karyotyping (SKY) to combine Fourier spectrography, CCD imaging, and light microscope. Here, the specially prepared illuminant could stimulate the emission spectra from each chromosome. Each pixel element could be turned into three types of spectral regions, i.e., red spectral region (650–750 nm), green spectral region (550–650 nm), and blue spectral region (475–550 nm), after being changed by the interferometer and fourier spectrography. Then the spectral regions could be changed into the digital signals. As each chromosome was comprehensively measured, these digital signals could be converted into the simulated color images which were assigned to each chromosome, so as to sort out the different chromosomes. mFISH and SKY further improve the assessment on cytogenetics of pernicious disease through provision of more karyotype and aberrant chromosome-related data [18–20]. However, technique limitations also occur. For example, the translocation, inversion, and intrachromosomal aberration inside the same chromosome are undetected. The expensive experimental materials (probe), experimental setup, and analytical software are demanded. So, mFISH shall combine with array CGH to bring the superiority thereof into full play. For instance, mFISH is used to detect the translocation and marker chromosome of complex nucleus; CGH is used to detect the unbalanced area, so that both deficiency discovery and augment are made available to offer better convenience to the research.

Gene Chip Technology

For the gene chip technology, a lot of molecular identification probes (gene or gene segment) are orderly fixed to the surface of the tiny solid-phase supporters (silicon wafer, slide, nylon membrane slice, and ceramic chip), so as to hybridize with the target gene in the marked specimen as per the principle of base pairing. Finally, the instrument (laser focused fluorescent scanning instrument) could be adopted to carry out the qualitative and quantitative examining on the visualized signal intensity speedily, simultaneously, and efficiently. In this case, thousands upon thousands of genetic expressions and coadjustment thereof could be analyzed at the same time [21].

As per the components of probe, the gene chip is mainly divided into two types: cDNA chip (also called as cDNA array) and DNA chip (also called as nucleotide chip or array). The former is mainly used for gene expression analysis, and the latter is used for gene expression spectrum analysis or gene mutation and mononucleotide polymorphism (SNP) testing [22–24]. As per the usage, the gene chip is also divided into expression spectrum chip, sequencing chip, diagnosing chip, and fingerprint chip.

CDNA Chip Technology

CDNA chip technology was established by Schena in Stanford University [22]. Here, as enlarged by PCR, the special cDNA is directly dotted on the chip through the manipulator, so that it could be hatched with fluorescently labeled mRNA from cell, tissue, or other biological samples. These transcripts will be hybridized with complementary cDNA on the chip, so that based on the analysis of signal intensity for hybridization, the gene with differential expression could be chosen (see the Fig. 5.1 as follows).

On the strength of cDNA chip technology, the gene expression-related data could be sufficiently obtained from time to time, so as to lay a solid foundation on revealing the function of these genes. On the other hand, the quantity of mRNA could basically reflect the protein level of current cell, so as to facilitate the effective and systematic assessment on the protein content inside the cell.

Due to the above merits of cDNA chip, it is widely used in the research on cell metabolism, disease mechanism, drug screening, and active mechanism. For the disease diagnosis, cDNA chip is generally used in the classification of cancer. For example, Alizadeh used cDNA chip

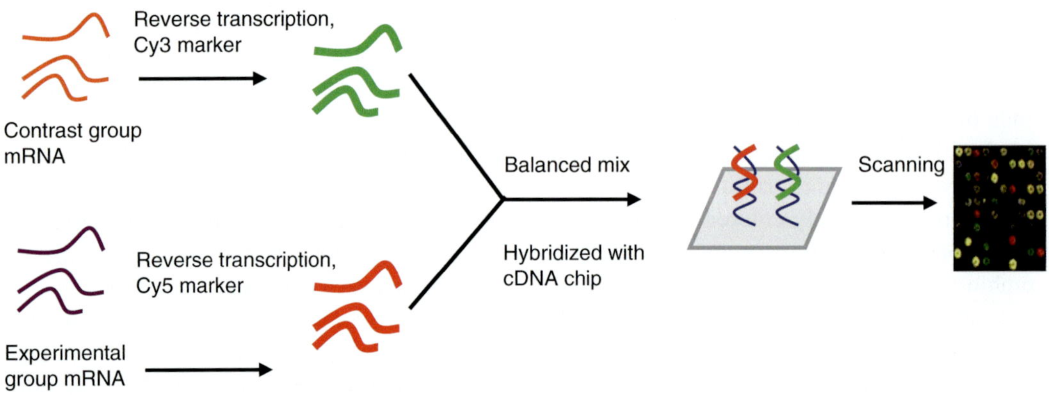

Fig. 5.1 Main procedures of cDNA technology

with nearly 15,000 genes to classify the huge diffusive B-cell lymphoma [25]. Also, Okabe adopted cDNA chip with 23,040 genes to analyze the primary liver cancer tissue and normal tissue, so as to find out 165 upregulated genes and 170 downregulated genes. In addition, 19 genes with change of expression were used to distinguish the HBV-caused hepatocellular carcinoma and HCV-infected hepatocellular carcinoma [26].

With the fast growth of proteomics, the transcriptomics and proteomics are combined to become the new method for seeking the molecular markers. For example, Seliger [27] adopted cDNA chip and proteomics to search out annexin A4, tubulin α-1A chain, and ubiquitin carboxyl-terminal hydrolase L1, the candidate molecular markers of kidney cell cancer.

SNP Chip Technology

SNP (single-nucleotide polymorphism): The traditional SNP shall be examined through gel electrophoresis. The SNP chip technology introduces the in situ synthesis of single nucleotide or microprinting to orderly fix a lot of DNA segments on the surface of solid-phase supporter, so as to form the probe array which is hybridized with the labeled specimen. Here, the hybridized signals are examined to realize the fast, effective, and collateral polymorphic information analysis. The chip technology platform includes microarray, fiber film microdot, and sheet glass array chip of which the density reaches hundreds or millions of probes.

Common types:

1. As one of the methods adopted to examine quantitative DNA, TaqMan probe chip combines the real-time examining with chip technology, so that not only the common quantitative examining, sensitivity, and real-time examining are merged together, but the parallelized analysis under high flux reactor is also considered. However, the PCR augment synchronizes TaqMan probe enzyme to cause the increase of non-specificity signals. Thus, it shall be further studied to demonstrate whether such technique is suitable to the SNP chip with low and middle densities.
2. Single-base extension (SBE) is mainly used for research and development of low-density chip as well as the accurate screening of randomly chosen SNP positions [28, 29]. For another single-base extension technique, the extension marker reaction is completed, and the specific type of allele is tested as per the level of matching. As compared with SNP stream, SBE primer design only demands one type of fluorescent light. Thus, examining on abrupt change of SNPs is not limited.
3. Ligation-rolling circle amplification (L-RCA)-based low-flux reactor chip: padlock probe cyclization of T4 joining enzyme or thermal arrest joining enzyme medium as well as point mutation of sensitive and differential DNA series. The circular probe series could be hybridized for distinguishing after rolling circle augment and enzymes. Design of L-RCA

and complexity of gene order may affect the flux reactor, so that the classification of chip with high flux reactor is unable to be met.

4. High flux reactor chip with Golden Gate TM: Golden Gate TM achieves the highest-flux reactor for current preparation of SNP chip, so as to reach one million. However, it only demands 250 ng for the genome. This multiple inspection level could meet the demands for gene classification testing as far as possible. Thus, the precision ratio of gene classification could reach 96.64 %. However, such technique is only suitable to the SNP examining under two condition changes. Only 60 % of SNP could be detected [30, 31]. For the full-genome scanning, this technique could detect SNP label. The content of genetic information is more than that of the GeneChip Human Mapping 100 K Array chip.

With the fast growth of SNP chip technology in massive parallelism, high flux reactor, miniaturization, and automation, this technique could be used to search the new SNP positions and realize the pinpointing of SNP positions in genome. The large-scale SNP classification shall be supported by the accurate and reliable test method. However, the research and development of SNP chip technology could be the important method for molecular diagnosis, clinical examination, clinical treatment, and new drug development in the future [32]. The development of SNP chip and gene polymorphism research hereof has not only improved the individualized medical detection technique but also provided the diagnosis basis for the use of individualized medicine, so as to facilitate the growth of small-sized diagnosing market [33].

DNA Methylation Test Method

DNA Methylation Chip

As one of the most common changes of epigenetics, DNA methylation is crucial to the normal cell development and texture stability. It shows that the methylation in the promoter or the first exon-extron CpG causes the deactivation of gene expression.

The examining methods for methylation marker are mainly divided into two types: examination after chemical modification and examination after modification of methylation-sensitive restriction enzymes. The first examining method was created by Frommer [34]. Based on the former one, Gitan [35] developed methylation-specific oligonucleotide microarray, i.e., MSO microarray. For MSO, a pair of probe series with GC (AC) shall be designed to respectively identify the methylation and non-methylation probe series, which then are fixed on the supporter. The targeted segment is treated with bisulfite; the non-methylation cytosine is changed to uracil. When methylation is unchanged, PCR augment is conducted. The 3′-end of product shall be provided with fluorescein label and then hybridized with the probe. As the fluorescence intensity after hybridization is tested, the level of methylation in the series to be tested shall be judged. This method is one of the commonly used DNA methylation chips. As per this method, the detailed research has been conducted for the promoter area of such genes as estrogen receptor (ER), p16, and adenomatous polyposis coli (APC) [36, 37]. However, MSO is unable to obtain the data concerning each CpG position. Also, the criss-crossing may occur in the probe. As a result, the false-positive rate is high. So, the comparison shall be established.

Examination after modification of methylation-sensitive restriction enzymes includes differential methylation hybridization (DMH), methylation-sensitive arbitrarily primed PCR (MS-AP-PCR), methylated CpG island amplification (MCA), and restriction landmark genomic scanning (RLGS). DMH is used in the differential methylation hybridization of the entire genome as well as the differential methylating pedigree between cancer tissue and normal structure. It is similar to mRNA expression spectrum or cDNA array. So, it belongs to CpG island array. Cross et al. [38] created the affinity substrate with methylating CpG binding domain, so as to separate CpG island series from the human genome DNA. Mse I enzyme identifies TTAA position. Here, genome DNA enzyme could be cut into the segments of which the size is less than 200 bp, while the area enriched with CpG islands is not cut. Then, as both ends of enzyme segment are connected with the joint, the endoenzyme with sensitive methylation such as BstU I, Hpa II, and Hha I DNA segments could be used. DNA segment with methylation is not cut due to the protection of methylation so as to achieve the joint-PCR augment; however, the segment without methylation is unable to be enlarged. Afterwards, the fluorescence labeling, hybridization, image, and data handling procedure are exactly similar to those of expression spectrum chip [39]. This method is simple but effective, so that it could be used to discriminate the tumor. Currently, DMH has been successfully used in examining the methylation spectrum of oophoroma. However, the popularization of this technique is restricted owning to the finiteness of enzyme location and specialty of instrument.

The different methylation spectra reflect the different phases or types of tumor. High methylation position of CpG islands is related to the occurrence of tumor. Therefore, it could be deemed as the unique marker for special tumor haplotype. Currently, it is widely used in the examining of various tumors such as non-Hodgkin's lymphoma, lung cancer, and oophoroma. Also, high flux reactor screening of methylation could detect the abnormal gene expression mode of such diseases as malignant tumor. Thus, it is helpful to ascertain the tumor formation mechanism, so as to provide the effective monitoring and prediction on non-methylation drug reaction in chemotherapy.

Restriction Landmark Genome Scanning (RLGS)

RLGS is a high flux reactor DNA methylation parsing technique which combines MS-RE (methylation-sensitive restriction endonuclease) with the two-dimensional gel electrophoresis [40]. The technical principle is based on the divergence of sensitivity on CpG position with or without methylation during the application of restriction enzyme. The sequence information is not demanded ahead of time. So, it is suitable to the examination on thousands of CpG islands within the entire genome, so as to seek the methylation gene of new CpG islands.

Here, the sensitive restriction enzyme with methylation could be used to learn about the methylation condition of entire gene. Also, GC-rich restriction enzyme could be used to obtain a plurality of landmarks on CpG islands near the promoter. However, the shortcoming is that due to the restriction enzyme, the position of examining is limited by that of restriction enzyme; also, the insufficient restriction enzyme could produce false positive. In addition, the deactivation of tumor suppressor genes due to methylation of promoter CpG islands is closely related to the occurrence of tumor, so that it is important to learn the changes of methylation of tumor suppressor gene CpG islands [2].

Procedures of RLGS [41–44]: Specimen DNA is digested through landmark enzyme which is crucial to RLGS. In general, methyl-sensitive Not I (GC↓GGCCGC) or Asc I (GG↓CGCGCC) is used due to low cutting rate and at least two available CGP positions. After cutting, the end is marked with ^{32}P-dCTP and ^{32}P-dGTP. Also, digestion is conducted through EcoRV (methyl insensitivity and cutting rate are higher than that of Not I) to produce the shorter Not I-Eco RV segment, which is extended via 1D electrophoresis. Then the segment is digested within the gel via Mbo I, so as to further produce the shorter Not I-Mbo I segment, which is extended in 2D electrophoresis. Then RLGS map is made. Analysis of virtual RLGS: for the organism with fully interpreted genome, RLGS figure could be independently simulated to make comparison with the real RLGS to identify the stain (for details, see Ref. [44]). As compared, the lost or subdued signal points in the specimen mean CpG islands with high methylation (excluding the loss of DNA). To the contrary, the newly appeared or enhanced signal points mean CpG islands with low methylation (excluding the DNA augment).

The potential application could include (1) polymorphism screening and gene mapping research, (2) mark gene research, (3) research on gene structure and methylation of cancer tissue and clone mouse, and (4) varietal appraisal of crops.

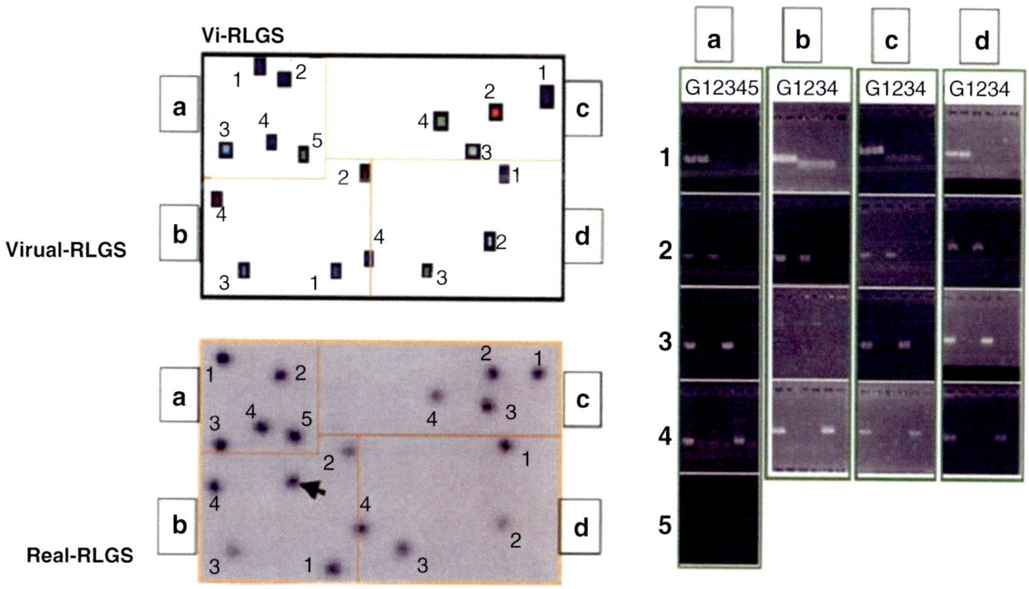

Fig. 5.2 Comparison between simulated RLGS and real RLGS (Reprint from *Nucleic Acids Res*, Ref. [44])

Peripheral Blood DNA as Well as Related Microsatellite DNA and Tumor-Specific DNA (RNA)

Peripheral blood DNA, also called as free DNA, plasma DNA, or serum DNA, is composed of double-bond DNA, single-bond DNA, or the mixture thereof. It exists by means of free DNA and DNA-protein. The circulated DNA level in the healthy human body is very low, accounting for around 3.6–5.0 ng/ml which may be sourced from death of cells. Most of DNA segments are less than 180 bps [45]. The cytology research shows that the above DNA segments are found through the cultivation liquid which is induced by the apoptotic cells, while most of DNA segments are more than 10,000 bps for the cultivation liquid induced by the necrobiosis. For the tumor patients, the content of peripheral blood DNA is always increased; also, the component hereof is complicated. This is related to the physiological parameters of pathology. It is said that this may be caused by the death of tumor cells, splitting of circulated tumor cell or focal transfer, or DNA released by the tumor cell to peripheral circulation such as shedding of protein on the surface [46–48] (Fig. 5.2).

The common measuring method for peripheral blood DNA includes the total content of peripheral blood DNA; category and content of tumor metastasis-related microsatellite DNA and tumor-specific DNA (RNA) and percentage thereof to total content of DNA. Changes of above factors often occur earlier than the tumor markers such as AFP and CEA. Therefore, they are important to the early tumor diagnosis, tumor metastasis after operation, and curative effect assessment. Gabriella et al. [49] tested DNA from 43 bottles of healthy human plasma and 84 bottles of human plasma from non-small-cell carcinoma of the lung patients, so as to find out that the plasma DNA concentration in the control group was 18 ng/ml, while the plasma DNA of lung cancer patients at Ia and Ib, respectively, reached 320 ng/ml and 344 ng/ml. According to the follow-up survey on 38 lung cancer patients with pneumonectomy, the mean concentration of plasma DNA for 35 patients without recurrence was 34 ng/ml, while for the three patients with increased plasma DNA for 2–20 times after operation, two patients died from hepatic metastasis after the operation and one patient suffered from partial recurrence after 2 years. Oliver et al. [50] adopted real-time fluorescent quantization PCR to test plasma DNA of 46 healthy humans and 185 patients with non-small-cell carcinoma of the lungs before or after chemotherapy, so as to find out that circulated DNA concentration of patients with steady conditions was decreased as compared with that before treatment, while plasma DNA of patients with exacerbation was increased. Chao et al. [51] conducted dynamic monitoring on circulation of plasma DNA of the cancer patient after chemotherapy to discover that the plasma DNA was temporarily raised within 2 weeks after the beginning of chemotherapy. Afterwards, plasma DNA was under stabilized descent.

5.1.2.2 Proteomics

Good Separating of Complicated Proteomics and Examining of Low-Abundance Protein

Two-Dimensional Electrophoresis (2DE)-Based Protein Expression Spectrum

The protein separating in 2DE includes the isoelectrofocusing electrophoresis of which the protein mixture is separated as per the ups and downs of isoelectric point along the first direction as well as the SDS-PAGE electrophoresis of which the protein mixture is separated as per the size of molecular weight along the second direction. 2DE display method is used in gel staining (Coomassie Brilliant Blue), metal reagent (silver staining) or total protein staining, sugar protein, or phosphorylated protein. Also, the protein could be diverted to the membrane through Western blot, so as to conduct the immunology testing or other analysis. The currently used gel scanning equipment is the density scanner, phosphor screen, or fluorescent scanner. Also, image analysis software (Gel Image and PDQuest) is used to conduct the analysis such as protein spot searching, quantifying, background deduction, and punctual matching. In this case, the protein with differential expression could be discovered.

Difference in Gel Electrophoresis (DIGE) [52]: On the basis of traditional two-dimensional gel electrophoresis, the multi-fluorescence analysis is combined to jointly separate a plurality of samples with different fluorescent labels. The fluorophore used for labeling all belongs to the same class with similar molecular structure; also, the molecular weight thereof is the same and provided with positive charge, so that as reaction with remained lysine of peptide chain, all the samples could be transferred to the same position, so as to substantially improve the accuracy, dependability, and repeatability of the result. The sensitivity of such method could compare with that of silver staining and SYPRO Ruby. Here, the protein of 100–200 pg could be observed.

Non-2DE-Based Protein Expression Spectrum

1. Two-dimensional liquid phase chromatography and mass spectra (2DLC-MS) [53]: the multidimension chromatographic resolution could be used with the mass spectra to make up for the display deficiency of two-dimensional electrophoresis and mass spectra to the protein with low abundance, hydrophobicity, alkalinity, and maximum and minimum. Here, the mixed proteolysis is properly under chromatographic separation. Then MS/MS analysis is made for peptide segment so as to realize the albumin evaluation (also called Shotgun). So far, the most representative analysis is strong cation exchange (SCX)-reverse phase (RP). The peptide segments are firstly divided into groups on the SCX column as per electrostatic interaction. Then, by means of gradient, the components from SCX column are directly sampled on the reversed-phase column. According to the acting force of peptide segment and hydrophobic interaction, the above components are eluted by the mobile phase from chromatographic column. Finally, the mass-spectrometric detection is used to test the peptide segment.
2. Surface-enhanced laser desorption ionization time-of-flight mass spectrometry (SELDI-TOF-MS) [54, 55] is composed of protein chip, flight mass spectrum, and analytical software. The protein chip is divided into chemical surface and biological surface. Also, the protein chip with chemical surface is divided into lyophobic surface and water-wetted surface, weak cation and strong anion

exchange surface, metal ion coupling surface, and specific combination surface. The protein chip with biological surface is divided into antigen-antibody, reception body-lagan, DNA-protein, and enzyme. The chip with chemical surface adopts fewer specimens and could be directly used in the analysis on serum, body fluid, and urine. So, it is easy for automatic operation under high flux reactor to evaluate well on the hydrophobic albumin with low abundance. For the currently appeared combination of ClinProt's liquid chip with mass spectrum, peptide series could be detected directly.

3. Labeling technique-based protein expression spectrum: (i) isotope-coded affinity tags (ICAT) [56] is based on the use of cold labeling reagent and unique analytical apparatus. The structure of tagging reagent is the biotin tag joint reactive group. Here, biotin tag is designed to separate the peptide segment. The joint is divided into two types: tritium labeling for joint in D8-ICAT and hydrogen (unlabeled) for the joint in D0 ICAT. The reactive group could be connected with SH of remained cysteine in peptide segment. ICAT reagent (D8 or D0) is reacted with the equal protein to be analyzed, to achieve ICAT albumin which is under proteolysis after equal blending to achieve the mixture of peptide segment. As purified by avidin column, the mixture of peptide segment could form ICAT marked peptide. Also, molecular weight and intensity (D0/D8) of D8-ICAT and D0-ICAT peptide could be analyzed by MS to arrive the difference of the same peptide segments in different specimens. Moreover, MS-MS could be used to conduct sequencing analysis on peptide with differential expression. (ii) Amino acid-coded mass tagging (AACT) [57] is also called SILAC of which the fundamental principle is the same as that of ICAT. The major difference is that AACT is the cold tagged amino acid in the cell culture group to be analyzed, i.e., based on biosynthetic method, the synthetic protein could be provided with grade tag. Then, the cells incubated by normal amino acid are blended equally and under enzymolysis. Finally, MS analysis is used to analyze the difference of the same peptide segments in the different specimens. This technique could improve the accuracy of MALDI TOF/TOF mass spectrometer to sequential analysis of peptide segment. (iii) Isobaric tags for relative and absolute quantization (iTRAQ) [58]: the fundamental principle is the same as that of ICAT. However, the adopted marker joint is made up of reporting group (114–117), balancing group (31–28), and amino acid reactive group. Here, the total mass number is the same. Then, the different protein specimens shall be marked. The proportion of specific protein to each specimen could be obtained after the composite specimen is analyzed by the mass spectrum. As per the rule of analysis and difference of protein, the protein with differential expression could be made available for future research.

Protein Evaluation and Characteristic Analysis Thereof

1. Western blot [59]

   Evaluation on proteinic expression: in order to avoid the false positive of protein with differential expression and increase the confidence level of observed data, the protein shall be transferred to the solid-phase supporter, i.e., membrane (nitrocellulose filter or PVDF membrane), for immunodetection, staining, and other solid analysis as the SDS-PAGE is over. The modifiable albumin such as sugar protein could be tested through development process, combined techniques of agglutinin, and sugar protein fluoroscopic examination. The testing level depends on the glycosyl level of protein. In case of phosphorylated protein, the antibody of serine phosphate, phosphothreonine, and phosphotyrosine could be adopted for testing.

2. Immunoprecipitation

   It is based on antibody-antigen reaction; the immunoprecipitation is divided into immunoprecipitation, joint immunoprecipitation, and tandem affinity purification (TAP). The basic steps of joint immunoprecipitation and immunoprecipitation are the same, but not the difference in the pretreatment. TAP could be used in the purification of protein complex. The principle thereof is that the gene (bait protein) is connected to two tagged genes to form the fusion gene which stains saccharomycete or mammal cell strain. Such fusion is under quadratic chromato-purification with the coupled albumin glue column which combined with the tagged protein, so that research could be conducted for the separation and purification of protein complex under approximate natural conditions as well as the succeeding protein-to-protein interaction [60].

3. Evaluation on protein functions

   It is mainly based on genetic manipulation, including gene compensation and gene deletion. For the gene compensation, the expression vector of protein gene is constructed and transferred, and then the gene expression control, cellular metabolism, and change of cell behavior are observed; The gene was knocked in to form the transgenic animal or organism model, so as to learn about various changes of transgenic borganism as a whole. The gene deletion includes the application of antisense nucleic acid, RNA interference (RNAi), RNA enzyme, and single nucleotide bonded with the gene promoter. At the transcriptional and posttranscriptional levels, the gene expression is "cancelled and reduced" or knockout is used to produce the organism with gene defect. Here, research is conducted on the gene control, signal method, and metabolism of cell and organism "cancelled and reduced."

Research on Tumor Protein Molecule Marker of Serum and Histiocyte

1. The tumor serum marker is divided into two types: one is the spontaneous antibody produced due to tumor antigen's stimulation on the immunity of organism, and the other is the albumin tagged molecule which is derived from the tumor and closely related to the development of tumor. In view of these two tumor serum markers with different properties, SERPA and two-dimensional gel electrophoresis-mass-spectrometric technique in proteomics could be respectively adopted to screen the tumor-related antibody and albumin in the serum.

1. Serum proteome analysis (SERPA)

   It is a new technique formed via the combination of proteomics with immunology, so as to achieve the high flux reactor screening and evaluation of tumor antigen and antibody thereof [61, 62]. The fundamental principle of SERPA is that two-dimensional gel electrophoresis is used to separate the tumor tissue or total protein of cell, which is under Western blotting. Then it is hybridized with the sero-immunity of tumor patients to realize the color rendering. In this case, the tumor antigen could be ascertained when the reaction points on the two-way gel are evaluated by the mass spectrum. For this technique, there is no need to create the expression library, so that a lot of serum specimens of the patients could be analyzed. Meanwhile, the frequency of tumor antibody occurrence could be calculated. It is more important that the modificatory proteantigen after translation could be found. Therefore, since this technique is invented, it is immediately used in the screening and judgment of various tumor antigens for kidney cancer, lung cancer, and breast cancer [63, 64]. Le Naour [64] adopted this technique to find that eight kinds of albumin are provided with the specific tumor antibody in the serum of over 10 % liver cancer patients.

2. Two-dimensional gel electrophoresis-mass spectroscopy of serum and tumor-related albumin tagged molecule: the two-dimensional gel electrophoresis-mass spectroscopy of serum faces a lot of difficulties. Firstly, the abundance of albumin in the serum could have the large divergence of quantity degree of 10^{12}. For example, albumin and immunoglobulin could account for 60–97 % of total serum protein, while the potential albumin acting as the disease-related marker only accounts for less than 1 % thereof [65, 66]. So, it is crucial to remove the albumin with high abundance in

the serum, so as to conduct the two-dimensional gel electrophoresis-mass spectroscopy for the serum. The other difficulty of two-dimensional gel electrophoresis-mass spectroscopy of serum is that the big individual variation exists among the serum specimens. Therefore, the serum in the same group could be firstly mixed to ensure the dependability of difference among the groups. Finally, Western blotting could be adopted to further verify the screened albumin markers, so as to guarantee the reliability of the result.

3. SELDI-TOF-MS: it is widely used in such fields as tumor, new drug development, infectious disease, and mental sickness. It could refer to the research result of tumor diagnosis from Lancet in 2002 and the early diagnosis [67] jointly launched by FDA and NCI on oophoroma. As compared with the traditional CA 125 index (positive predictor only accounts for 35 %), a plurality of indices for protein fingerprint reaches the sensitivity of 100 %, and positive predictor achieves 94 %. Now this method is already used in small-cell carcinoma of the lung [68], prostatic cancer [69], kidney cancer [70], breast cancer [71], and neck tumor [72]. Currently, this technique has been introduced into China, e.g., it is used in carcinoma of urinary bladder [73], glioma, pancreatic cancer, blood diseases, and chronic liver diseases, including hepatitis, hepatocirrhosis, liver cancer, and metastasis and recurrence [74]. However, such measurement has strict requirements for the specimen. Also, the limitations exist due to the instable system and subsequent software analysis.

2. Selection of tumor biological marker via the proteomics of cell and tissue

Comparative proteomics compares dynamic variation and divergence of protein expression at each stage of tumor tissue and normal tissue, tumor tissue, and cancer peripheral tissue or disease as well as specifies the modified conditions, tissue distribution, tissue specificity, and testing sensitivity. Meanwhile, the review and foreseeable research shall be substantially conducted to test the probability of protein molecule as the tumor marker. Also, the comparison could be made with the serum proteomics. Now HSP 27 is exemplified herein. Two-way gel electrophoresis (2DE) is used o separate the HCC tissue with metastasis and six HCC tissue protein without metastasis. In addition, 16 albumin points with significant difference could be tested, including S100 Ca-binding protein (S100), HSP 27, and keratin 18 (CK 18). It is verified that the expression level of HSP 27 is closely related to the latent energy of liver cancer metastasis [75]. The research on serum proteomics further verified that HSP 27 could be used as the potential liver cancer-related biological marker [76].

In terms of medical service, the proteomics could be helpful for the research on pathogenesis, early diagnosis, and treatment of human diseases. Based on the comparison, the analysis could be made on the differential expression of entire protein within the normal tissue and abnormal histiocyte as well as the cell at the different phases of disease. The evaluation and quantitative analysis could be conducted for the albumin with differential expression to find out the new markers which are related to the disease, so as to offer new methods and basis for the human disease study. Also, the target spot for oncotherapy could be made available.

5.2 Polymolecular Classification Model of Tumor Molecular Marker

5.2.1 The Expression Difference of Molecular Marker

According to the comparative study, the expression difference of gene, protein, or metabolite could be obtained under different pathological conditions, e.g., the molecular marker with expression difference, which shall follow the conditions below.

5.2.1.1 Verification on the Expression Difference of Molecular Markers

RT-PCR or real-time PCR is used to study the expression of mRNA through semiquantitative or quantitative method, or Western blot or immunohistochemistry (including chip technology), and immunofluorescence cytochemistry to study the expression of protein level and verify the expression results of chip.

5.2.1.2 Bioinformatic Analysis on Expression Difference of Molecular Markers

Cluster analysis, PPI analysis, database-oriented Meta-analysis or HTML-based aggregate analysis is commonly used in the early diagnosis, prediction and prognosis of potential biological marker.

5.2.2 Methods for Ascertaining the Tumor Biological Marker

Chip technologies of genome and transcriptomics as well as mass-spectrometric technique of proteomics and metabonomics are the commonly used real-time test methods with high flux reactor. Such test methods are core to the screening of disease molecular markers. Here, the mass data are sorted out through bioinformatic parsing technique. The establishing of disease classification model shall follow the steps: normalization of data, selection of features and sorting algorithm, and mathematical model testing.

5.2.2.1 Normalization of Data

The influencing factors such as "technique" and "biology" may exist during the experiment. So, the normalization of raw data shall be conducted before the comparison of various observed data, so as to reduce the difference among the experiments.

For gene chip test, "housekeeping gene" is always used as the control point, so that the proportion of control point to sample point could be adopted to reduce the error of "technique." For the error of "biology," it could be optimized by the replicated experiment. For specific calculation, the normalization of gene chip data is always realized through lowness. Afterwards, SAM software (significant analysis of microarray) is used to sort out the differential expression of gene and conduct the cluster analysis thereof.

During the mass-spectrum test, the later processing of data is relatively complicated. As the peptidome-based original spectrogram is obtained, alignment of the spectra shall be firstly conducted. Here, the intensity of the same peak in the same sample shall be kept in line during various measurements. Besides the built-in software kit of commercialized software, the software with more universality on the file format is developed by some study team, so as to overcome the compatible problems of analytical software [77]. After the spectrogram is calibrated, denoising and normalization shall be still carried out. The denoising includes removal of substrate, electronic jamming, and random ion motion as well as calibrating of spectrogram baseline [78, 79]. Normalization shall remove the systematic error caused by specimen or instrument. In general, the average value or median of adopted peak is for reference [80]. Then, the mass-to-charge ratio and intensity of each peak could be effectively measured. Next, the Biomarker Pattern Software (BPS) is mostly used to sort out the difference of peaks.

5.2.2.2 Selection of Features or Sorting Algorithm

Based on gene chip technology and mass-spectrometric technique, the researcher could obtain a lot of gene and peptide expression-related data. If one or more expressions are obviously different in various specimens, such gene- or peptide-based disaggregated model may boast very strong discriminability in diagnosis or prediction of disease. The chosen marker (also called property) is generally provided with following features: pathological meaning is available for discrimination or classification of disease. Also, the interactive messages are made available among the properties. So, the number of properties shall be reduced as far as possible to achieve high efficiency. Therefore, the selection of markers plays a vital role in the accuracy of disease classification model.

The existing feature selection algorithm is divided into two types:

Filter: the properties are sorted, so that several properties at the highest rank are chosen. Wrapper: sorting algorithm is embedded into the selective process of features, so that the results of classification are the selection criterion which is observed to choose the best feature subset. For the studies on multifactor cancer disaggregated model, the Wrapper is commonly used for feature selection.

The sorting algorithm means that the targets to be identified are sorted as certain category in the feature space via some computational methods. The elementary operation is that the training samples are used to ascertain and optimize the sorting algorithm. Thus, such algorithm could reach the highest precision ratio in the training sample set, so as to obtain the related disaggregated model; then, the above disaggregated model could be used to sort out the specimen. Currently, the multifactor cancer disaggregated model, particularly SELDI-TOF-MS data-based disaggregated model, adopts decision tree [81–92], which has fewer nodes and is subject to the specific peak, so as to prompt the further research on the single molecular marker. The other major merit of decision tree is that the composite sample with different properties or even the numerical value or nonnumerical value-based composite sample could be processed. Therefore, as the SELDI-TOF-MS and existing clinical indices are used as aggregate analysis, the strong operability is available. Other common sorting algorithms include artificial neural network [93, 94] and support vector machine [95]. The former is suitable to a lot of specimen but may suffer from "overstudy," thus causing a large gap between training set and test set; the latter is based on stricter mathematical theory and has the overall optimality, but it is more suitable to small-scale specimens; also, only two kinds of classified algorithm are available [96].

For the study on gene chip-based disaggregated model, prediction analysis for microarrays (PAM) [97, 98], nearest mean [99], classifier of nearest centroid [97], k-nearest neighbor [100, 101], log linear [102], multidimensional ranking [103], and compound covariate predictor [24] are adopted besides decision tree [104], artificial neural network, and support vector machine [103, 105] as per stated above. It is difficult to judge the superior and inferior of different sorting algorithms in terms of mathematical foundation. The appropriate method is that based on the same sample set, the results of different sorting algorithms are compared to choose the most appropriate disaggregated model [95, 97] of special incident; or, as per the mutual authentication among different algorithms, the model with highest precision ratio could be created for the classification of special incidents.

5.2.2.3 Test on Disease Classification Model

The multiple regression analysis [106, 107], ROC tracing analysis [101, 103, 108], foreseeable verification [24, 97, 102, 109], and review verification are usually adopted for the test on a disease classification model.

1. Multiple regression analysis is the analytic method used for studying the correlation between dependent variable (diagnostic summary) and various arguments (molecular markers) as well as among various arguments. For tumor diagnosis, the contributions of each molecular marker to the function of disaggregated model as well as the correlation between the molecular markers could be learned through the multiple regression analysis. This will guide the future research on the development, metastasis, and recurrence of tumor as well as prognosis and survival rate. As the most used regression algorithm, logistic and Cox adopt the method of maximum likelihood for parameter estimation. Logistic is suitable to the dependent variable belonging to grouped data, so that quantitative analysis and research could be made for the influence of each factor to the dependent variable; Cox is mainly used in the survival analysis, so as to effectively analyze such special dependent variable (survival time of patient). The

multiple regression analysis could be realized through various types of common computer software such as SPSS and Excel.

2. ROC, the abbreviation of receiver operating characteristic, is a sensitivity- and specificity-based analytic method used to reflect the accuracy of disaggregated model via "area under the curve (AUC)". Also, it could be quantitative method used to evaluate the contributions of single molecular tag to the classified diagnosis model and polymolecular aggregate analysis, so as to improve the overall efficiency. The operation thereof could be achieved by SPSS and Excel.
3. For disaggregated models of cancer, double-blind regression of sample set is widely used, e.g., the comparison between overall survival, OS, and disease-free survival (DFS) in the life table. For the tumor metastasis research, comparison of tumor metastasis rate is taken into special account. Also, foreseeable verification on the survival rate of patient is reported. However, due to the difficulty in actual operation, the verification on cancer prediction of disaggregated model via follow-up survey on high-risk population is still not reported. Yet, it is necessary to carry out the foreseeable research on the polymolecular model which is useful in the prediction, diagnosis, and clinical outcome or prognosis.

5.3 Colorectal Cancer and Hepatic Metastasis Molecular Marker Thereof

5.3.1 Common Tumor Molecular Marker of Colorectal Cancer

The sick rate of colorectal cancer in China has been rising. The 5-year survival rate thereof only accounts for 50 %. CEA and carbohydrate antigen (CA 199) are the two common colon cancer markers, which are mainly used in evaluating the curative effect and monitoring the recurrence of tumor at the late period. So, they do not produce the major significance to the screening of colon cancer at the early stage. Currently, the serological diagnosis indices with high sensitivity and specificity for diagnosis of colorectal cancer are unavailable. Therefore, it is necessary to find out the new tumor marker.

Shiwa et al. [110] discovered the protein with the molecular weight of 12KD in the cell strain of colon cancer. Here, the mass-spectrometric technique is adopted to identify the protein of 12KD as α-prothymosin, which may be the biological marker to diagnose the colon cancer. Lawrie et al. [111] analyzed the proteomics for cell line LIM 1215 of colon cancer, so as to identify 92 membrane proteins and offer the "target ion" to evaluate albumin with low abundance. Simpson et al. [112] also analyzed LIM 1215 and established membrane protein database, so as to further study the development of colorectal cancer.

Studying on cell line HCT 116 of colon cancer with high metastasis, Ahmed et al. [113] discovered that plasma urokinase plasminogen activator (uPA) and the reception body (uPAR) thereof may be the significant factors which cause the deterioration or metastasis of colon cancer, so they not only help in establishing the signaling molecule proteomics database for uPAR but also become the new method for diagnosis and treatment of colon cancer. Stierum et al. [114] analyzed the Caco-2 proteomics of colorectal cancer cell line and detected 11 kinds of protein related to the reproduction and disintegration hereof. The research shows that FABL, CH 60, GTA 1, TCTP, and NDKA albumin are closely related to the colorectal cancer. Thus, it will be helpful to verify the molecular mechanism concerning the occurrence and development of colorectal cancer.

Xu et al. [115] used SELDI protein chip to analyze the serum specimen of colorectal cancer patient, so as to set up seven models. Each model is made up of a plurality of distinctive albumin peaks. The precision ratio in phase for the patient before operation reached 78.72 % to the minimum and 86.67 % to the maximum. Roboz et al. [116] chose the hydrophobicity chip (H4) to find out albumin of m/z 8942 shows high expression and albumin of m/z 9300 shows low expression. Also, Petricoin et al. [117] made the comparative study on colorectal cancer and polypus to find a 13.8×10^3 protein, which is expressed via both colorectal cancer and polypus. So, it is meaningful to the early screening of colorectal cancer.

Friedman analyzed 12 specimens for colorectal cancer tissue and normal tissue to obtain more than 1,500 distinctive albumin points. As per the mass-spectrum evaluation, 52 kinds of protein with abnormal expression, including cytokeratin, annexin IV, creatine kinase, and fatty-acid-binding protein, are found, so as to greatly enrich the protein database of colorectal cancer tumor [118].

Chaurand et al. [119] analyzed mucosa of both normal colon and colon cancer to find out that 100A8, S100A9, and S100A11 in the Ca-binding protein family of cancer tissue were increased, so as to prompt that these three kinds of protein were the specific markers of colon cancer.

Stulik et al. [120, 121] found that the content of EF-2, Mn-SOD, and nm 23 was particularly high in colon cancer; also, the changes of nine kinds of protein were the same in the cancer tissue and adenoma tissue, namely, expression decrease of L-psoriasis-related albumin and carbonic anhydrase and expression increase of S100A11, PPIASE alkalinity mutant, attached element III and VI, DDA H, CK 18, and inhibin, so as to demonstrate the correlation between change of these albumin and development of colorectal cancer.

Roblick et al. [122] analyzed the specimens of normal tissue, adenoma tissue, cancer tissue, and tumor metastasis tissue of sigmoid carcinoma patient via 2DE, peptide mass fingerprinting, PMF, and MS and carried out the comparison for the individual patient as well as between the patients, so as to find out the abnormal expression of 112 albumin points, among which 72 proteins were evaluated. Here, 46 were increased, but 26 were decreased.

Pei Haiping et al. [123] found that apolipoprotein A1 with differential expression, calreticulin precursor, glutathione-s transferring enzyme (GST-s), liver-type fatty-acid-binding protein, and heat shock protein 27 could be chosen as the candidate biological markers for early diagnosis of colorectal cancer.

An Ping et al. [124] found that loss of calmodulin, DNase 262 precursor protein, and α-mannosidase and the increase of apolipoprotein are related to the occurrence of colorectal cancer and hepatic metastasis.

Tachibana et al. [125] conducted proteome analysis on primary tumor and metastatic tumor of colon cancer so as to obtain Apo A1 (apolipoprotein A1). Also, as per the further research on RT-PCR and immunohistochemistry, expression of Apo A1 in the primary tumor is much lower than that in metastatic tumor. Expression of Apo A1 is related to the pernicious degree of colonic adenocarcinoma. Therefore, Apo A1 could be chosen as the potential marker for enhancement of tumor invasiveness.

5.3.2 Molecular Markers for Hepatic Metastasis of Colorectal Cancer

The hepatic metastasis of colorectal cancer pertains to secondary or metastatic liver cancer. Therefore, the research on molecular markers thereof shall include gene level and genomics, protein expression and proteomics, and immunohistochemistry and also the synthetic study on gene, protein, clinical patho- and physiological index, and biostatistics.

5.3.2.1 Research on Gene Level and Genomics

For the research on polygene chip, Lin et al. [126] adopted whole genomics chip, statistical analysis, and significance analysis of microarrays (SAM) to analyze 48 cases of primary colorectal cancer and 28 cases of hepatic metastasis, so as to identify 778 genes with differential expression in primary tumor and metastasis hereof. The genetic analysis shows that as compared with primary tumor, tissue remodeling and immunological reaction-related genes were increased during metastasis, while reproduction- and oxidative phosphorylation-related genes were decreased. The real-time PCR demonstrated that the increase of osteopontin, versican, ADAM 17, CKS 2, PRDX 1, CXCR 4, CXCL 12, and LCN 2 with differential expression as well as tissue remodeling and immunological reaction-related genes is associated to the transfer of invasiveness to the new location. The above genes could facilitate the growth of tumor. However, the decrease of reproducing-related genes demonstrated that as compared with primary tumor, the reproducing in metastasis was reduced.

As per the analysis on gene expression spectrum at different phases of metastatic colorectal cancer and nonmetastatic colorectal cancer, TGF-β inhibitor BAMBI is only increased in nearly half of metastatic primary tumor and metastatic carcinoma in terms of 115 gene tags with differential expression [127]. Also, BAMBI inhibited the channel of TGF signal B and increased the transfer of cancer cell; β-catenin co-activated BCL 9-2 in channel Wnt. Gene expression of BAMBI could be used to predict the metastasis. Meanwhile, it was reported that the expression of FGF-1 and FGF-2 in various cancers was related to the harmful prognosis of the tumor patients. Sato et al. [128] used quantitative and real-time reverse transcription PCR to make the comparison between 202 cases of colorectal cancer tissue and associated normal tunica mucosa, so as to find out expression of FGFR-2 was decreased. The analysis on the relation between clinical patho-characteristics and gene showed that the increase of FGFR-1 in hepatic metastasis was related to the hepatic metastasis.

The non-chip gene expression is adopted to study the tumor metastasis-related genes. For example, MMP-7 from cancer cell participates in invasiveness metastasis of tumor cell via destroying the basilar membrane. The epidemiology shows that the increase of IGF-1 is related to colorectal cancer. Oshima et al. [129] adopted RT-PCR to study MMP-7, IGF-1, IGF-2, IGF-1R, and β-actin mRNA of the cancer tissue and nearby normal tunica mucosa in 205 cases of untreated colorectal cancer: gene expression of MMP-7 and IGF-1R was increased, and gene expression of IGF-1 was decreased; IGF-1R was related to the invasiveness of vein and hepatic metastasis, so that they were the useful prediction indices for hepatic metastasis of colorectal cancer.

The research shows that the transcription factors EphA 4 and EphB 2 participate in the occurrence and development of various cancers. Oshima et al. [130] adopted RT-PCR and clinical pathology to analyze the specimens of cancer tissues and nearby normal tunica mucosa in 205 cases of untreated colorectal cancer, so as to find out the increase of EphA 4 and decrease of EphB 2 were related to hepatic metastasis. However, the correlation is unavailable between the gene expression of EphA 4 and that of EphB 2. Here, the increase of EphA 4 and decrease of EphB 2 could be used to predict the hepatic metastasis of colorectal cancer.

Akashi et al. [131] adopted inverse transcription of PCR to study CEA mRNA in the leading venous blood before the resection in 80 cases of colorectal cancer treatments: 80 % (28/35) CEA mRNA were positive and free from hepatic metastasis. According to Cox risk model, the lymphatic metastasis was the only factor to predict the recurrence of hepatic metastasis. However, the research did not demonstrate CEA mRNA in the leading venous blood was provided with high prediction during hepatic metastasis, but the cancer cells in the leading venous blood were three key elements and initial steps of hepatic metastasis.

It is reported that Osteopontin (OPN) in the tumor is the phosphorylated protein which is related to the occurrence of tumor. As per the study on transcription of colorectal cancer, Rohde et al. [132] found the high expression of OPN genetic transcription. Also, real-time reverse transcription of PCR, multivariate analysis, and immunohistochemistry were adopted to analyze 13 cases of normal colon cancer tissues, nine cases of adenoma, 120 cases of primary colorectal cancer, and ten cases of hepatic metastasis, so as to discover the remarkable increase of OPN in the primary colon cancer and hepatic metastasis.

Rubie et al. [133] adopted Q-RT-PCR and ELISA to analyze six cases of UC, eight cases of colorectal adenoma (CRA), 48 cases of colorectal cancer at different stages, and 16 cases of colorectal cancer hepatic metastasis (CRLM) simultaneously or at different times. The results showed that IL-8 expression was related to the occurrence and development of colorectal cancer and hepatic metastasis. As compared with CRA and UC, IL-8 in CRC specimen was obviously overexpressed; also, compared with CRA tissue, IL-8 was increased by 30 times; IL-8 has a close relation with tumor grading; in addition, as compared with primary colorectal cancer tissue, expression of IL-8 in CRLM is higher than the normal level by 80 times.

Miyagawa et al. [134] adopted the end-mark methods of deoxyribonucleoside monophosphate transferring enzyme to analyze the paraffin embedding tissue of 70 cases of colorectal cancer hepatic metastasis after excision, so as to find the number of dead cancer cells and expression of tumor gp 96 affecting the number of CD 83-positive cell at the outlying part of cancer invasiveness. Here, CD 83-positive cell was the key factor to predict the hepatic metastasis of colorectal cancer.

5.3.2.2 Research on Expression of Protein and Proteomics

The high flux reactor and real-time research on proteomics is focused on the rule of dynamic variation under different pathological and physiological conditions, so as to find out the molecules with differential expression and choose disease-related molecular markers. The molecular markers of colorectal cancer hepatic metastasis could be sorted out via the technique of proteomics.

Shi et al. [135] adopted 35S-methionine and 2DE-MS to conduct the comparative study on synthetic proteome of colorectal cancer (CRC) hepatic metastasis and normal colon mucosa under culture in vitro for 16 h, so as to find out that the main constituent of newly synthetic protein was made up of cytoplasmic protein with low abundance and traditional secreted protein. Thirty two kinds of protein with differential expression were displayed hereby, among which desmocollin-2 was increased, while fibrinogen gamma chain was decreased. Thus, the further research may discover the serum markers of colorectal cancer hepatic metastasis.

Katayama et al. [136] adopted 2D-DIGE and LC/MS/MS with maleimide CyDye fluorescein labels to study the change of albumin in CRC metastasis (protopathic SW 480 and SW 620 of lymphatic metastasis in the same patient). For in vivo studies on metastasis, two cell lines were injected to the spleen of nude mice, so as to reveal that nine obviously increased albumin were available in SW 620 as compared with SW 480. The test on in vivo metastasis shows that α-enolase and triosephosphate isomerase were related to metastasis of these two cell lines.

Pei et al. [137] adopted two-dimensional gel electrophoresis of ionization time-of-flight mass spectrometry and immunoblotting to study the fresh tumor and related normal tunica mucosa of non-LNM CRC and LNM CRC. Also, proteomics, tissue chip technology, and immunity histochemical stain were obtained from non-LNM CRC and LNM CRC of 40 CRC specimens with paraffin-embedded technique to identify four proteins with differential expression. There were 25 proteins with differential expression in the normal tunica mucosa and CRC tissue. As compared with non-LNM CRC, heat shock protein-27 (HSP-27), glutathione S-transferase, GST, and Annexin II in LNM CRC were increased, while liver fatty-acid-binding protein (L-FABP) was decreased, so as to prompt the LNM risk in CRC.

Kang et al. [138] adopted differential proteomics, Western blot, and immunohistochemistry to identify 34 unique differential albumins from the primary tumor of 14 cases of hepatic metastasis or non-hepatic metastasis CRC as well as a differential protein cluster, consisting of 17 proteins throughout PI3K/AKT pathway; also, three albumin tags from proteomics of CRC 105 and normal specimen; phosphorylated IkB-α, TNF-α, and MFAP 3 L are related to the hepatic metastasis so as to distinguish the CRC patients with high hepatic metastasis risk. In addition, according to the nude mice model used for hepatic metastasis of RKO and HT 29 in colon cancer, the protein tag from the channel PI 3 K/AKT may become the biological marker of colorectal cancer hepatic metastasis.

Pierobon et al. [139] adopted reverse-phase protein microarrays and laser micro-slitting technology to obtain CRC tumor tissues which were concentrated upon the functional protein-based channel (signal network). Also, comparative study was made on the differential expression of the patients with CRC or non-recurred CRC. The results showed that the activation of EGFR and that of COX 2 signal passages were quite different, so as to become the prognostic tools, which were used to guide the potential treatment.

As increased in many tumor cases of human, cyclooxygenase-2 (COX-2) was used to adjust angiogenesis through inducting the blood vessel production. Nakamoto et al. [140] adopted immunohistochemistry. Spearman rank test analyzed 44 specimens of primary tumor tissues as well as COX-2, VEGF-A, VEGF-C, TP, and MVD of relevant hepatic metastasis tissue: the primary tumor is proved with the same COX-2, VEGF-A, TP, and immunological unresponsiveness of MVD as those of relevant hepatic metastasis tumor. The immunological unresponsiveness of COX-2 was higher in hepatic metastasis, while VEGF-A was higher in the primary tumor. The immunological unresponsiveness of COX-2 and VEGF-A in both primary tumor and metastatic tumor were correlated. Also, the expression of COX-2, VEGF-A, TP, and MVD of primary tumor and colorectal cancer liver metastasis presents the positive correlation, which was helpful to predict the angiogenesis via primary tumor analysis as well as administrate personalized cancer treatment.

Melle et al. [141] adopted ProteinChip (SELDI) to analyze the result spectrum of 17 cases of colon cancer hepatic metastasis. As compared with CRC and HCC, 49 signals with differential expression were found. Also, based on the immunodepletion, Ca-binding protein S100A6 was found to accurately set the position in the cell via immunohistochemistry as well as Ca-binding protein S100A11 to identify the different tumors.

5.3.2.3 Level of Immunohistochemistry

The application of immunohistochemistry includes tissue chip, traditional immunohistochemistry and Western blot, and related statistics which are adopted to study on the potential biological markers of colorectal cancer hepatic metastasis.

Fang et al. [142] adopted tissue microarray (TMA) to test the biological markers (β-catenin, CD44v7, c-myc, cyclin D1, estrogen receptor β, mitogen-activated protein kinase/extracellular signal-regulated kinase, maspin, matrix metalloproteinase-7 (MMP7), p53, Pin1, PPARγ (peroxisome proliferator-activated receptor-gamma), survivin, T-cell transcription factor 4 (TCF4), transforming growth factor β receptor II (TGF-βRII), TGF-β, TROP2, and Wnt) in 620 cases of colorectal cancer. As per clinical data, risk regression analysis on COX was made. The result showed that all the markers in the tumor were increased. Also, Kaplan-Meier analysis showed that increase of TROP 2, MMP 7, and survivin lowered the survival rate. Survivin and TROP 2 were the meaningful prediction indices for the patients with low survive rate. Meanwhile, TROP 2 and MMP 7 are closely related with recurrence of tumor and hepatic metastasis.

For the research on adherent molecules and related signal path molecules, Ochiai et al. [143] adopted immunohistochemistry and array training for nine predicted or prognosis molecular (p53) of hepatic metastasis, so to study 439 cases of CRC patients and find out the combination of dysadherin, E-cadherin and matrilysin could predict the hepatic metastasis; thus, the high sensitivity and potential clinical application were provided. Meanwhile, Choi et al. [144] adopted immunochemistry staining to compare the expression of SRF, E-cadherin, and β-catenin in 43 groups of primary colorectal cancer and hepatic metastasis, so as to discover that the expression of SRF was obviously increased, while the expression of E-cadherin was obviously lowered. The overexpression of SRF in SW 480 reduced E-cadherin, increased the unphosphorylated β-catenin, and enhanced cytoplasmic movement and invasiveness. So, SRF have an important role in the metastasis of colorectal cancer.

As immunohistochemistry and Western blot were adopted, Pancione et al. [145] made the comparative study on β-catenin, PPARγ (peroxisome proliferator-activated receptor-γ), cyclooxygenase 2, and NF-kB in 72 cases of mucosa with rectal cancer or without cancerization. It was discovered that the expression spectrum was related to 5-year survival rate of patients. According to the test on 18.1 % tumor, the survival rate of patients with β-catenin was low, while expression of PPARγ in protoplasm/core showed favorable prognosis. The decrease and deficiency of β-catenin and PPARγ were closely related to TAM invasiveness, hepatic metastasis, and short lifetime of tumor, but negatively correlated to NF-kB to prompt that the decrease of β-catenin and PPARγ was the prognostic index of CRC. Thus, it was good for sorting out the patients with high fatality rate.

Delektorskaya et al. [146] adopted immunohistochemistry to analyze the specific expression, distribution, and interplay between adhesion molecules of E-cadherin, β-catenin, and CD-44v6 proteins in hepatic metastasis and lymphatic metastasis of colorectal cancer to evaluate the latent energy of colorectal cancer cell metastasis. For metastasis of colorectal cancer, E-cadherin was decreased or disappeared; for metastasis of at least 80 % colorectal cancer, immunological reaction and core translocation of β-catenin's cytoplasm metastasis were increased. Change of E-cadherin and β catenin could be used as the prognostic indices for colorectal cancer. Also, no correlation was tested between expression of CD-44v6 protein and latent energy of tumor cell metastasis.

Increase of FAK, Src, and paxillin may increase the latent energy of colorectal cancer cell metastasis. de Heer et al. [147] adopted immunohistochemistry to study 104 cases of colorectal cancer under follow-up survey and made quantitative investigation on FAK, Src, and paxillin in 68 cases of colorectal cancer to find that the tumor recurrence time was shorter if both FAK and Src were increased. Thus, high level of FAK and Src predicted the recurrence of colorectal cancer and remote metastasis thereof.

It is reported that the decrease of vascular endothelium adhesion molecule P-selectin expression is related to the melanoma tumor. Peeters et al. [148] adopted immunostaining series such as colorectal tissue specimen (including normal colorectal tissue, un-transitionary primary tumor, and hepatic metastasis of primary cancer). The result shows that the P-selectin is decreased due to colorectal cancer's escape from inflammation recovery, so as to increase canceration risk.

Noike et al. [149] adopted immunohistochemistry and multivariate analysis to study on 84 cases of HMCRC resection. Here, the expression of Trx-1, VEGF, and Ref-1 was not found in the remaining tumor. Also, it was found that Trx-1 was an independent prediction factor, while the expression of VEGF and Ref-1 was related to the overexpression of Trx 1, which were all related to the harmful prediction factors of HMCRC.

For cell strain or animal model, Wang et al. [150] adopted three colorectal cancer cell strains, HT-29c, HT-29d, and WiDr, to set up the nude mice metastasis model via the application of ELISA, IHC, and FACS, so as to find out that there was a positive correlation between the level of uPA and PAI-1 and metastasis potency of tumor cell; also, PI 3-kinase was related to the development and metastasis of tumor.

Wang et al. [151] developed orthotopic transplantation model of white rat CRC and related SW 480 CRC cell subcloning M5 of high hepatic metastasis and compared the difference of gene expression between M5 and SW 480, so as to find out the decrease of SATB 2 (special AT-rich sequence-binding protein 2) in M5. Meanwhile, immunohistochemistry was used to analyze 146 cases of tumor specimen of colorectal cancer, so as to display the decrease of SATB 2 which was related to the tumor and lymph invasiveness, remote metastasis, Dukes classification, and prognosis. As shown in single-factor and multi-factor analysis sheet for existence, SATB 2 was the prognosis indices of new CRC.

Oue et al. [152] adopted immunostaining ELISA to test the expression and distribution of Reg IV (Regenerating islet-derived family, member 4) in CRC as well as the content thereof in the serum. The conclusion was that the concentration of serum Reg IV before operation was the prediction indices for harmful existence. The concentration of serum Reg IV could predict HMCRC.

PRL-3 (phosphatase of regenerating liver3) is the molecular related to hepatic metastasis of CRC. Peng et al. [153] adopted hybrid tumor technique to prepare PRL-3 antibody, and then ELISA and immunoblotting were used to ascertain the specificity thereof; the PRL-3 in the normal colorectal epithelium was analyzed through immunohistochemistry, logistic regression, and existence analysis to discover that expression rate of PRL-3 was apparently higher than that in the primary colorectal cancer and normal colorectal epithelium. The expression of PRL-3 was related to the hepatic metastasis of colorectal cancer, so as to shorten the survival time. The first research demonstrated that PRL-3 was the potential marker of hepatic metastasis of colorectal cancer, so as to produce the negative effect on the prognosis of colorectal cancer patient. PRL-3mRNA was raised in the specimen of colorectal cancer metastasis. Li et al. [154] chose 1,400 hybridoma clones of special mAbs for each PRL. Also, two specially hybridized clones were obtained for PRL-3 and the other two specially hybridized cell strains for PRL-1. Then various methods were used to verify the reaction specificity of PRL-3 and single PRL-1-antibody. The expression of PRL-3 in 10 % specimens of primary colorectal cancer showed that the expression of PRL-3 may be the initial stage of transition process; these mAbs would become the markers used for assessing the clinical diagnosis of tumor invasiveness. Also, Hatate et al. [155] studied 107 primary focal resections to find that there was negative correlation between expression of PRL-3 and prognosis; pN factor, CEA, and CA 19-9 could be used with PRL-3 as the independent prediction factor. The hepatic metastasis from PRL-3 may be mediated via lymphatic metastasis and deemed as the marker of serum tumor.

As a β-galactoside-binding protein, galectin-3 is related to a lot of biological processes such as adhesion, identification, reproduction, disintegration, and death of cell. By means of immunohistochemistry, clinical pathology, and statistical concept, Tsuboi et al. [156] analyzed the expression of galectin-3, β-catenin, and Ki-67 in 108 cases of colorectal cancer as well as the expression of galectin-3 on the tumor surface and invasiveness. When the expression of galectin-3 at the outlying invasiveness was lower than that on the tumor surface, the remarkable hepatic metastasis appears. β-catenin on the tumor surface was related to hepatic metastasis and neoplasm staging. The decrease of galectin-3 expression was related to the invasiveness and metastasis of colorectal cancer. Therefore, the expression of galectin-3 may participate in the invasiveness, metastasis, and reproduction of colorectal cancer.

Maspin could repress the invasiveness and metastasis of malignant tumor. Zheng et al. [157] used tissue chip and CD 34 antibody marked immunostaining to study maspin and capillary density (MVD) in 119 cases of colorectal adenoma (CRA), 22 cases of relay pleomorphic adenoma, 118 cases of relay pleomorphic non-cancer mucosa, and 67 cases of patients with metastases as well as the clinical parameters of tumor (including p53, Ki-67 and tenascin, MVD, and survival data). Analysis on Kaplan-Meier revealed that the expression of maspin was not related to the survival time of cancer. Also, maspin was increased during the cancerization of colorectal adenoma. Low expression of Maspin could enhance the activity of cancer cells through the degrading of extracellular matrix and closely related to CRA hepatic metastasis.

Connective tissue growth factor (CTGF) is related to the occurrence and development of tumor. Lin et al. [158] adopted immunohistochemistry staining to test 119 CRC specimens. Meanwhile, transfection of CTGF via liposome was adopted. The invasiveness and hepatic metastasis of BALB/c mouse were tested. The genetic analysis was made for CTGF in the signal channel of β-catenin/T-cell factor. The result shows that CTGF was the key moderator for invasiveness and metastasis of CTGF, so as to well predict CRC at phase II and phase III.

Saito et al. [159] adopted EIA, single\multivariate analysis, and COX risk regression model to analyze 205 cases of colorectal cancer (109 cases of intestinal cancer, 96 cases of colon cancer, 52 cases of hepatic metastasis, and 153 cases of non-hepatic metastasis), so as to find out that the average serum laminin (668.0 ± 274.7 ng/ml) of hepatic metastasis was remarkably higher than that of non-hepatic metastasis. The serum laminin before operation was the marker to predict the colorectal cancer.

Monocyte chemoattractant protein-1 (MCP-1) plays the role in the development of tumor. Yoshidome et al. [160] adopted clinical stages and immunohistochemistry to test MCP-1, Angiopoietin-2, CD 68, and CD 34(capillary density MVD was tested) in 87 cases of CRC patients. MCP-1 with high expression accompanied high MVD and was related to Angiopoietin-2; the expression thereof was increased with the progress of clinical stages. The cytological test indicated that there was positive relation between increase of MCP-1mRNA and high potency of cell metastasis. The single-factor analysis showed that transfer time, tumor size, number of metastasis, and MCP-1 were the meaningful prognosis factors. The multiple factor analysis verified the expression of MCP-1 was the prognosis factor not related to the survival. MCP-1 in CRC may be related to the angiopoiesis; also, it was the index to predict the recurrence of CRC hepatic tumor resection.

Angiopoietin, Ang-2, and VEGF are key moderators for angiogenesis of tumor. Ochiumi et al. [161] adopted immunohistochemistry and anti-CD 34 immunohistochemistry staining to analyze the expression of Ang-2 and VEGF and tumor vs microvessel density (MVD) at the CRC tumor invasive positions during the progressive stage of 152 cases of excision. The recursive multivariate analysis on 5-year survival after operation indicated that the expression of lymphatic metastasis, VEGF, and Ang-2 was the meaning indices of harmful prognosis. The result shows that co-expression of Ang-2and VEGF may cause the tumor angiogenesis which was the factor to predict the development of CRC.

Yokomizo et al. [162] studied the expression of FasL in 67 cases of colorectal cancer to discover 48 cases presented as FasL positive; for FasL negative, only one case has hepatic metastasis; FasL was unavailable in the case of vein invasiveness. It was prompted that FasL may be the prediction factor for vein invasiveness and hepatic metastasis.

Fujimoto et al. [163] adopted single argument and multivariate analysis to assess the relation of clinical pathology and immunohistochemistry (including the age, gender, tumor localizing, overall size, type of tissue, disintegrated outlying invasiveness, invasiveness depth, lymph invasiveness, vein invasiveness, lymphatic metastasis, CD 10, MUC 2, and human gastric mucin) with hepatic metastasis in 505 cases of colorectal cancer excision patients at T2/T3/T4 stage, so as to find that overall size, type of tissue, disintegrated outlying invasiveness, invasiveness depth, lymph invasiveness, vein invasiveness, lymphatic metastasis, and CD 10 were related to the hepatic metastasis. CD 10 of colorectal cancer was the best prediction for hepatic metastasis in colorectal cancer.

Hayashi et al. [164] studied the hepatic tumor and apoptotic index (AI) and proliferation index (PI) of peripheral hepatic tissue in 43 cases of resected colorectal cancer hepatic metastasis as well as TGF-β1, TGF-βRII, and Fas and FasL of immunohistochemistry, so as to find that except value PI, other parameters were raised; enhanced expression of TGF-β1 appears at the interface near the tumor metastasis and liver parenchyma. Enhanced expression of TGF-β1 and death of liver cells around the liver parenchyma tumor showed that TGF-β1 was substantial in the hepatic metastasis of colorectal cancer.

For the relationship between inflammation and tumor metastasis, Auguste et al. [165] demonstrated that upon entering the liver, the metastatic tumor cell stimulated TNF-α release and epidermal cells adhesive reception body under mediation of stellate cells of the liver, e.g., inflammatory reaction due to increase of E-selectin. Afterwards, the author (Auguste) utilized the immunohistochemistry focusing microscope and three-dimensional reconstruction technique as well as human colorectal cancer CX-1 and mouse cancer cell H-59 to analyze the subsequent interaction among tumor endothelial cells in terms of time and space. The result shows that the metastatic tumor cell could change the expression of new endothelial cell reception body of liver vas capillare. Thus, it was good for adhesion and vascular of cell.

The researchers are not enough to the changes of anticancer drug-related metabolizing enzyme. For example, the activated 5-FU is composed of dihydropyrimidine dehydrogenase (DPD), orotate phosphoribosyltransferase (OPRT), thymidylate synthase (TS), thymidine kinase (TK), thymidine phosphorylase (TP), and deoxyuridine triphosphatase (dUTPase). Kawahara et al. [166] adopted immunohistochemistry to compare the expression of 5-FU enzyme in 20 cases of colorectal cancer without metastasis and in 35 cases of colorectal cancer with remote metastasis: dUTPase and TK were increased, but DPD was decreased; for 35 cases of remote metastasis, OPRT, TS, and dUTPase were obviously increased; dUTPase was the most possible index for metastasis of colorectal cancer.

5.3.2.4 Synthetic Study

Various methods are adopted. For instance, gene and genome, protein and proteomics, and single or multi-molecular immunology are used for joint testing. Afterwards, statistics and epidemiology are adopted to study the metastasis of colorectal cancer.

Zhou et al. [167] made the retrospective analysis on 197 cases of colorectal cancer hepatic metastasis: hepatic metastasis resection, concentration of serum CEA (sCEA) as well as the number and size of hepatic metastasis were the key factors to predict the hepatic metastasis of colorectal cancer. In addition, PI value could be also used in predicting the hepatic metastasis of colorectal cancer. Takagawa et al. [168] adopted multivariate analysis to study 638 cases of sCEA before operation to find that the optimal critical value was 10 ng/ml; also, the recurrence and survival rates of 92 cases of TNM at stage II and III were obviously different before and after he serum critical value. Mehrkhani et al. [169] used Cox regression to analyze 1,090 cases of colorectal cancer resection in 1999–2002. Here, recurrences of colorectal cancer or new supplementary chemotherapy were removed, so that the level of preoperative CEA could predict the survival rate of colorectal cancer patient after operation.

The degrading of extracellular matrix is the intrinsic procedure for invasiveness and development of cancer, among which matrix metalloproteinases (MMP)-2 and MMP-9 and their natural suppressors participated in this process. Waas et al. [170] adopted zymogram, ELISA, ROC curve, and Kaplan-Meier to analyze plasma proMMP-2 and proMMP-9 and TIMP-1 in 57 cases of hepatic metastasis before and after resection. The obtained data were compared with 51 cases of healthy control group and 94 cases of primary CRC. The plasma proMMP-2 and proMMP-9 and TIMP-1 before operation were useless to the diagnosis or prediction of colorectal cancer hepatic metastasis, while CEA was proved to be the better marker in the diagnosis and prediction-related test. According to the follow-up survey, it was seemed that the low-level proMMP in the long and middle term was related to the recurrence hereof.

CEA and CA 19-9 in the colorectal cancer patients are often increased. Sasaki et al. [171] adopted single argument and multivariate to analyze sCEA, CA 19-9, and other clinical data of 90 cases of colorectal cancer hepatic metastasis before and after hepatectomy. It was found that the increase of sCA 19-9 was the danger signal of hepatic metastasis. Thus, it may assist the prediction on outside hepatic metastasis of colorectal cancer patient. Iwasaki et al. [172] adopted Cox risk regression model to review 80 cases of liver or lung metastasis of colorectal cancer, so as to find that sCEA was obviously different during the lung metastasis. However, no difference thereof was found during hepatic metastasis. Katoh et al. [173] adopted multivariance to make retrospective analysis on the relationship between clinical variables (including value CA 19-9 before operation, peritoneum diffusion, invasive depth, age, hepatic metastasis scope, pathological lymphatic metastasis, and sexual distinction as well as aftertreatment, blood transfusion during pre-operation, and lymph node dissection) and survival rate in 162 cases of CRC IV, so as to find out that aftertreatment, blood transfusion during pre-operation, CA 19-9, hepatic metastasis scope, and peritoneum diffusion were independent factors for prediction. The illative CA 19-9, remote metastasis, and partial progress were three definite variables. Delektorskaya et al. [174] studied primary colorectal cancer markers such as β-catenin, MMP 9, collagen IV, and laminin in CRC, so as to prompt that high expression of MMP 9 at outlying invasiveness and β-catenin in the cancer cell nucleus and high concentration of laminin in the hyalomitome were obviously related to the lack of collagen IV in the membrane basilaris. Such changes showed the high potency of colorectal gland cancer invasiveness. Therefore, these indices could be used to predict the clinical progress and CRC risk of colorectal cancer.

The recent studies indicated that interaction of CXCR 3/chemotactic factors in the CRC cytoplasmic movement was one of the cancerous transition processes. Cambien et al. [175] adopted the human CRC HT 29 and rat C26 with CXCR 3 as well as the AMG 487, the blocking agent of CXCR 3. CXCR 3 inductive lagan and migration and growth of CRC cells could be interdicted by AMG 487. The test showed precaution of AMG 487 and control of CXCR 3in lymphonodi pulmonales and tumor could remarkably repress the lung metastasis of human and mouse's CRC, while the hepatic metastasis was not affected. Rubie et al. [176] adopted real-time PCR, IHC, and Western blot to compare 25 cases of UC, eight cases of CRA, and 48 cases of CRC at the different stages as well as 16 cases of CRLM and CXCR 1–4 which is the chemotactic factor for resection of colorectal cancer: CXC 1, 2, and 4 were increased in all CRC; CXCR 3 was only overexpressed in CRLM; expression of CXCR 4 mainly appeared on the tumor cell of CRC; and tumor of CRLM invaded the outlying liver cells.

The expression of Sialyl LewisX synthesizing-related GnT-V is related to hematogenous metastasis and harmful prognosis. Murata et al. [177] established the overexpression of GnT-V in human colon cancer cell line DLD-1 and WiDr. SLeX (Sialyl LewisX) was the ligand of E-selection. High expression of GnT-V induced the expression of SLeX in the colon cancer cell, so as to enhance the hypophloeodal adhesive attraction of vascular of remote organs (liver and lung) to guide the metastasis of colon cancer cell. Suppression of GnT-V reactivity may stop the metastasis of colon cancer through the decrease of SLeX expression. The metastasis of cancer cell was provided with the similar characteristics with those available for lymphocyte's entry to inflamed tissue. Sialyl LewisX (SLeX) on the lymphocyte membrane was the adhesive molecular of activated vascular endothelial cell in the inflammation area – the lagan of selection. The increase of C2 GnT1 reactivity may increase the synthesizing of C2-O-SLeX so as to substantially increase the adhesion between lymphocyte and vascular endothelial cell. St Hill et al. [178] adopted 113 cases of primary colorectal cancer, 10 cases of colorectal tumor, 46 metastasis liver cancer, 28 cases of normal colon tissues, and 5 cases of normal hepatic tissue to test the changes of C2-O-SLeX (CHO-131 testing) in the canceration and metastasis of rectal adenocarcinoma as well as the expression of C2 GnT1 mRNA in 20 cases of normal, 15 cases of ordinary, and 2 cases of disintegrated colorectal cancer as well as 5 cases of normal colon tissues. The result showed that 70% colorectal cancer and 87% metastatic liver cancer presented hyperergy to CHO-131 while no reaction on colorectal tumor and normal colon and liver. Meanwhile, C2 GnT1 in the colorectal cancer was higher than that in the normal colorectal tissues by 15 times, so as to indicate that high expression of C2-O-SLeX was the marker to predict the early colorectal cancer.

Uner et al. [179] adopted ELISA to study 64 cases of colorectal cancer (32 cases of male patients and 32 cases of female patients) as well as 16 cases of healthy persons, so as to discover that concentration of sE-selectin in patients with colorectal cancer hepatic metastasis was obviously increased; however, no correlation is available with other parameters (age, stage, disintegration, or primary tumor positioning). It was verified that sE-selectin was related to the overall survival rate. Concentration of sE-selectin may not be deemed as the marker to predict the metastasis of colorectal cancer. However, the high expression of sE-selectin was helpful to the diagnosis of hepatic metastasis.

Uemura et al. [180] studied the relationship between the expression of sialidase (NEU1) and potency of metastasis. When HT-29 of NEU1 was injected to the mouse, it was found that hepatic metastasis was obviously decreased. Also, in vitro cytoplasmic movement and invasiveness and adhesion were suppressed. Major molecular change includes decrease of sialic acid in integrin β4. The desialylation was accompanied by decreased phosphorylation of the integrin followed by attenuation of focal adhesion kinase and Erk1/2 pathway. NEU1 could cause the decrease of MMP 7. GalNAc α-o-benzyl, an inhibitor of O-glycosylation was used to treat the cell, so as to show that positive integrin β4 of PNA was increased with the decrease of phosphorylating to prompt that iNEU1's integrin β4 guided signal transmitter caused the suppression on metastasis.

Vascular adhesion protein-1 (VAP-1) is the endothelial cell molecule for controlling the penetrating power of lymphocyte tissue. VAP-1 (sVAP-1) in the colorectal cancer patient is obviously higher than that in the healthy control group. Also, it is related to the remote hepatic metastasis and TMN grading. The further study shows that sVAP-1 before operation prompted the poor prognosis. sVAP-1 is an independent index to predict the lymph node and hepatic metastasis [181].

The research on pernicious phenotype-related blood coagulation system is concerned. Illemann et al. [182] studied the phenotype of urokinase-type PA (uPA) and plasminogen activator inhibitor-1 (PAI-1) thereof. For all the 14 cases of primary intestinal cancer, the expression of uPAR, uPA mRNA, and PAI-1 was increased at the front part of invasiveness. For five cases of hepatic metastasis, the expression of uPAR, uPA mRNA, and PAI-1 was similar to that of primary carcinoma. Another nine cases of hepatic metastasis were related to the necrobiosis of focal metastasis. Two different types of expression in the hepatic metastasis were closely related to the different clinical tumor growths, so as to indicate that it may play a role in the treatment of colon cancer.

For the research on TGF/Smad signals, mutation or decrease, increase, and metastasis of Smad 4 are directly related to the harmful prognosis. It was reported that Smad 7 induced tumor and death via blocking TGF-β. Halder et al. [183] adopted spleen injection model, genome DNA polymerase chain reaction, and immunohistochemistry to discover the migration of Smad 7 to the liver, so as to induce the hepatic metastasis. In this case, the cells were highly increased by means of spindle-shaped poor differentiation. For hepatic metastasis, the increase of TGF-βRII was related to phosphorylation and aggregation of Smad 2. The expression of claudin-1, claudin-4, and E-cadherin was increased. The blocking of TGF-β/Smad channel in the colon cancer cells induced the metastasis. Thus, the signal approach of Smad played an important role in the suppression on colon cancer.

The allopolyploidy and dimerization of (human epidermal growth factor 2, HER 2) caused activation of EGFR/HER 1. The Amphiregulin (AR) of EGFR may be related to the colorectal cancer. Yamada et al. [184] adopted immunohistochemistry and multivariate analysis to study the expression of AR, EGFR, and HER 2 in 106 cases of primary colorectal cancer and 16 cases of liver metastasis to find that AR was the independent factor to predict the hepatic metastasis of colorectal cancer.

Murad et al. [185] analyzed the immunity expression of p53, Ki-67, and p16 and molecular marker in 49 cases of hepatic metastasis of colorectal cancer which did not affect the other organs. Also, according to the clinical data (age, gender, size of hepatic metastasis or largest focus, resection, compromised satellite-like nodules, and resectional section of tumor) of the patient, it was found that immunity expression of p53 was related to the shortest disease free survival. Ki-67 was unrelated to the decrease of disease-free lifetime and survival. Immunity expression of p16 was synchronized to the hepatic metastasis. The expression of markers with 5-FU and leucovorin after operation was unrelated to the disease-free lifetime. The molecular markers are helpful to the evaluation on the hepatic metastasis of colorectal cancer.

The tumor-infiltrating lymphocytes (TILs) have an important role in the primary colorectal cancer. Wagner et al. [186] adopted polychrome cells and interferon γ stain to analyze 16 cases of the hepatic metastasis of colorectal cancer and relevant normal hepatic tissue to find that the metastasis were obviously increased in CD (+), among which hepatic metastasis was remarkably increased in the active (CD 4(+)CD 25(+)). Also, it demonstrated that the metastasis occurred in CD 69(+), CD 25(+) with higher proportion and active CD 107a(+) CD 8(+) TIL with cell toxicant. CD 4(+) and CD 8(+) TIL were under selective activation during the hepatic metastasis.

Table 5.1 Colorectal cancer hepatic metastasis-related molecules

Classification of research	Colorectal cancer hepatic metastasis-related molecules	References
Genomics and gene	CEA BAMBI FGFR-1 IGF-1R OPN versican ADAM17 CKS2 PRDX1 CXCR4 CXCL12 LCN2 IL-8 EphA4 EphB2	[126–134]
Proteomics and protein	Desmocollin-2 α-enolase triosephosphate isomerase HSP-27 GST pIkB-α TNF-α MFAP3L COX-2 VEGF-A TP S100A6 S100A11 Annexin II L-FABP FNγ	[135–141]
Immunohistochemistry	TROP2 MMP7 (dysadherin, E-cadherin, matrilysin) E-cadherin β-catenin NF-kB PPARγ (FAK, Src) Trx-1 VEGF Ref-1, PI3K SATB2 Reg IV PRL-3 galectin-3 Maspin P-selectin CTGF laminin MCP-1(Ang-2, VEGF) FasL CD10 TGF-β1 E-selectin dUTPase	[142–166]
Others	CEA CA19-9 β-catenin MMP 9 CoIV LN CXCR3 SLeX C2-O-SLeX GnT-V NEU1 sVAP-1 sE-selectin uPAR uPA PAI-1 Smad7 Amphiregulin (AR) p16 proMMP-2	[167–187]

Sasaki et al. [187] studied the absolute counting, clinical pathology, and long-term prediction on white cell of peripheral blood of colorectal cancer hepatic metastasis patient with hepatectomy. The univariate analysis showed that the patients were more interrelated to the poor 5-year survival if the number of peripheral mononuclear cells >300/mm^3; multivariate analysis showed that the number of peripheral blood mononuclear cells before operation >300/mm^3 and CEA level (>10 ng/ml) before operation were the cancer-related independent survival factors after hepatectomy. The number of peripheral mononuclear cells and white cells and neutrophilic granulocyte before operation was related to the interval of colorectal and liver surgical department or CEA value before operation but unrelated to the number of tumor cells. The absolute number of peripheral blood mononuclear cells >300/mm^3 was the independent factor to predict the survival rate related to the colorectal cancer hepatic metastasis patients after hepatectomy.

See Table 5.1 on the colorectal cancer hepatic metastasis-related molecules obtained via different research platforms.

References

1. Cho JY, Sung HJ. Proteomic approaches in lung cancer biomarker development. Expert Rev Proteomics. 2009;6(1):27–42.
2. Sun S, Lee NP, Poon RT, et al. Oncoproteomics of hepatocellular carcinoma: from cancer markers' discovery to functional pathways. Liver Int. 2007;27(8):1021–38.
3. Gebhart E, Liehr T. Patterns of genomic imbalances in human solid tumors. Int J Oncol. 2000;16(2): 383–99.
4. Kelly L, Clark J, Gilliland DG. Comprehensive genotypic analysis of leukemia: clinical and therapeutic implications. Curr Opin Oncol. 2002;14(1): 10–8.
5. Walther A, Johnstone E, Swanton C, et al. Genetic prognostic and predictive markers in colorectal cancer. Nat Rev Cancer. 2009;9(7):489–99.
6. Kallioniemi A. CGH microarrays and cancer. Curr Opin Biotechnol. 2008;19(1):36–40.
7. Shah SP. Computational methods for identification of recurrent copy number alteration patterns by array CGH. Cytogenet Genome Res. 2008;123(1–4):343–51.
8. Lockwood WW, Chari R, Chi B, et al. Recent advances in array comparative genomic hybridization technologies and their applications in human genetics. Eur J Hum Genet. 2006;14(2):139–48.
9. Bejjani BA, Shaffer LG. Application of array-based comparative genomic hybridization to clinical diagnostics. J Mol Diagn. 2006;8(5):528–33.
10. Shinawi M, Cheung SW. The array CGH and its clinical applications. Drug Discov Today. 2008; 13(17–18):760–70.
11. Costa JL, Meijer G, Ylstra B, et al. Array comparative genomic hybridization copy number profiling: a new tool for translational research in solid malignancies. Semin Radiat Oncol. 2008;18(2):98–104.
12. Harada T, Chelala C, Crnogorac-Jurcevic T, et al. Genome-wide analysis of pancreatic cancer using microarray-based techniques. Pancreatology. 2009;9(1–2):13–24.
13. Pinkel D, Straume T, et al. Cytogenetic analysis using quantitative, high-sensitivity, fluorescence hybridization. Proc Natl Acad Sci. 1986;83(9): 2934–8.
14. Ried T, Baldini A, Rand TC, et al. Simultaneously visualization of seven different DNA probes by in

situ hybridization using fluorescence and digital imaging microscopy. Proc Natl Acad Sci. 1992;89: 1388–92.
15. Nederlof PM, van de Flier S, Vrolijk J, et al. Fluorescence ratio measurements of double-labeled probes for multiple in situ hybridization by digital imaging microscopy. Cytometry. 1992;13:839–45.
16. SpeciherM R, Gwyn BS, Ward DC. Karyotyping human chromosomes by combinatorial multi-fluor FISH. Nat Genet. 1996;12:368–75.
17. Schrock E, du Manoir S, Veldman, et al. Multicolor spectral karyotyping of human chromosomes. Science. 1996;273:494–7.
18. Kearney L. Multiplex-FISH (M-FISH): technique, developments and applications. Cytogenet Genome Res. 2006;114:189–98.
19. Eils R, Uhrig S. An optimized, fully automated system for fast and accurate identification of chromosomal rearrangements by multiplex-FISH (M-FISH). Cytogenet Cell Genet. 1998;82:160–71.
20. Uhrig S, Schuffenhauer S, et al. Multiplex-FISH for pre- and postnatal diagnostic applications. Am J Hum Genet. 1999;65(2):448–62.
21. Marshall A, Hodgson J. DNA chips: an array of possibilities. Nat Biotchol. 1998;16:27–8.
22. Schena M, Shalon D, Davis RW, et al. Quantitative monitoring of gene expression patterns with a complementary DNA microarray. Science. 1995;270: 467–70.
23. Lipshutz RJ, Fodor SP, Gingeras TR, et al. High density synthetic oligonucleotide arrays. Nat Genet. 1999;21:20–4.
24. Ye QH, Qin LX, Forgues M, et al. Predicting hepatitis B virus-positive metastatic hepatocellular carcinomas using gene expression profiling and supervised machine learning. Nat Med. 2003;9:416–23.
25. Alizadeh AA, Eisen MB, Davis RE, et al. Distinct types of diffuse large B-cell lymphoma identified by gene expression profiling. Nature. 2000;40: 503–11.
26. Okabe H, Satoh S, Kato T, et al. Genome-wide analysis of gene expression in human hepatocellular carcinomas using cDNA microarray: identification of genes involved in viral carcinogenesis and tumor progression. Cancer Res. 2001;61:2129–37.
27. Seliger B, Dressler SP, Wang E, et al. Combined analysis of transcriptome and proteome data as a tool for the identification of candidate biomarkers in renal cell carcinoma. Proteomics. 2009;9:1567–81.
28. Mandoiu II, Prajescu C. High-throughput SNP genotyping by SBE/SBH. IEEE Trans Nanobioscience. 2007;6:28–35.
29. Cunha BA, Esrick MD, Larusso M. Staphylococcus hominis native mitral valve bacterial endocarditis (SBE) in a patient with hypertrophic obstructive cardiomyopathy. Heart Lung. 2007;36:380–2.
30. Shen R, Fan JB, Campbell D, et al. High-throughput SNP genotyping on universal bead arrays. Mutat Res. 2005;573:70–82.
31. Van Heek NT, Clayton SJ, Sturm PD, et al. Comparison of the novel quantitative ARMS assay and an enriched PCR-ASO assay for K-ras mutations with conventional cytology on endobiliary brush cytology from 312 consecutive extrahepatic biliary stenoses. J Clin Pathol. 2005;58: 1315–20.
32. Dalma-Weiszhausz DD, Murphy Jr GM. Single nucleotide polymorphisms and their characterization with oligonucleotide microarrays. Psychiatr Genet. 2002;12:97–107.
33. Haihui S, Huasheng X. Polymorphyism and drug metabolism of cytochrome P450gene. Int Genet. 2008;31(3):206–12.
34. Frommer M, McDonald LE, Millar DS, et al. A genomic sequencing protocol that yields a positive display of 5-methylcytosine residues in individual DNA strands. Proc Natl Acad Sci U S A. 1992;89(5):1827–31.
35. Gitan RS, Shi H, Chen CM, et al. Methylation-specific oligonucleotide microarray: a new potential for high-throughput methylation analysis. Genome Res. 2002;12(1):158–64.
36. Gao L, Cheng L, Zhou JN, et al. DNA microarray: a high throughput approach for methylation detection. Colloids Surf B Biointerfaces. 2005;40(3–4): 127–31.
37. Bibikova M, Chudin E, Wu B, et al. Human embryonic stem cells have a unique epigenetic signature. Genome Res. 2006;16(9):1075–83.
38. Cross SH, Charlton JA, Nan X, et al. Purification of CpG islands using a methylated DNA binding column. Nat Genet. 1994;6(3):236–44.
39. Versmold B, Felsberg J, Mikeska T, et al. Epigenetic silencing of the candidate tumor suppressor gene PROX1 in sporadic breast cancer. Int J Cancer. 2007;121(3):547–54.
40. Rush L, Plass C. Restriction landmark genomic scanning for DNA methylation in cancer: past, present and future applications. Anal Biochem. 2002;307(2):191–201.
41. Songfa Z, Feng Y, Cheng H, et al. Research on genome CpG methylation detection. Int J Genet. 2006;29(3):201–17.
42. Hatada I, Hayashizaki Y, Hirotsune S, et al. A genomic scanning method for higher organisms using restriction sites as landmarks. Proc Natl Acad Sci U S A. 1991;88(21):9523–7.
43. Hyashizaki Y, Watanabe S, editors. Restriction landmark genomic scanning (RLGS). Tokyo: Springer; 1997.
44. Matsuyama T, Kimura MT, Koike K, et al. Global methylation screening in the Arabidopsis thaliana and Mus musculus genome: applications of virtual image restriction landmark genomic scanning (Vi-RLGS). Nucleic Acids Res. 2003;31(15):4490–6.
45. Nobuyasu S. Characterization of circulating DNA in healthy human plasma. Clin Chim Acta. 2008; 387:55–8.
46. Sabine J. DNA fragments in the blood plasma of cancer patients: quantitations and evidence for their origin from apoptotic and necrotic cells. Cancer Res. 2001;61:1659–65.

47. Ugur D, et al. Frequent copresence of methylated DNA and fragmented nucleosomal DNA in plasma of lymphoma patients. Clin Chim Acta. 2003;335:89–94.
48. Ning R, et al. The prognostic value of circulating plasma DNA level and its allelic imbalance on chromosome 8p in patients with hepatocellular carcinoma. J Cancer Res Clin Oncol. 2006;32:399–407.
49. Gabriella S, et al. Analysis of circulating tumor DNA in plasma at diagnosis and during follow-up of lung cancer patients. Cancer Res. 2001;61:4675–8.
50. Oliver G, et al. Circulating deoxyribonucleic acid as prognostic marker in Non small-cell lung cancer patients undergoing chemotherapy. Clin Oncol. 2004;22:4157–64.
51. Chao CH, et al. Quantification of circulating cell-free DNA in the plasma of cancer patients during radiation therapy. Cancer Sci. 2009;100:303–9.
52. Mayrhofer C, Krieger S, Allmaier, et al. DIGE compatible labeling of surface proteins on vital cells in vitro and in vivo. Proteomics. 2006;6(2):579–85.
53. Choi KS, Song L, Park YM, et al. Analysis of human plasma proteome by 2DE- and 2D nanoLC-based mass spectrometry. Prep Biochem Biotechnol. 2006;36(1):3–17.
54. Hutchens TW, Yip TT. New desorption strategies for the mass spectrometric analysis of macromolecules. Rapid Commun Mass Spectrom. 1993;7:576–80.
55. Seibert V, Wiesner A, Buschmann T, et al. Surface-enhanced laser desorption ionization time-of-flight mass spectrometry (SELDI TOF-MS) and proteinchip technology in proteomics research. Pathol Res Pract. 2004;200:83–94.
56. Fauq AH, Kache R, Khan MA, et al. Synthesis of acid-cleavable light isotope-coded affinity tags (ICAT-L) for potential use in proteomic expression profiling analysis. Bioconjug Chem. 2006;17(1):248–54.
57. Shui WQ, Liu YK, Fan HZ, et al. Enhancing TOF-TOF-based novo sequencing for high throughput identification with amino acid coded mass tagging. J Proteome Res. 2005;4:83–90.
58. Ross PL, Huang YN, Marchese JN, et al. Multiplexed protein quantitation in saccharomyces cerevisiae using amine-reactive isobaric tagging reagents. Mol Cell Proteomice. 2004;3(12):1154–69.
59. Ledue TB, Garfin D, et al. Immunofixation an dimmunoblotting. In: Rose NR, de Conway ME, Folds JD, editors. Manual of clinic laboratory microbiology. 5th ed. Washington, DC: American Society for Microbiology; 1997. p. 54–64.
60. Puig O, Caspary F, Rigaut G, et al. The tandem affinity purification (TAP) method: a general procedure of protein complex purification. Methods. 2001;24:218–29.
61. Naour FL, Brichory F, Beretta L, et al. Identification of tumor-associated antigens using proteomics. Technol Cancer Res Treat. 2002;1:257–62.
62. Lichtenfels R, Kellner R, Bukur J, et al. Heat shock protein expression and anti-heat shock protein reactivity in renal cell carcinoma. Proteomics. 2002;2:561–70.
63. Brichory FM, Misek DE, Yim AM, et al. An immune response manifested by the common occurrence of annexins I and II autoantibodies and high circulating levels of IL-6 in lung cancer. Proc Natl Acad Sci U S A. 2001;98:9824–9.
64. Le Naour F, Misek DE, Krause MC, et al. Proteomics-based identification of RS/DJ-1 as a novel circulating tumor antigen in breast cancer. Clin Cancer Res. 2001;7:3328–35.
65. Le Naour F, Brichory F, Misek DE, et al. A distinct repertoire of autoantibodies in hepatocellular carcinoma identified by proteomic analysis. Mol Cell Proteomics. 2002;1:197–203.
66. Jutao F, Yinkun L, Zhi D. Screening of spontaneous antibody of liver cancer via serum proteomics. China Hepatopathy Mag. 2005;13(11):832–5.
67. Petricoin EF, Ardekani A, Hitt P, et al. Use of proteomic patterns in serum to identify ovarian cancer. Lancet. 2002;359(2):572–7.
68. Yanagisawa K, Yu S, Xu BJ, et al. Proteomic patterns of tumor subsets in non-small-cell lung cell. Lancet. 2003;362(9382):433–9.
69. Ornstein DK, Rayford W, Fusaro VA, et al. Serum proteomic profiling can discriminate prostate cancer from benign prostates in men with total prostate specific antigen levels between 2.5 and 15.0ng/ml. J Urol Oncol. 2004;172:1302–5.
70. Junker K, Gneist J, Melle C, et al. Identification of protein pattern in kidney cancer using proteinchip arrays and bioinformatics. Int J Mol Med. 2005;15(2):285–90.
71. Hudelist G, Margit P-Z, Christian SF, et al. Use of high-throughput protein array for profiling of differentially expressed proteins in normal and malignant breast tissue. Breast Cancer Res Treat. 2004;86(3):281–91.
72. Scott G, Quynh-Thu L, et al. The use of plasma surface-enhanced laser desorption/ ionization time-of-flight mass spectrometry proteomic patterns for detection of head and neck squamous cell cancers. Clin Cancer Res. 2004;10:4806–12.
73. Chen YD, Zheng S, Yu JK, et al. Artificial neural networks analysis of surface-enhanced laser desorption/ ionization mass spectra of serum protein pattern distinguishes colorectal cancer from healthy population. Clin Cancer Res. 2004;10:8380–5.
74. Huangcheng FJ, Jian Z. Research on serum protein molecular markers related to the cancer embolus formation of portal vein of hepatocellular carcinoma. Chin Med J (Engl). 2005;85(11):781–5.
75. Song HY, Liu YK, Feng JT, et al. Proteomic analysis on metastasis-associated proteins of human hepatocellular carcinoma tissues. J Cancer Res Clin Oncol. 2006;132(2):92–8.
76. Feng JT, Liu YK, Song HY, et al. Heat shock protein 27: a potential biomarker for hepatocellular carcinoma identified by serum proteome analysis. Proteomics. 2005;5(17):4581–8.
77. Wong J, Cagney G, Cartwright H. SpecAlign-processing and alignment of mass spectra datasets. Bioinformatics. 2005;21(9):2088–90.

78. Shin H, Mutlu M, Koomen JM, et al. Parametric power spectral density analysis of noise from instrumentation in MALDI TOF mass spectrometry. Cancer Inform. 2007;3:317–28.
79. Shin H, Markey MK. A machine learning perspective on the development of clinical decision support systems utilizing mass spectra of blood samples. J Biomed Inform. 2006;39(2):227–48.
80. Cruz-Marcelo A, Guerra R, Vannucci M, et al. Comparison of algorithms for pre-processing of SELDI-TOF mass spectrometry data. Bioinformatics. 2008;24(19):2129–36.
81. Cui J, Kang X, Dai Z, Huang C, et al. Prediction of chronic hepatitis B, liver cirrhosis and hepatocellular carcinoma by SELDI-based serum decision tree classification. J Cancer Res Clin Oncol. 2007; 133(11):825–34.
82. Schwegler EE, Cazares L, Steel LF, et al. SELDI-TOF-MS profiling of serum for detection of the progression of chronic hepatitis C to hepatocellular carcinoma. Hepatology. 2005;41(3):634–42.
83. Scarlett CJ, Saxby AJ, Nielsen A, et al. Diagnostic potential of SELDI-TOF MS in malignant bile duct stricture. Hepatology. 2006;44(3):658–66.
84. Lim JY, Cho JY, Paik YH, et al. Diagnostic application of serum proteomic patterns in gastric cancer patients by ProteinChip surface-enhanced laser desorption/ionization time-of-flight mass spectrometry. Int J Biol Markers. 2007;22(4):281–6.
85. Liu XP, Shen J, Li ZF, et al. A serum proteomic pattern for the detection of colorectal adenocarcinoma using surface enhanced laser desorption and ionization mass spectrometry. Cancer Invest. 2006; 24(8):747–53.
86. Yang SY, Xiao XY, Zhang WG, et al. Application of serum SELDI proteomic patterns in diagnosis of lung cancer. BMC Cancer. 2005;20(5):83.
87. Xu G, Xiang CQ, Lu Y, et al. SELDI-TOF-MS-based serum proteomic screening in combination with CT scan distinguishes renal cell carcinoma from benign renal tumors and healthy persons. Technol Cancer Res Treat. 2009;8(3):225–30.
88. Navaglia F, Fogar P, Basso D, Tonidandel L, Fadi E, Zambon CF, Bozzato D, Moz S, Seraglia R, Pedrazzoli S, Plebani M. Pancreatic cancer biomarkers discovery by surface-enhanced laser desorption and ionization time-of-flight mass spectrometry. Clin Chem Lab Med. 2009;47(6):713–23.
89. Cheng L, Zhou L, Tao L, et al. SELDI-TOF MS profiling of serum for detection of laryngeal squamous cell carcinoma and the progression to lymph node metastasis. J Cancer Res Clin Oncol. 2008; 134(7):769–76.
90. Wei YS, Zheng YH, Liang WB, et al. Identification of serum biomarkers for nasopharyngeal carcinoma by proteomic analysis. Cancer. 2008;112(3): 544–51.
91. Zhou L, Cheng L, Tao L, et al. Detection of hypopharyngeal squamous cell carcinoma using serum proteomics. Acta Otolaryngol. 2006;126(8):853–60.
92. Ho DW, Yang ZF, Wong BY, et al. Surface-enhanced laser desorption/ionization time-of-flight mass spectrometry serum protein profiling to identify nasopharyngeal carcinoma. Cancer. 2006;107(1):99–107.
93. Ward DG, Cheng Y, N'Kontchou G, et al. Changes in the serum proteome associated with the development of hepatocellular carcinoma in hepatitis C-related cirrhosis. Br J Cancer. 2006;94(2):287–92.
94. Cao SM, Guo X, Chen FJ, et al. Serum diagnosis of head and neck squamous cell carcinoma using surface-enhanced desorption ionization mass spectrometry and artificial neural network analyses. Ai Zheng. 2007;26(7):767–70.
95. Au JS, Cho WC, Yip TT, et al. Deep proteome profiling of sera from never-smoked lung cancer patients. Biomed Pharmacother. 2007;61(9):570–7.
96. Qi XN. Support vector machines and application research overview. Comput Eng. 2004;30:10.
97. Shen Q, Shi WM, Kong W. New gene selection method for multiclass tumor classification by class centroid. J Biomed Inform. 2009;42(1):59–65.
98. Oberthuer A, Berthold F, Warnat P, et al. Customized oligonucleotide microarray gene expression-based classification of neuroblastoma patients outperforms current clinical risk stratification. J Clin Oncol. 2006;24(31):5070–8.
99. Roepman P, Schuurman A, Delahaye LJ, et al. A gene expression profile for detection of sufficient tumour cells in breast tumour tissue: microarray diagnosis eligibility. BMC Med Genomics. 2009;2(1):52.
100. Rosenfeld N, Aharonov R, Meiri E, et al. MicroRNAs accurately identify cancer tissue origin. Nat Biotechnol. 2008;26(4):400–1.
101. Kawamura T, Mutoh H, Tomita Y, et al. Cancer DNA microarray analysis considering multi-subclass with graph-based clustering method. J Biosci Bioeng. 2008;106(5):442–8.
102. Trolet J, Hupé P, Huon I, et al. Genomic profiling and identification of high-risk uveal melanoma by array CGH analysis of primary tumors and liver metastasis. Invest Ophthalmol Vis Sci. 2009;50(6): 2572–80.
103. Hewett R, Kijsanayothin P. Tumor classification ranking from microarray data. BMC Genomics. 2008;9(2):21.
104. Botting SK, Trzeciakowski JP, Benoit MF, et al. Sample entropy analysis of cervical neoplasia gene-expression signatures. BMC Bioinforma. 2009;10:66.
105. Murakami Y, Yasuda T, Saigo K, et al. Comprehensive analysis of microRNA expression patterns in hepatocellular carcinoma and non-tumorous tissues. Oncogene. 2006;25(17):2537–45.
106. Jiang H, Deng Y, Chen HS, et al. Joint analysis of two microarray gene-expression data sets to select lung adenocarcinoma marker genes. BMC Bioinforma. 2004;5:81.
107. Jiang DF, Gao J, Zhao NQ (2005) Microarray data analysis for breast cancer. Fudan Univ J Med Sci 32(2):167–72.

108. Patwa TH, Li C, Poisson LM, et al. The identification of phosphoglycerate kinase-1 and histone H4 autoantibodies in pancreatic cancer patient serum using a natural protein microarray. Electrophoresis. 2009;30(12):2215–26.
109. Moriya Y, Iyoda A, Kasai Y, et al. Prediction of lymph node metastasis by gene expression profiling in patients with primary resected lung cancer. Lung Cancer. 2009;64(1):86–91.
110. Shiwa M, Nishimura Y, Wakatabe R, et al. Rapid discovery and identification of a tissue specific tumor biomarker from39 human cancer cell lines using the SELDI protein chip platform[J]. Biochem Biophys Res Commun. 2003;309(1):18–25.
111. Lawrie LC, Curran S, McLeod HL, et al. Application of laser capture microdissection and proteomics in colon cancer [J]. MolPat hol. 2001;54(4):253–8.
112. Simpson RJ, Connolly LM, Eddes JS, et al. Proteomic analysis of the human colon carcinoma cell line (LIM1215): development of a membrane protein database. Electrophoresis. 2000;21(9):1707–32.
113. Ahmed N, Oliva K, Wang Y, et al. Proteomic profiling of proteins associated wit h urokinase plasminogen activator receptor in a colon cancer cell line using an antisense approach[J]. Proteomics. 2003; 3(3):288–98.
114. Stierum R, Gaspari M, Dommels Y, et al. Proteome analysis reveals novel proteins associated wit h proliferation and differentiation of t he colorectal cancer cell line Caco22[J]. Biochim Biophys Acta. 2003;1650(1–2):73–91.
115. Xu WH, Chen YD, Hu Y, et al. Preoperatively molecular staging with CM10 ProteinChip and SELD I2TOF2MS for colorectal cancer patients. J Zhejiang Univ Sci B. 2006;7(3):235–40.
116. Roboz J, Mal H, Sung M, et al. Protein profiles of serum in colon cancer by SEIDL – TOF mass spectrometry [R]. Proeomic: Poster Session AACR; 2002.
117. Petricoin EF, Liotta LA. SELDI-TOF-based serum proteomic pattern diagnostics for early detection of cancer [J]. Curr OpinBiotechnol. 2004;15(1):24–30.
118. Friedman D, Hill S, Keller J, et al. Proteome analysis of human colon cancer by two-dimensional difference gel electrophoresis and mass spectrometry. Proteomics. 2004;4(3):793–811.
119. Chaurand P, DaGue BB, Pearsall RS, et al. Profiling proteins from azoxymethane induced colon tumors at the molecular level by matrix assisted laser desorption/ ionization mass spectrometry. Proc Natl Acad Sci U S A. 2001;1(10):1320–6.
120. Stulik J, Koupilova K, Osterreicher J, et al. Protein abundance alterations in matched sets of macroscopically normal colon mucosa and colorectal carcinoma. Electrophoresis. 1999;20(18):3638–46.
121. Stulik J, Hernychova L, Porkertova S, et al. Proteome study of colorectal carcinogenesis. Electrophoresis. 2001;22(14):3019–25.
122. Roblick UJ, Hirschberg D, Habermann JK, et al. Sequential proteome alterations during genesis and progression of colon cancer [J]. Cell Mol Life Sci. 2004;61(10):1246.
123. Haiping P, Zhu H, Liang Z, et al. Application of two dimension electrophoresis and mass-spectrometric technique to sort out the differential protein expression between carcinoma of large intestine and normal intestinal tissue [J]. China Gen Surg. 2005;10(14):7482752.
124. Ping A, Yu B, Shiyong L. Proteomics research on occurrence and hepatic metastasis of carcinoma of large intestine [J]. China Surg Dep Mag. 2004; 42(11):668–71.
125. Tachibana M, Ohkura Y, Kobayashi Y, et al. Expression of apolipoprotein A1 in colonic adenocarcinoma [J]. Anticancer Res. 2003;23(5b): 4161–7.
126. Lin HM, Chatterjee A, Lin YH, et al. Genome wide expression profiling identifies genes associated with colorectal liver metastasis. Oncol Rep. 2007;17(6): 1541–9.
127. Fritzmann J, Morkel M, Besser D, et al. A colorectal cancer expression profile that includes transforming growth factor β inhibitor BAMBI predicts metastatic potential. Gastroenterology. 2009;137(1):165–75.
128. Sato T, Oshima T, Yoshihara K, et al. Overexpression of the fibroblast growth factor receptor-1 gene correlates with liver metastasis in colorectal cancer. Oncol Rep. 2009;21(1):211–6.
129. Oshima T, Akaike M, Yoshihara K, et al. Clinicopathological significance of the gene expression of matrix metalloproteinase-7, insulin like growth factor-1, insulin-like growth factor-2 and insulin-like growth factor-1 receptor in patients with colorectal cancer: insulin-like growth factor-1 receptor gene expression is a useful predictor of liver metastasis from colorectal cancer. Oncol Rep. 2008;20(2):359–64.
130. Oshima T, Akaike M, Yoshihara K, et al. Overexpression of EphA4 gene and reduced expression of EphB2 gene correlates with liver metastasis in colorectal cancer. Int J Oncol. 2008;33(3):573–7.
131. Akashi A, Komuta K, Haraguchi M, et al. Carcinoembryonic antigen mRNA in the mesenteric vein is not a predictor of hepatic metastasis in patients with resectable colorectal cancer: a long term study. Dis Colon Rectum. 2003;46(12):1653–8.
132. Rohde F, Rimkus C, Friederichs J, et al. Holzmann B,Siewert JR, Janssen KP. Expression of osteopontin, a target gene of de-regulated Wnt signaling, predicts survival in colon cancer. Int J Cancer. 2007;121(8):1717–23.
133. Rubie C, Frick VO, Pfeil S, et al. Schilling MK Correlation of IL-8 with induction, progression and metastatic potential of colorectal cancer. World J Gastroenterol. 2007;13(37):4996–5002.
134. Miyagawa S, Soeda J, Takagi S, et al. Prognostic significance of mature dendritic cells and factors associated with their accumulation in metastatic liver tumors from colorectal cancer. Hum Pathol. 2004;35(11):1392–6.

135. Shi HJ, Stubbs R, Hood K. Characterization of de novo synthesized proteins released from human colorectal tumour explants. Electrophoresis. 2009;30(14):2442–53.
136. Katayama M, Nakano H, Ishiuchi A, et al. Protein pattern difference in the colon cancer cell lines examined by two-dimensional differential in-gel electrophoresis and mass spectrometry. Surg Today. 2006;36(12):1085–93.
137. Pei H, Zhu H, Zeng S, et al. Proteome analysis and tissue microarray for profiling protein markers associated with lymph node metastasis in colorectal cancer. J Proteome Res. 2007;6(7):2495–501.
138. Kang B, Hao C, Wang H, et al. Evaluation of hepatic-metastasis risk of colorectal cancer upon the protein signature of PI3K/AKT pathway. J Proteome Res. 2008;7(8):3507–15.
139. Pierobon M, Calvert V, Belluco C, et al. Multiplexed cell signaling analysis of metastatic and nonmetastatic colorectal cancer reveals COX2-EGFR signaling activation as a potential prognostic pathway biomarker. Clin Colorectal Cancer. 2009;8(2):110–7.
140. Nakamoto RH, Uetake H, Iida S, et al. Correlations between cyclooxygenase-2 expression and angiogenic factors in primary tumors and liver metastasis in colorectal cancer. Jpn J Clin Oncol. 2007;37(9): 679–85.
141. Melle C, Ernst G, Schimmel B, et al. Colon-derived liver metastasis, colorectal carcinoma, and hepatocellular carcinoma can be discriminated by the Ca(2+)-binding proteins S100A6 and S100A11. PLoS One. 2008;3(12):3767.
142. Fang YJ, Lu ZH, Wang GQ, Pan ZZ, et al. Elevated expressions of MMP7, TROP2, and survivin are associated with survival, disease recurrence, and liver metastasis of colon cancer. Int J Colorectal Dis. 2009;24(8):875–84.
143. Ochiai H, Nakanishi Y, Fukasawa Y, et al. A new formula for predicting liver metastasis in patients with colorectal cancer: immunohistochemical analysis of a large series of 439 surgically resected cases. Oncology. 2008;75(1–2):32–41.
144. Choi HN, Kim KR, Lee JH, et al. Serum response factor enhances liver metastasis of colorectal carcinoma via alteration of the E-cadherin/β-catenin complex. Oncol Rep. 2009;21(1):57–63.
145. Pancione M, Forte N, Sabatino L, et al. Reduced β-catenin and peroxisome proliferator-activated receptor-gamma expression levels are associated with colorectal cancer metastatic progression: correlation with tumor-associated macrophages, cyclooxygenase 2, and patient outcome. Hum Pathol. 2009;40(5):714–25.
146. Delektorskaya VV, Perevoshchikov AG, Golovkov DA, et al. Expression of E-cadherin, β-catenin, and CD-44v6 cell adhesion molecules in primary tumors and metastasis of colorectal adenocarcinoma. Bull Exp Biol Med. 2005;139(6):706–10.
147. de Heer P, Koudijs MM, van de Velde CJ, et al. Combined expression of the non-receptor protein tyrosine kinases FAK and Src in primary colorectal cancer is associated with tumor recurrence and metastasis formation. Eur J Surg Oncol. 2008;34(11):1253–61.
148. Peeters CF, Ruers TJ, Westphal JR, et al. Progressive loss of endothelial P-selectin expression with increasing malignancy in colorectal cancer. Lab Invest. 2005;85(2):248–56.
149. Noike T, Miwa S, Soeda J, et al. Increased expression of thioredoxin-1, vascular endothelial growth factor, and redox factor-1 is associated with poor prognosis in patients with liver metastasis from colorectal cancer. Hum Pathol. 2008;39(2): 201–8.
150. Wang M, Vogel I, Kalthoff H. Correlation between metastatic potential and variants from colorectal tumor cell line HT-29. World J Gastroenterol. 2003;9(11):2627–31.
151. Wang S, Zhou J, Wang XY, et al. Down- regulated expression of SATB2 is associated with metastasis and poor prognosis in colorectal cancer. J Pathol. 2009;219(1):114–22.
152. Oue N, Kuniyasu H, Noguchi T, et al. Serum concentration of Reg IV in patients with colorectal cancer: overexpression and high serum levels of Reg IV are associated with liver metastasis. Oncology. 2007;72(5–6):3713–80.
153. Peng L, Ning J, Meng L, et al. The association of the expression level of protein tyrosine phosphatase PRL-3 protein with liver metastasis and prognosis of patients with colorectal cancer. J Cancer Res Clin Oncol. 2004;130(9):521–6.
154. Li J, Guo K, Koh VW, Tang JP, et al. Generation of PRL-3 and PRL-1 specific monoclonal antibodies as potential diagnostic markers for cancer metastasis. Clin Cancer Res. 2005;11(6):2195–204.
155. Hatate K, Yamashita K, Hirai K, et al. Liver metastasis of colorectal cancer by protein-tyrosine phosphatase type 4A, 3 (PRL-3) is mediated through lymph node metastasis and elevated serum tumor markers such as CEA and CA19-9. Oncol Rep. 2008;20(4): 737–43.
156. Tsuboi K, Shimura T, Masuda N, et al. Galectin-3 expression in colorectal cancer: relation to invasion and metastasis. Anticancer Res. 2007;27(4B):2289–96.
157. Zheng H, Tsuneyama K, Cheng C, et al. Maspin expression was involved in colorectal adenoma-adenocarcinoma sequence and liver metastasis of tumors. Anticancer Res. 2007;27(1A):259–65.
158. Lin BR, Chang CC, Che TF, et al. Connective tissue growth factor inhibits metastasis and acts as an independent prognostic marker in colorectal cancer. Gastroenterology. 2005;128(1):9–23.
159. Saito N, Kameoka S. Serum laminin is an independent prognostic factor in colorectal cancer. Int J Colorectal Dis. 2005;20(3):238–44.
160. Yoshidome H, Kohno H, Shida T, et al. Significance of monocyte chemoattractant protein-1 in angiogenesis and survival in colorectal liver metastases. Int J Oncol. 2009;34(4):923–30.

161. Ochiumi T, Tanaka S, Oka S, et al. Clinical significance of angiopoietin-2 expression at the deepest invasive tumor site of advanced colorectal carcinoma. Int J Oncol. 2004;24(3):539–47.
162. Yokomizo H, Yoshimatsu K, Ishibashi K, et al. Fas ligand expression is a risk factor for liver metastasis in colorectal cancer with venous invasion. Anticancer Res. 2003;23(6D):5221–4.
163. Fujimoto Y, Nakanishi Y, Sekine S, et al. CD10 expression in colorectal carcinoma correlates with liver metastasis. Dis Colon Rectum. 2005;48(10):1883–9.
164. Hayashi H, Kohno H, Ono T, et al. Transforming growth factor-β1 induced hepatocyte apoptosis; a possible mechanism for growth of colorectal liver metastasis. Acta Oncol. 2004;43(1):91–7.
165. Auguste P, Fallavollita L, Wang N, et al. The host inflammatory response promotes liver metastasis by increasing tumor cell arrest and extravasation. Am J Pathol. 2007;170(5):1781–92.
166. Kawahara A, Akagi Y, Hattori S, et al. Higher expression of deoxyuridine triphosphatase (dUTPase) may predict the metastasis potential of colorectal cancer. J Clin Pathol. 2009;62(4):364–9.
167. Zhou ZW, Ren JQ, Wan DS, et al. Multivariate regressive analysis of prognosis of liver metastasis from colorectal cancer. Ai Zheng. 2006;25(9):1149–52.
168. Takagawa R, Fujii S, Ohta M, et al. Preoperative serum carcinoembryonic antigen level as a predictive factor of recurrence after curative resection of colorectal cancer. Ann Surg Oncol. 2008;15(12):3433–59.
169. Mehrkhani F, Nasiri S, Donboli K, et al. Prognostic factors in survival of colorectal cancer patients after surgery. Colorectal Dis. 2009;11(2):157–61.
170. Waas ET, Wobbes T, Ruers T, et al. Circulating gelatinases and tissue inhibitor of metalloproteinase-1 in colorectal cancer metastatic liver disease. Eur J Surg Oncol. 2006;32(7):756–63.
171. Sasaki A, Kawano K, Inomata M, et al. Value of serum carbohydrate antigen 19-9 for predicting extrahepatic metastasis in patients with liver metastasis from colorectal carcinoma. Hepatogastroenterology. 2005;52(66):1814–9.
172. Iwasaki A, Shirakusa T, Yamashita Y, et al. Characteristic differences between patients who have undergone surgical treatment for lung metastasis or hepatic metastasis from colorectal cancer. Thorac Cardiovasc Surg. 2005;53(6):358–64.
173. Katoh H, Yamashita K, Kokuba Y, et al. Surgical resection of stage IV colorectal cancer and prognosis. World J Surg. 2008;32(6):1130–7.
174. Delektorskaya VV, Golovkov DA, Kushlinskii NE. Clinical significance of levels of molecular biological markers in zones of invasive front-line of colorectal cancer. Bull Exp Biol Med. 2008;146(5):616–9.
175. Cambien B, Karimdjee BF, Richard-Fiardo P, et al. Organ-specific inhibition of metastatic colon carcinoma by CXCR3 antagonism. Br J Cancer. 2009;100(11):1755–64.
176. Rubie C, Kollmar O, Frick VO, et al. Differential CXC receptor expression in colorectal carcinomas. Scand J Immunol. 2008;68(6):635–44.
177. Murata K, Miyoshi E, Ihara S, et al. Attachment of human colon cancer cells to vascular endothelium is enhanced by N-acetylglucosaminyltransferase V. Oncology. 2004;66(6):492–501.
178. St Hill CA, Farooqui M, Mitcheltree G, et al. The high affinity selectin glycan ligand C2-O-SLeX and mRNA transcripts of the core 2 β-1,6-N-acetylglucosaminyltransferase (C2GnT1) gene are highly expressed in human colorectal adenocarcinomas. BMC Cancer. 2009;9:79.
179. Uner A, Akcali Z, Unsal D. Serum levels of soluble E-selectin in colorectal cancer. Neoplasma. 2004;51(4):269–74.
180. Uemura T, Shiozaki K, Yamaguchi K, et al. Contribution of sialidase NEU1 to suppression of metastasis of human colon cancer cells through desialylation of integrin β4. Oncogene. 2009;28(9):1218–29.
181. Toiyama Y, Miki C, Inoue Y, et al. Circulating form of human vascular adhesion protein-1 (VAP-1): decreased serum levels in progression of colorectal cancer and predictive marker of lymphatic and hepatic metastasis. J Surg Oncol. 2009;99(6):368–72.
182. Illemann M, Bird N, Majeed A, et al. Two distinct expression patterns of urokinase, urokinase receptor and plasminogen activator inhibitor-1 in colon cancer liver metastasis. Int J Cancer. 2009;124(8):1860–70.
183. Halder SK, Rachakonda G, Deane NG, et al. Smad7 induces hepatic metastasis in colorectal cancer. Br J Cancer. 2008;99(6):957–65.
184. Yamada M, Ichikawa Y, Yamagishi S, et al. Amphiregulin is a promising prognostic marker for liver metastasis of colorectal cancer. Clin Cancer Res. 2008;14(8):2351–6.
185. Murad JC, Ribeiro Jr U, Safatle-Ribeiro AV, et al. Evaluation of molecular markers in hepatic metastasis of colorectal adenocarcinoma. Hepatogastroenterology. 2007;54(76):1029–33.
186. Wagner P, Koch M, Nummer D, et al. Detection and functional analysis of tumor infiltrating T-lymphocytes (TIL) in liver metastasis from colorectal cancer. Ann Surg Oncol. 2008;15(8):2310–7.
187. Sasaki A, Kai S, Endo Y, Iwaki K, et al. Prognostic value of preoperative peripheral blood monocyte count in patients with colorectal liver metastasis after liver resection. J Gastrointest Surg. 2007;11(5):596–602.

6 Genetic Diagnosis on Hepatic Metastasis from Colorectal Cancer

Suzhan Zhang

Early diagnosis is one of the bottlenecks to cure the hepatic metastasis of colorectal cancer (CRC). About 15–25 % patients are diagnosed with hepatic metastasis when the primary tumor is detected, while 25 % CRC patients will suffer from metachronous hepatic metastasis [1]. Currently, the diagnoses for synchronous hepatic metastasis of colorectal cancer mainly counts on preoperative examination and/or exploratory intraoperation; when necessary, biopsy is performed to determine hepatic metastasis of cancer; the diagnoses for metachronous hepatic metastasis mainly count on regular follow-up reexaminations by means of such imaging checks as ultrasound, CT, MRI, and PET and cancer embryo antigen (CEA). However, genetic diagnosis still remains at the exploratory stage of laboratory, so it is far away from clinical application.

6.1 Common Markers for Hepatic Metastasis of Colorectal Cancer

6.1.1 Cancer Embryo Antigen (CEA)

CEA is a kind of sugar protein with the molecular weight of 180 kDa, which exists in the mucous epithelium of embryonic stomach and bowel and cell surface of some malignant tumors. As a relatively mature tumor marker, CEA plays a critical role in the diagnoses for hepatic metastasis of colorectal cancer, though sensitivity and specificity are not quite high.

The research on CEA in the peripheral blood serum was made earliest. At the primary diagnoses of colorectal cancer, the positive rate of serum CEA is not high at all. Usually, we can predict the occurrence of metastasis upon the rise of serum, but the prognosis is quite poor. Generally speaking, the half-life of CEA is 3–4 days. If CEA fails to fall to the normal level 1 month after the operation, occult metastasis or early relapse can be anticipated; if CEA falls to the normal level and then rise after the operation, it is related to metastasis by 75 %; even if the patient's CEA is not high before the operation, it is meaningful to take postoperative examination. Once Abir et al. [2] summarized several prospective studies (see Table 6.1). It is said that the abnormal rise of serum CEA is 4–10 months earlier than the clinical detection of recurred metastasis, and the positive rate can reach 70 % and above. Hence, reexamination of serum CEA at the interval of 2–3 months is an effective means to detect recurred metastasis at the early stage. In addition, the symptoms of hepatic metastasis are usually not obvious, while the symptoms of local relapse can be anticipated, so the value of serum CEA is superior to that of local relapse in terms of hepatic

S. Zhang
The Second Affiliated Hospital of Zhejiang University School of Medicine, Zhejiang, China
e-mail: zhangscy@tom.com

X. Qin et al. (eds.), *Multidisciplinary Management of Liver Metastases in Colorectal Cancer*,
DOI 10.1007/978-94-017-7755-1_6

Table 6.1 Value of CEA in peripheral blood serum for the diagnoses of hepatic metastasis of colorectal cancer

Researcher	Caseload	Duration of median follow-up survey (year)	Relapse prompted by CEA (%)	Hepatic metastasis prompted by CEA (%)	The rise of CEA is earlier than relapse/metastasis (month)
McCall	311	4.5	58	80	6
Moertel	1,217	6	59	70	4.5
Ohlsson	160	6.8	41	66	6
Engaras	132	5	88	100	8
Makela	106	5	31	43	Not clear

metastasis prompts. However, CEA in the peripheral blood serum is not featured with the specificity of hepatic metastasis, so it can only generally prompt the recurrence and/or metastasis of colorectal cancer.

In 1989, Yeatman et al. [3] pioneered to report the value of measuring the level of bile CEA inside the gallbladder for the diagnoses of hepatic metastasis of colorectal cancer. Among 17 patients with single and multiple hepatic metastasis, the level of bile CEA was 4.7–259 times higher than that of serum CEA ($P=0.0009$). The hepatic metastasis less than 1 cm^3 may generate 9–41 ng/ml bile CEA. Li Destri et al. [4] examined intraoperative bile CEA, preoperative serum CEA, and lymph node involvement among 89 cases after the radical operation for colorectal cancer and follow-up survey last for 3 years. Hepatic metastasis occurred in 11 cases, 9 of which had higher level of bile CEA (5 ng/ml). Among the rest of 78 cases, 73 cases had the normal level of bile CEA, so the ratio of sensitivity, specificity, and accuracy for the anticipation of hepatic metastasis can, respectively, reach 81.8 %, 93.6 %, and 92.1 %. Owing to a few caseloads, this study failed to contribute to serum CEA and lymph node involvement. Tuech et al. [5] examined the level of bile CEA in three groups, the hepatic metastasis group ($n=35$), the non-hepatic metastasis group ($n=154$), and the contractive group ($n=23$), and the level of CEA was shown as follows: the hepatic metastasis group > the non-hepatic metastasis group > the contrastive group. The follow-up survey was made for the non-hepatic metastasis group for 3 years. Hepatic metastasis occurred in 22 cases, and the patients with the bile CEA >5 ng/ml were more subject to hepatic metastasis than those with the normal level of CEA (18/95 vs. 4/59). Kanellos et al. [6] made a 5-year follow-up survey for 73 cases with colorectal cancer. Thirteen cases suffered from hepatic metastasis and the level of bile CEA was abnormal. However, among the 60 cases with no tumor, the abnormity of bile CEA occurred in 32 cases, so the rate of false positive was quite high.

Based on the current research on bile CEA, the time to collect bile is in the course of the operation for primary colorectal cancer as a rule, but right now the bigger tumor exists in the body, and bile CEA secreted from the liver, the upmost organ to remove CEA in the body, is bound to be impacted by the primary tumor. So, the examination of bile CEA along with the primary tumor may influence the accurate diagnoses of hepatic metastasis and invasion could hardly be avoided during postoperative examination of bile CEA. Therefore, it is hard to realize clinical application to a great extent.

Besides peripheral blood serum and bile, scholars have also examined the level of CEA in the portal vein blood [6], vena mesenterica, duodenal juice and exudate from abdominal cavity, etc. However, further development is hindered due to the difficulty in sampling and early diagnosis as well as lower positive rate.

6.1.2 CEA-mRNA and Cytokeratin (CK)-mRNA

Tumor cells in blood circulation are considered as one of the markers to anticipate hematogenous dissemination and distant metastasis of tumor, so it is feasible to examine tumor cells in blood circulation for the risk evaluation of hepatic metastasis of colorectal cancer or early diagnosis. However, owing to fewer tumor cells in blood circulation, relevant test methods request higher sensitivity and specificity. Currently, the reverse transcription PCR (RT-PCR) technology, originated from the classic PCR, is widely applied to detect a certain gene at the mRNA level. A tumor cell can be detected from 10^6 to 10^7 normal cells, so such technology is obviously superior to traditional cytomorphology, immunohistochemistry, cytogenetics, and flow cytometer. If the RT-PCR technology is applied to examine the circulating tumor cells, the objective gene should be featured with the specificity in tumor tissue. Most common solid tumor lacks the genes with tumor specificity, so currently tissue specificity or tumor-related target gene is selected for examination. CEA and CK are mainly applied as the target gene for the colorectal cancer. CEA can be almost detected on any epithelia including cancer cell, while CK is the component protein of the interzonal fiber of epithelia as well as reliable marker for the differentiation of epithelium; for example, CK_{19} and CK_{20} exist in the malignant tumor related to glandular epithelium. Given the unstable condition of mRNA in the cell's external environment, it is assumed that tumor cells exist if CEA-mRNA or CK-mRNA is detected in the blood of colorectal cancer patients.

Xu et al. [7] reported the positive rate of CEA, CK_{20}, and CK_{19}-mRNA by 35.8, 28.3, and 41.9 % among 168 colorectal cancer patients. Iinuma et al. [8] examined CEA-mRNA and CK20-mRNA in the peripheral blood and the blood of tumor drainage area among 167 colorectal cancer patients: the positive rate of CEA-mRNA and/or CK_{20}-mRNA in the peripheral blood was 10.2 % (17/167), while that in the blood of tumor drainage area was 34.1 % (57/167). CEA-mRNA and CK_{20}-mRNA expressions are obviously correlated with the depth of tumor infiltration, vein encroachment, lymphatic metastasis, hepatic metastasis, and other clinical pathogenesis by stages. Also, both the survival time free from diseases and the total lifetime of positive patients are lower than those of negative patients. Moreover, CEA-mRNA and CK_{20}-mRNA expressions in the blood of tumor drainage area belong to independent prognosis factors. Other scholars [9] also concluded similar findings. Also, some scholars [10] conducted CEA and CEA-mRNA monitoring on the patients after the resection of hepatic metastasis per month. As compared with CEA, CEA-mRNA can more sensitively prompt the postoperative relapse and metastasis at the earlier stage.

However, this method has higher false negative and false positive rate. The reasons for false negative may consist in the following: (1) Tumor cells are featured with heterogeneity and the expression of the same target gene may differ on different patients or different tumor cells of the same patient, thus resulting in low or no expression in some samples. Therefore, the combined examination with several target genes will be helpful to increase the detectable rate; (2) exfoliation or dissemination of tumor cells is intermittent, so single blood sampling is hard to find it out. If the condition permits, more blood sampling can be taken. The reasons for false positive may consist in (1) the increase of pseudo genes in hemocyte, (2) DNA contamination in the process of RNA extraction or the increase of DNA pieces due to chemotherapy, (3) CEA and CK expression of some regenerated infant cells or preexisting variant cells and low expression of non-epithelia, (4) cross contamination among samples and the contamination of skin epithelia when drawing blood, etc., and (5) other existing subclinical malignant tumors [11]. In addition, similar to CEA in the peripheral blood serum, CEA-mRNA and CK-mRNA examinations are not featured with the specificity of hepatic metastasis, so it is more suitable for risk evaluation and prompt of hepatic metastasis rather than diagnoses.

6.1.3 C-met Gene and Hepatic Growth Factor

C-met is the gene to encode hepatic growth factor receptor (HGFR). As a kind of cross membrane receptor protein tyrosine kinase, c-met mainly exists in the epithelial tissue. The ligand of HGFR is the hepatic growth factor/scatter factor (HGF/SF), but the combination of HGFR and HGF/SF can lead to the phosphorylation of HGFR, thus activating tyrosine kinase and tyrosine phosphorylation of many substrate proteins, and then the biological effect comes into being. In addition, excessive expression of c-met genes in many malignant tumors plays a vital role in the occurrence, growth, angiopoiesis, and metastasis of tumors. As a kind of multifunctional cell factor, HGF can induce epithelia and many tumor cells to split, move, and invade as well as develop angiogenesis. High expression of c-met and HGF in tumor tissue can form positive feedback, thus leading to indeterminate growth and invasion of tumors [12, 13].

Di Renzo et al. [14] discovered that excessive expression of c-met protein, 5–50 times the normal level, exists in 50 % primary colorectal cancer and 70 % hepatic metastasis. This phenomenon occurs at each stage of colorectal cancer, so it may stimulate the metastasis thereof. Xu Jianmin et al. in China [15] also reported that the expression of c-met protein in primary tumor and synchronous hepatic metastasis is more than that in primary tumor with no hepatic metastasis ($P<0.05$); but the expression of c-met protein in metachronous hepatic metastasis is not at odds with that in primary tumor with no hepatic metastasis or synchronous hepatic metastasis. Lately, Zeng et al. [16] made use of the quantitative PCR/joining enzyme reaction technology to directly examine c-met gene copy number in the tissue sample. This study collected 247 pairs of primary colorectal cancer/normal intestinal mucosa and 147 pairs of hepatic metastasis/normal hepatic tissue. The c-met gene copy number in normal intestinal mucosa and hepatic tissue is similar, while that in primary tumor is apparently higher than that in normal tunica mucosa and the c-met gene copy number in hepatic metastasis is apparently higher than that in normal hepatic tissue ($P<0.001$). Moreover, the c-met gene copy number in hepatic metastasis is apparently higher than that in primary tumor ($P<0.0001$). The rate of c-met gene amplification in the patients with local tumor is only 2 % (3/177), while that in the patients with other distant metastases and the patients with hepatic metastasis, respectively, reaches 9 % (6/70, $P<0.02$) and 18 % (25/147, $P<0.01$). After the operative treatment for hepatic metastasis, the patients with c-met gene amplification may have a shorter 3-year survival rate ($P=0.07$).

Shi Weijian et al. in China [17] reported 52 cases of colorectal cancer, whose serum HGF was apparently higher than that of healthy persons. Higher HGF value was closely related to later clinical stadium. Seventeen cases with hepatic metastasis had higher HGF than those with no hepatic metastasis. Yoon et al. [18] kept monitoring plasma HGF of 26 cases with hepatic metastasis, whose preoperative HGF was apparently higher than healthy persons. Three days after the resection, plasma HGF began to rise. Three months later, plasma HGF recovered to the preoperative level. During the 19-month median follow-up survey, ten patients suffered relapse, which might be associated with higher preoperative HGF ($P=0.021$).

The positive feedback between c-met gene products and HGF doesn't belong to the specificity of colorectal cancer or hepatic metastasis, which widely exists in a great variety of tumors.

6.1.4 Matrix Metalloproteinase (MMP) and Tissue Inhibitors of Metalloproteinases (TIMP)

Matrix metalloproteinase (MMP) is a series of hydrolytic enzyme that is featured with high autopolyploid and can degrade extracellular matrix, but such metal ions as calcium and zinc are needed as the accessory factor and that is what its name stems from; MMP can degrade various proteins in extracellular matrix and destroy tumor cells, so it is deemed as the protective screen against tumor cell invasion. MMP, as the main proteolytic enzyme in the process, plays a critical role against tumor cell invasion and metastasis. Extracellular matrix is mainly composed of basilar membrane and interstitial substance; the former is made of membrana basilaris collagen, i.e., type IV collagen, which is the protective screen against tumor cell invasion and metastasis. In view of type IV collagenase (MMP-2 and MMP-9) that can degrade this protective screen, there are quite a lot of research resources available. Tissue inhibitors of metalloproteinases (TIMP) are the main repressors of MMP, so the degree of degradation as well as tumor cell invasion and metastasis depends on the dynamic equilibrium of MMP and TIMP [19].

Currently, most of studies aim at primary tumor or metastasis, for example, German scholars [20], reported that the expression of MMP-1, MMP-2, MMP-3, and MMP-12 in hepatic metastasis was apparently lower than those in primary colorectal cancer; also, the tumors with high expression of MMP-7, TIMP-1, and TIMP-2 were less sensitive to 5-FU chemotherapy, while the tumors with high expression of MMP-2, MMP-9, MMP-11, and MMP-14 were quite sensitive to chemotherapy.

However, the studies on MMP and TIMP in blood are relatively less. Waas et al. [21] reported the examination results on MMP-2, MMP-9, and TIMP-1 in the plasma of 57 patients with hepatic metastasis, 94 patients with no hepatic metastasis, and 51 healthy persons. The level of MMP-2 in the patients with hepatic metastasis was lower than that of the healthy persons, while the TIMP-1 thereof was higher than the healthy persons ($P < 0.001$); the difference between the groups with or without hepatic metastasis was not obvious at all; after the resection of hepatic metastasis, MMP-2 still remained at the lower level, which might be related to relapse. Actually, the diagnoses and prognosis value of MMP-2, MMP-9, and TIMP-1 are inferior to CEA, so they are not ideal markers. Ishida et al. [22] examined the level of MMP-9 in the peripheral and portal vein plasma of the patients with colorectal cancer and discovered that the level of MMP-9 in peripheral blood was irrelevant to various clinical pathogeneses; on the contrary, the level of MMP-9 in portal vein blood was associated with tumor pathogenesis type, Dukes stages, hepatic metastasis, and lymphatic metastasis. The level of MMP-9 in the portal vein blood of the patients with hepatic metastasis was apparently higher than that with no hepatic metastasis ($P < 0.01$). Moreover, the ratio of MMP-9 in portal vein blood to peripheral blood was meaningful to anticipate the relapse of hepatic metastasis. The higher the ratio, the higher the probability of relapse would be. If the critical ratio was set at 1.6, the ratios of sensitivity, specificity, and accuracy can, respectively, reach 77.8 %, 81.3 %, and 80.8 %.

Theoretically speaking, the change of dynamic equilibrium between MMP and TIMP, higher MMP and lower TIMP, is essential to the successful tumor cell invasion and metastasis, but this phenomenon cannot be verified in quite a number of studies on hepatic metastasis from colorectal cancer. Some findings are even the opposite. This may be associated with the complexity of MMP-TIMP system, the selection of samples, sampling time and caseload, etc., so further studies shall be made available.

6.1.5 Vascular Endothelial Growth Factor (VEGF)

Vascular endothelial growth factor (VEGF) is a kind of heparin-binding growth factor related to the specificity of vascular endothelial cell, which can stimulate the splitting, reproduction, and movement of endothelial cells and enhance vascular permeability, thus helping the growth of vasculogenesis. So, VEGF plays a vital role in the growth of angiogenesis.

Alabi et al. reported that higher level of VEGF-A in preoperative serum was related to relapse after the operation of colorectal cancer [23]; VEGF-C was quite lower in the patients with distant metastasis [24]. Ding Wei et al. [25] examined the level of VEGF in peripheral and portal vein blood of 101 cases with colorectal cancer and discovered that the level of VEGF was apparently higher than that of the healthy persons; the level of VEGF in portal vein blood with synchronous hepatic metastasis was apparently higher than that with no hepatic metastasis; the level of VEGF in portal vein blood on all the patients with hepatic metastasis was higher than 250 μg/L, and the proportion of hepatic metastasis on the patients with VEGF higher than 250 μg/L was 67.6 %. Also, sensitivity was 100 % and specificity was quite higher. But some scholars [26] propose objection, the level of preoperative VEGF on 18 cases with postoperative relapse, 21 cases with hepatic metastasis, and 40 cases with the survival time over 5 years free from diseases, and the level of VEGF on 28 healthy persons was divided into four sets. No significant difference was found on any two sets.

6.1.6 E-cadherin

E-cadherin (E-cad) is the hypotype of transmembrane protein in the cadherin protein molecular family. The expression of E-cad is on the epithelial surface of normal large intestinal mucosae, and the major functions thereof are to mediate adherence among epithelia and maintain normal morphological structure of tissue. The hepatic metastasis from colorectal cancer originates from the breakdown of complete epithelium, and then tumor cells pass through epithelium, blood, or lymphatic system and finally arrive at the liver. E-cad is essential for the completeness of epithelium, thus preventing the occurrence of metastasis.

Elzagheid et al. conducted tissue-related research [27] and discovered that the expression of E-cad on the cell membrane of primary tumor was apparently higher than that of metastasis; the patients with metastasis had higher E-cad and the expression of E-cad in hepatic metastasis was higher than other metastases. Moreover, higher E-cad in the cytoplasm of primary tumor was associated with shorter DFS. Upon a small sample-based research on the soluble E-cad in serum [28], the soluble E-cad in serum in the patients with colorectal cancer and benign diseases was higher than healthy persons; the concentration thereof was related to T stages rather than N and M stages. Among the patients with hepatic metastasis, the concentration of E-cad was related to the level of serum CEA. Currently, there is no report on large sample-based research on soluble E-cad.

6.1.7 Interleukin-6 and Interleukin-8 (IL-6 and IL-8)

As the multifunctional cytokine produced by mononuclear macrophage, lymphocyte, and nonlymphocyte, IL-6 is the sugar protein which is composed of 212 amino acids and provided with the molecular weight of 21 kDa. As the protein with the molecular weight of 8.4–8.9 kDa, IL-8 is composed of 72–77 amino acids and produces strong chemotaxis on the cells with specific and nonspecific immunological reaction. Both IL-6 and IL-8 are the key cell factors participating in the inflammatory reaction of organism. In recent years, the research showed that they also took part in the growth, invasiveness, and metastasis of tumor.

In 1994, Ueda et al. [29] found the level of IL-6 and IL-8 in the colorectal cancer patient before operation was apparently higher than those in the healthy person. The concentration of IL-6 and IL-8 was related to that of CA199. Also, the concentration of IL-6 and IL-8 in the hepatic metastasis patient was apparently higher than those without the hepatic metastasis. The further research also proved it [30, 31] and showed that the expression of IL-8 in the normal intestinal mucosa, primary tumor, and hepatic metastasis tissue was successively raised. The high expression of IL-8 in the primary tumor caused the high risk of hepatic metastasis. In addition, the Japanese specialists [32] reported the higher level of IL-8 in Dukes' C tumor venous blood meant the high risk of hepatic metastasis after operation.

6.1.8 Macrophage Migration Inhibitory Factor (MIF)

In 1966, MIF was discovered. As the lymphokine is produced from activated thymus-dependent lymphocytes, MIF could repress the macrophage during in vitro test. MIF is the multifunctional protein which is composed of cell factor, neuroendocrine hormone, and enzyme property. In recent years, it was found that MIF participated in the reproducing and disintegration of cells.

Also, it is closely related to the evolution, angiogenesis, and metastasis of tumor. Repression of p53's antitumor function may be one of the mechanisms for tumor promotion [33].

He Xingxiang et al. [34] reported that the expression of MIF in colorectal cancer tissue was apparently higher than that in the normal intestinal tissues around the cancer. The expression of MIF in primary tumor of hepatic metastasis and serum was higher than that in the person without hepatic metastasis. Also, MIF level in the serum was the independent risk factor to affect the hepatic metastasis (OR = 1.25, 95 % CI = 1.02–1.52, P = 0.03). Meanwhile, the animal experiment was used to certify MIF depressant could reduce the tumor load of tumor-bearing mouse.

6.2 Application of New Technique in the Genetic Diagnosis on Colorectal Cancer Hepatic Metastasis

6.2.1 Application of Proteomics in the Colorectal Cancer Hepatic Metastasis

With the smooth implementation of human genome project, the protein-based proteomics has gradually become one of the most vital fields in life sciences [35]. The protein rather than nucleic acid is the specific executor and reflector of vital movement. Therefore, the research at the level of proteomics is demanded on such aspects as pathogenesis of colorectal cancer hepatic metastasis as well as sensitive and specific markers used in clinical treatment.

2-DE is the method mainly used in the proteomics. According to the different electric charges, the protein specimen is separated through isoelectric focusing, so that various proteins are further separated via different molecular weights. By the use of silver staining, 3,000 protein points are obtained from one gel. Then image analysis is conducted via software to screen out the protein with differential expression, and the mass spectrometric techniques such as MALDI-TOF-MS are used to decode [36]. In terms of colorectal cancer hepatic metastasis, current researches are still not enough. Bai Xue et al. [37] adopted the above methods to compare the protein expression of primary tumor and hepatic metastasis of colorectal cancer, so as to find 46 differential protein points and make the assessment on 20 protein points hereof. The result showed the expression of activator protein factor 2B and adenosylmethionine mutant was decreased in the hepatic metastasis. The expression of zinc finger protein 64 homologue, guanylic acid interchange factor 4, human arginase, human glutathione S-transferring enzyme A3, and tumor necrosis factor α-induced protein 9 was increased during the hepatic metastasis. Zhang Yingnan et al. [38] also used the similar methods to find the high expression of Cdc 42 in the hepatic metastasis. Also, Western hybridization was used to verify that the positive rate of Cdc 42 was 100 % in the hepatic metastasis, while only 16 % in the primary tumor and no expression in the intestinal mucosa around the cancer. Li Zuguo et al. [39] used nude mice model and 2-DE successfully evaluated five remarkably increased proteins in serum after metastasis of SW480-EGFP: haptoglobin α chain, apoprotein A1, apoprotein E, immunoglobulin type K area VL chain, and transferrin.

In recent years, based on surface-enhanced laser desorption/ionization time-of-flight mass spectrometry (SELDI-TOF-MS), the protein fingerprint was used to diagnose various malignant tumors and screen out the new tumor markers. Based on the above technique, the protein chip series could combine with various proteins in the tested specimen via nonspecificity. When attacked by the laser in the mass spectrometer, various bonded proteins could be stimulated to form the gasified ions. Due to the different flight time of the ions with different mass-to-charge ratios, m/z, the ions could be reflected by the receiving device according to the difference, quantity, and strength thereof so as to form the relevant map for analysis and judgment (Fig. 6.1) [35]. As per the SELDI research result on colorectal cancer, it was still at the stage of pre-operation detection model establishing and preliminary screening of markers, while the hepatic metastasis-related studies were unavailable [40, 41].

Chen Yiding et al. from Tumor Research Institute of Zhejiang University [40] adopted

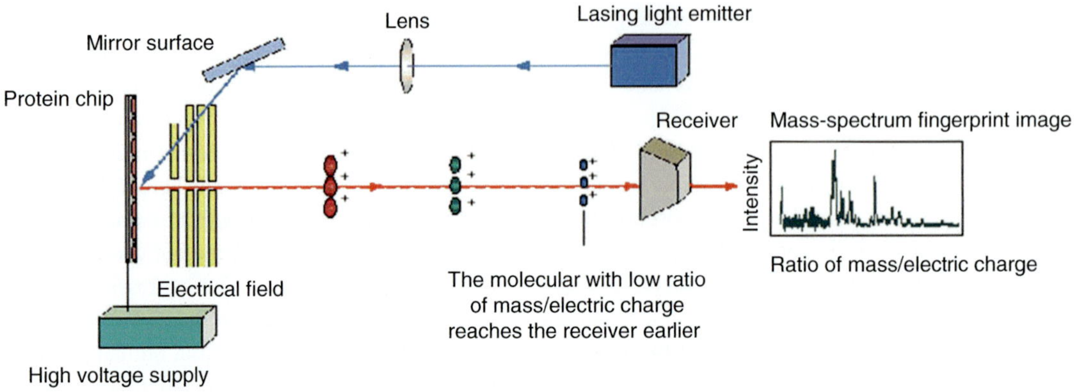

Fig. 6.1 Functional diagram of SELDI-TOF-MS (Reprint with permission from Shu [36])

SELDI-TOF-MS and H4 chip to test 42 patients at the stage of Dukes' A–C and 13 patients at the stage of Dukes' D, so as to find out three remote metastasis protein markers with mass-to-charge ratios of 5.5 kDa, 5.4 kDa, and 17.4 kDa and to find that the patients at the stage of D were obviously more than those without remote metastasis. Xu Wenhong et al. [42] adopted CM ten chip to set up the diagnosis model to judge Dukes'A–C and Dukes' D. Such model was composed of three protein peaks, namely, 6.9 kDa, 2.1 kDa, and 8.6 kDa. The precision ratio thereof reached 75.0 %. Shi Yijiu [43] analyzed 36 cases of SELDI patients with/without hepatic metastasis so as to establish the predictive model for hepatic metastasis of serum. Also, 44 patients with/without hepatic metastasis were used to conduct blind verification on the established model. The sensitivity and specificity of verification were, respectively, 75.0 % and 81.8 %.

6.2.2 Application of Gene Chip Technology in the Hepatic Metastasis of Colorectal Cancer

Since Affymetrix developed the first gene chip in the world in 1996, the gene chip technology was well accepted thanks to its high flux reactor, high velocity, and high automation. In recent years, this technique was widely used in the tumor research area. It not only provided powerful tools for the study on deactivation and activation of related gene in occurrence and development of tumor but acted as the new weapon to diagnose and treat the tumor [36].

Lin et al. [44] used this technique to compare the gene expression spectra of 48 primary tumor and 28 hepatic metastasis; also, 778 genes with differential expression in these two groups were found. The tissue reestablishing and immune response-related genes were increased in hepatic metastasis as compared with those in primary tumor. However, the genes related to cell multiplication and oxidative phosphorylation were decreased. The author adopted some genes hereof to verify via quantitative PCR: osteopontin, human versican, ADAM 17, CKS 2, PRDX 1, CXCR 4, CXCL 12, and LCN 2. Also, they were related to the invasive metastasis and clone of gene and tumor as the hepatic metastasis was increased. The decrease of cell multiplication-related gene may prompt the speed of cell multiplication in metastasis may slow down as compared with those in the primary tumor. Ki et al. [45] conducted entire genome analysis on the tissue specimen which was matched to normal tunica mucosa/primary tumor/hepatic metastasis. As the specific genes of organ were removed, 46 genes with hepatic metastasis were chosen; also, WNT 5A and carbonic anhydrase II hereof were verified. Meanwhile, the differential expression was found in 21 of above 46 genes in terms of primary tumor with/without hepatic metastasis. Nadal et al. [46] summarized a plurality of gene chip researches on hepatic metastasis

Table 6.2 Major hepatic metastasis genes currently selected by gene chip

Hepatic metastasis-related gene	Function	Expression of hepatic metastases (vs. primary tumor, IHC)
E-Cadherin	Adhesion	Decrease
EpCAM	Adhesion	Unclear
P-lectine and L-lectine	Adhesion	Unclear
CEA	Adhesion	Unclear
αvβ5	Adhesion and cell survival	Unclear
sLex and sLea	Adhesion	Increase
OPN	Adhesion, cell survival, and motion	Increase
ICAM-1	Adhesion	Unclear
VCAM-1	Adhesion	Unclear
CD44v6	Adhesion	Unclear
Cathepsin B	Invasiveness	Unclear
MMP-7	Invasiveness	Increase
MMP-2 and MMP-9	Invasiveness	Increase
Angiopoietin	Angiogenesis	Increase
EGFR	Growth	Equivalent
uPAR	Invasiveness, motion, and dormancy	Unclear
VEGF	Angiogenesis	Equivalent
TSP-1	Angiogenesis	Unclear
Angiostatin	Angiogenesis	Unclear
Endostatin	Angiogenesis	Unclear
dThdPase or PDECGF	Angiogenesis	Unclear
c-erbB-2	Growth	Unclear
c-Src/β-Arrestin 1	Growth	Unclear
FAS (CD95)	Death	Decrease
TRAIL (TRAIL-R1, TRAIL-R2, TRAIL-R3, and TRAIL-R4)	Death	Unclear
Nm23-H1 and Nm23-H2	Metastasis suppressor gene	Unclear
PRL-3	Motion and invasiveness	Increase

IHC immunohistochemistry

of colorectal cancer. Also, the major hepatic metastasis-related genes were listed currently (Table 6.2).

References

1. Ballantyne GH, Quin J. Surgical treatment of liver metastasis in patients with colorectal cancer. Cancer. 1993;71:4252–66.
2. Abir F, Alva S, Longo WE, et al. The postoperative surveillance of patients with colon cancer and rectal cancer. Am J Surg. 2006;192:100–8.
3. Yeatman TJ, Bland KI, Copeland 3rd EM, et al. Relationship between colorectal liver metastasis and CEA levels in gallbladder bile. Ann Surg. 1989;210:505–12.
4. Li Destri G, Lanteri R, Santangelo M, et al. Can biliary carcinoembryonic antigen identify colorectal cancer patients with occult hepatic metastasis? World J Surg. 2006;30:1494–9.
5. Tuech JJ, Pessaux P, Regenet N, et al. Detection of occult liver metastasis in colorectal cancer by measurement of biliary carcinoembryonic antigen concentration: a prospective study. J Surg Oncol. 2004;88:27–31.
6. Kanellos I, Zacharakis E, Demetriades H, et al. Value of carcinoembryonic antigen assay in predicting hepatic metastasis, local recurrence, and survival after curative resection of colorectal cancer. Surg Today. 2006;36:879–84.
7. Xu D, Li XF, Zheng S, et al. Quantitative real-time RT-PCR detection for CEA, CK20 and CK19 mRNA in peripheral blood of colorectal cancer patients. J Zhejiang Univ Sci B. 2006;7:445–751.
8. Iinuma H, Okinaga K, Egami H, et al. Usefulness and clinical significance of quantitative real-time RT-PCR to detect isolated tumor cells in the peripheral blood and tumor drainage blood of patients with colorectal cancer. Int J Oncol. 2006;28:297–306.
9. Miura M, Ichikawa Y, Tanaka K, et al. Real-time PCR (TaqMan PCR) quantification of carcinoembryonic antigen (CEA) mRNA in the peripheral blood of colorectal cancer patients. Anticancer Res. 2003;23:1271–6.
10. Kijima M, Togo S, Ichikawa Y, et al. Clinical significance of serum CEA protein and CEA mRNA after resection of colorectal liver metastasis. Anticancer Res. 2005;25:1327–32.
11. Hu Yue, Li Xufen, Zhang Suzhan. Test on expression of CK 19-mRNA in peripheral blood of lung cancer patient. Pract Cancer Mag. 2004;19:40–2.
12. Ide T, Kitajima Y, Miyoshi A, et al. The hypoxic environment in tumor-stromal cells accelerates pancreatic cancer progression via the activation of paracrine hepatocyte growth factor/c-Met signaling. Ann Surg Oncol. 2007;14:2600–7.
13. Jagadeeswaran R, Ma PC, Seiwert TY, et al. Functional analysis of c-Met/hepatocyte growth factor pathway in malignant pleural mesothelioma. Cancer Res. 2006;66:352–61.
14. Di Renzo MF, Olivero M, Giacomini A, et al. Overexpression and amplification of the met/HGF receptor gene during the progression of colorectal cancer. Clin Cancer Res. 1995;1:147–54.
15. Wei Ye, Xu Jianmin, Lu Xueyi. Application of c-met proto-oncogene in the hepatic metastasis of colorectal cancer. China Cancer Mag. 2006;16:993–7.

16. Zeng ZS, Weiser MR, Kuntz E, et al. c-Met gene amplification is associated with advanced stage colorectal cancer and liver metastasis. Cancer Lett. 2008;265:258–69.
17. Shi Weijian, Zhou Qiaoyun, Jiang Fenglian. Clinical value of serum hepatocyte growth factor in hepatic metastasis from colorectal cancer. Clin Oncol Mag. 2007;12:822–4.
18. Yoon SS, Kim SH, Gonen M, et al. Profile of plasma angiogenic factors before and after hepatectomy for colorectal cancer liver metastasis. Ann Surg Oncol. 2006;13:353–62.
19. Nelson AR, Fingleton B, Rothenberg ML, et al. Matrix metalloproteinases: biologic activity and clinical implications. J Clin Oncol. 2000;18:1135–49.
20. Gentner B, Wein A, Croner RS, et al. Differences in the gene expression profile of matrix metalloproteinases (MMPs) and their inhibitors (TIMPs) in primary colorectal tumors and their synchronous liver metastasis. Anticancer Res. 2009;29:67–74.
21. Waas ET, Wobbes T, Ruers T, et al. Circulating gelatinases and tissue inhibitor of metalloproteinase-1 in colorectal cancer metastatic liver disease. Eur J Surg Oncol. 2006;32:756–63.
22. Ishida H, Murata N, Tada M, et al. Determining the levels of matrix metalloproteinase-9 in portal and peripheral blood is useful for predicting liver metastasis of colorectal cancer. Jpn J Clin Oncol. 2003;33:186–91.
23. Alabi AA, Suppiah A, Madden LA, et al. Preoperative serum vascular endothelial growth factor-a is a marker for subsequent recurrence in colorectal cancer patients. Dis Colon Rectum. 2009;52:993–9.
24. Alabi AA, Suppiah A, Madden LA, et al. Preoperative serum levels of serum VEGF-C is associated with distant metastasis in colorectal cancer patients. Int J Colorectal Dis. 2009;24:269–74.
25. Ding Wei, Wang Jun, Han Gang. Clinical experimental study on early prediction of colorectal cancer metastatic liver disease. China Lab Diagn. 2007;11:647–9.
26. Roumen RM, Slooter GD, Croiset van Uchelen FA, et al. Preoperative serum vascular endothelial growth factor is not a marker for subsequent recurrence during long-term follow-up of colorectal cancer patients. Dis Colon Rectum. 2005;48:1070–5.
27. Elzagheid A, Algars A, Bendardaf R, et al. E-cadherin expression pattern in primary colorectal carcinomas and their metastasis reflects disease outcome. World J Gastroenterol. 2006;12:4304–9.
28. Wilmanns C, Grossmann J, Steinhauer S, et al. Soluble serum E-cadherin as a marker of tumor progression in colorectal cancer patients. Clin Exp Metastasis. 2004;21:75–8.
29. Ueda T, Shimada E, Urakawa T. Serum levels of cytokines in patients with colorectal cancer: possible involvement of interleukin-6 and interleukin-8 in hematogenous metastasis. J Gastroenterol. 1994;29:423–9.
30. Chung YC, Chang YF. Serum interleukin-6 levels reflect the disease status of colorectal cancer. J Surg Oncol. 2003;83:222–6.
31. Rubie C, Frick VO, Pfeil S, et al. Correlation of IL-8 with induction, progression and metastatic potential of colorectal cancer. World J Gastroenterol. 2007; 13:4996–5002.
32. Haraguchi M, Komuta K, Akashi A, et al. Elevated IL-8 levels in the drainage vein of resectable Dukes' C colorectal cancer indicate high risk for developing hepatic metastasis. Oncol Rep. 2002;9:159–65.
33. Hudson JD, Shoaibi MA, Maestro R, et al. A proinflammatory cytokine inhibits p53 tumor suppressor activity. J Exp Med. 1999;190:1375–82.
34. He XX, Chen K, Yang J, et al. Macrophage migration inhibitory factor promotes colorectal cancer. Mol Med. 2009;15:1–10.
35. Hu Yue, Zhang Suzhan. Current research and application of protein chip technology. Zhejiang Univ J (Med Ed). 2005;34:89–92.
36. Zheng Shu. Colorectal tumor: basic research and clinical practice. Beijing: People's Medical Publishing House; 2006.
37. Bai Xue, Li Shiyong, Yu Bo. Research on differential protein expression of primary tumor and hepatic metastasis of colorectal cancer. 2008;33: 487–9.
38. Zhang Yingnan, Li Shiyong, An Ping. Research on differential expression of proteomics in colorectal cancer hepatic metastasis and meaning thereof. China Stomach Intestine Surg Dep J. 2004;7:312–4
39. Li Zuguo, Zhao Liang, Liu Li. Observation on change of several proteins in the animal model serum of colorectal cancer metastasis. China Pathol Mag. 2007;36:48–52.
40. Chen YD, Zheng S, Yu JK, et al. Artificial neural networks analysis of surface-enhanced laser desorption/ionization mass spectra of serum protein pattern distinguishes colorectal cancer from healthy population. Clin Cancer Res. 2004;10:8380–5.
41. Hundt S, Haug U, Brenner H. Blood markers for early detection of colorectal cancer: a systematic review. Cancer Epidemiol Biomarkers Prev. 2007;16: 1935–53.
42. Xu WH, Chen YD, Hu Y, et al. Preoperatively molecular staging with CM10 protein chip and SELDI-TOF-MS for colorectal cancer patients. J Zhejiang Univ Sci B. 2006;7:235–40.
43. Shi Yijiu, Zhao Yun, Xu Jianmin. Application of surface enhanced laser desorption/ionization time-of-flight mass spectrometry to test colorectal cancer hepatic metastasis. China Tumor Mag. 2008;30: 910–3.
44. Lin HM, Chatterjee A, Lin YH, et al. Genome wide expression profiling identifies genes associated with colorectal liver metastasis. Oncol Rep. 2007;17: 1541–9.
45. Ki DH, Jeung HC, Park CH, et al. Whole genome analysis for liver metastasis gene signatures in colorectal cancer. Int J Cancer. 2007;121:2005–12.
46. Nadal C, Maurel J, Gascon P. Is there a genetic signature for liver metastasis in colorectal cancer? World J Gastroenterol. 2007;13:5832–44.

7 Diagnostic Value of Ultrasound in Metastatic Liver Cancer

Wenping Wang

Metastatic liver cancer is a common clinical disease. As the liver has a dual blood supply with abundance of blood flow, thus it is one of the most common sites for metastases of malignant tumors. About one-third of metastases of malignant tumors involve the liver. The common primary tumors derive from the gastrointestinal tract, pancreas, gallbladder, lung, nasopharynx, kidney, mammary gland, melanoma, etc. It was reported that 15–25 % of patients diagnosed with colorectal cancer are accompanied by liver metastases and a further 25–50 % of patients show delayed liver metastases 3–5 years after the operation for primary cancer. Therefore, early diagnosis of metastatic liver cancer has great significance for deciding treatment scheme and improving patient's survival time. At present, the imaging technique is the main noninvasive technology used in clinical diagnosis of metastatic liver cancer, including CT, MRI, nuclear medicine, PET/CT, ultrasound, etc., among which the ultrasound technology, which is characterized by accuracy noninvasiveness, simplicity, cheap, and conducting of repeat examination, has became the most preferred method of examination in clinical diagnosis of liver diseases.

W. Wang
Department of Medical Ultrasonics, Zhongshan Hospital affiliated to Fudan University, Shanghai, People's Republic of China
e-mail: wang.wenping@zs-hospital.sh.cn

7.1 Ultrasound Technology

Ultrasound examination technology is an efficient and practical examination technique developed after radiology and nuclear medicine technology. Currently, there are many types of ultrasound examination technologies being used in clinical practice, among which the most commonly used are as follows.

7.1.1 Conventional Gray-Scale Ultrasound

Conventional gray scale ultrasound is more commonly known as B-mode ultrasound and also a cross-sectional ultrasound, which is the most widely used technology in ultrasound examination. It shows in the form of two-dimensional image, also known as ultrasonography, with different brightness through signals (ultrasound term "echo") reflected by organs or lesions, and it's a two-dimensional cross-sectional image showing the anatomical organs or lesions in a real-time manner, i.e., continuous dynamic display of cross-sectional images. Clinical diagnosis is often made based on the change in echo and can be used for the detection and localization of lesions with which part of cases may give preliminary diagnoses.

X. Qin et al. (eds.), *Multidisciplinary Management of Liver Metastases in Colorectal Cancer*,
DOI 10.1007/978-94-017-7755-1_7

7.1.2 Color Doppler Ultrasound

Based on conventional gray-scale ultrasound to show signals reflected from moving blood in different colors by using the principle of the Doppler, the two-dimensional image presenting blood information of the organ or lesion, can use Pulse Doppler to detect colorful blood flow and thus to determine whether the blood flow is arterial or venous flow. It can also be used for the detection of hemodynamic parameters, such as velocity, resistance index (RI), etc., offering abundant information for qualitative diagnosis of lesions. Although it is a necessary complement to conventional gray-scale ultrasound, color Doppler ultrasound often reflects blood flow within thick-walled blood vessels and has difficulties in reelecting that in thin-walled blood vessels.

7.1.3 Contrast-Enhanced Ultrasound

Contrast-enhanced ultrasound is a new technology developed in recent years. By injecting specific ultrasound contrast agent and adopting matching contrast-enhanced ultrasound, it can be used to observe the enhancement and perfusion situation of blood flow in organs and lesions and presents in the form of two-dimensional and real-time images. Contrast-enhanced ultrasound makes diagnose based on the change in the upward enhancement and blood perfusion of liver tumor. Comparing with color Doppler ultrasound, it shows the blood flow in a more sensitive way. At present, this technology has been widely used for detection and diagnosis of intrahepatic space-occupying lesions, therapeutic follow-up after treatment, etc.

7.1.4 Interventional Ultrasound

It uses real-time feature of ultrasound, under the guidance of ultrasound image, to carry out local treatment including biopsy, radio frequency (RF), microwave, and percutaneous ethanol injection and has been part of the interventional imaging characterized by minimal invasiveness, accuracy and effectiveness.

7.1.5 Intraoperative Ultrasound

Put special ultrasound probe (mainly featuring small probe, high resolution, sterilizable, etc.) directly on the surface of the liver in abdominal surgery to detect lesions that are difficult to be detected by using common ultrasound, which helps to locate and determine the nature of lesions.

7.1.6 Laparoscopic Ultrasound

Put the tiny probe on laparoscopy by using laparoscopy and ultrasonic technology to scan the liver in operation so as to improve the success rate of laparoscopic operation.

7.2 Ultrasonographic Manifestations of Metastatic Liver Cancer

7.2.1 Conventional Gray-Scale Ultrasound

Metastatic liver cancer usually manifests in two-dimensional ultrasonograph as intrahepatic multiple space-occupying lesions. Since metastatic tumors derived from different tissues can present ultrasonographs and ultrasonographic manifestations with their own characteristics, clinical ultrasonography is often analyzed and diagnosed from the following aspects.

7.2.1.1 Morphology

Metastatic liver cancer usually manifests variedly in ultrasonographs with different morphologies. The small ones are mostly round in shape, while the larger ones are oval or irregular and may observe liver surface projections. Where there are relatively more metastases, the lesions may be diffusely distributed or integrated into mass. Areas of homogeneous high echogenicity with multiple nodules gathering at one lobe are like grapes in shape, therefore named "grape-like cluster."

7.2.1.2 Boundary

Most of them are clear and smooth and may be in irregular shape with the typical ones in the shape of "target ring," "bull-eye," or halo showing round-shape tumor and regular form; the internal is a high echo area which usually has echoless area in the center resulting from tumor necrosis and liquefaction; the periphery of high echo area is surrounded by a wide low-to-echoless area. "Target ring" is a characteristic of liver metastatic tumor and can be observed in a variety of tumor metastasis, among which the most commonly found is in gastrointestinal tumors.

7.2.1.3 Number

Metastatic liver cancer is characterized by multiple tumors. However, cases of solitary tumor have been showing increasing trend year by year. The former case characterized by multiple tumors may sometimes be distributed diffusely or infiltratively, presenting as (1) small liver metastases distributed diffusely (ultrasonograph indicates small intensive spot echoes distributed evenly, crude echo in the liver, unclear shape, and boundary of tumors showing hepatomegaly and deformation) and (2) "dark liver" (malignancies mostly seen in hematopoietic system in particular malignant lymphoma). The malignant cells proliferated diffusely and infiltratively in the liver result in the enlargement of the whole liver and reduction in the echo; thus low echo is observed in the liver, which is known as "dark liver."

7.2.1.4 Size

The diameter of metastatic liver cancer is varied from a few millimeters to tens of centimeters. The smallest one can be found in conventional gray-scale ultrasound. Five to 10 mm or so lesions are observed which may be related to many factors, such as tumor location; ultrasound of small lesions near liver capsule or diaphragm is difficult to be observed.

7.2.1.5 Internal Echo

According to the level of the lesion, it can be divided into the following types:

Hypoechoic Type

It is a typical lesion echo. Internal echo of tumor is lower than that of the liver parenchyma (Fig. 7.1) with uneven distribution, clear boundary, and multiple haloes, the manifestation of which is similar to that of the hyperechoic hepatocellular carcinoma, usually found in metastatic liver cancer, such as breast, stomach, esophagus, intestinal, and other adenocarcinomas.

Hyperechoic Type

The echo of lesion is higher than that of the liver parenchyma with the internal area presents hyperechoic area (Figs. 7.2a and 7.3), and the echo is either even or uneven both with commonly seen clear boundaries. Hyperechoic type is often found in gastrointestinal tract or urinary tract tumor metastasis.

Anechoic Type

The echo of lesion is similar with that of the endovascular (it's black in screen), called anechoic lesion. It mainly refers to the situation that large areas of liquefaction necrosis are observed in lesions and often seen in metastatic adenocarcinoma with secretory function. It has multilocular inner structure; the separate walls of different thicknesses may have papillary projections with clear boundary (Fig. 7.4). Anechoic type is often found in metastatic adenocarcinoma with secretory function or malignant stromal tumor in the nasopharynx, ovary, gastrointestinal organ, etc.

Mixed Type

The lesion is often large with mainly high echo in internal, irregular anechoic area around the center and clear boundary. This type may also show a high and low echo mix.

Calcified Type

It is mainly found in hyperechoic lesions of different shapes with attenuation in the rear and may

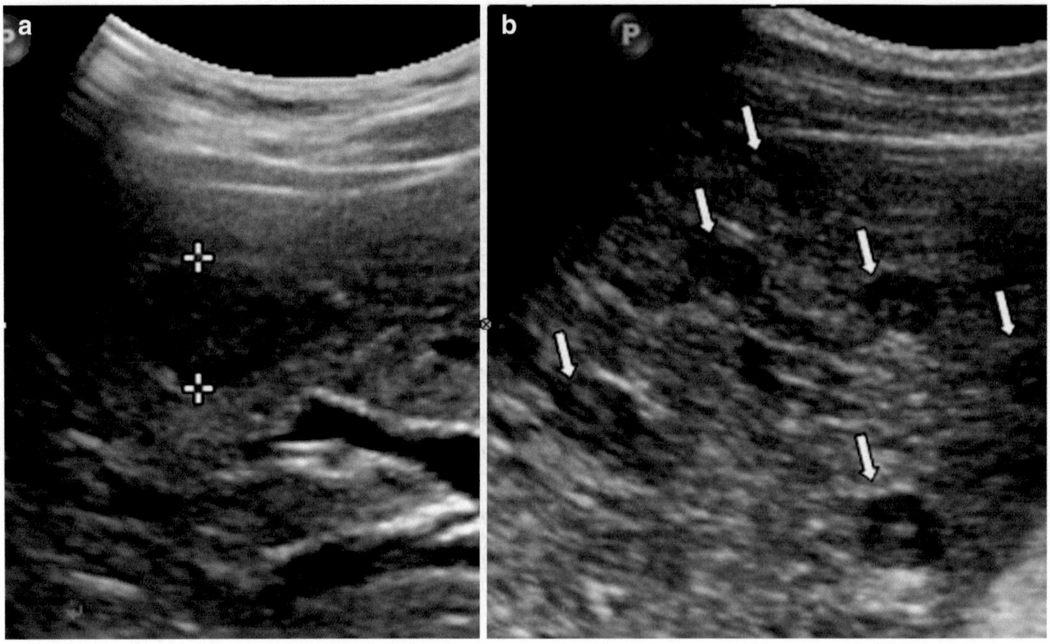

Fig. 7.1 (**a**) Single hypoechoic intrahepatic space-occupying lesion with clear boundary and regular shape. (**b**) Multiple hypoechoic intrahepatic space-occupying lesions (*arrow*) with the same size and round or oval shape

also be found in larger metastatic lesions, often seen in liver metastasis of gastrointestinal tract or ovarian tumor.

Posterior Echo

Mild attenuation of tumor posterior echo can be caused in metastatic liver cancer of large sound attenuation; while in tumors with greater necrosis and liquefaction, tumor posterior echo can be enhanced.

Intrahepatic Pipeline Structure

When the metastatic liver cancer is small or less, there will be no obvious change in the intrahepatic pipeline structure. But, when the lesions are larger and more, changes, such as compression, development, and an unclear display of portal vein, hepatic vein, and inferior vena cava, can occur. However, intravascular thrombosis is rarely seen. In addition, lesions in the hilar region often lead to expansion of intrahepatic bile duct.

Lymph Node Metastasis

Multiple enlarged lymph nodes can be presented near the hilum, pancreas (Fig. 7.2c), and abdominal aorta, which mainly belong to hypoechoic type that can be conglomerated.

Liver Parenchyma

Often shows liver parenchyma with homogeneous and fine echo because of having no liver cirrhosis background.

Primary Sites

If primary tumors are observed in the kidney, pancreas, bladder, accessories, etc., masses with abnormal echo can be found in these organs, which will provide positive support to decide that intrahepatic space-occupying lesions are metastatic lesions.

7.2.2 Color Doppler Ultrasound

Metastatic liver cancer often has a blood supply feature that the primary tumor has. Metastatic liver cancer derived from varied tissues with different levels of differentiation will present different color Doppler ultrasound manifestations, because of different blood supplies. Color Doppler ultrasound can show blood supply of hepatic tumors,

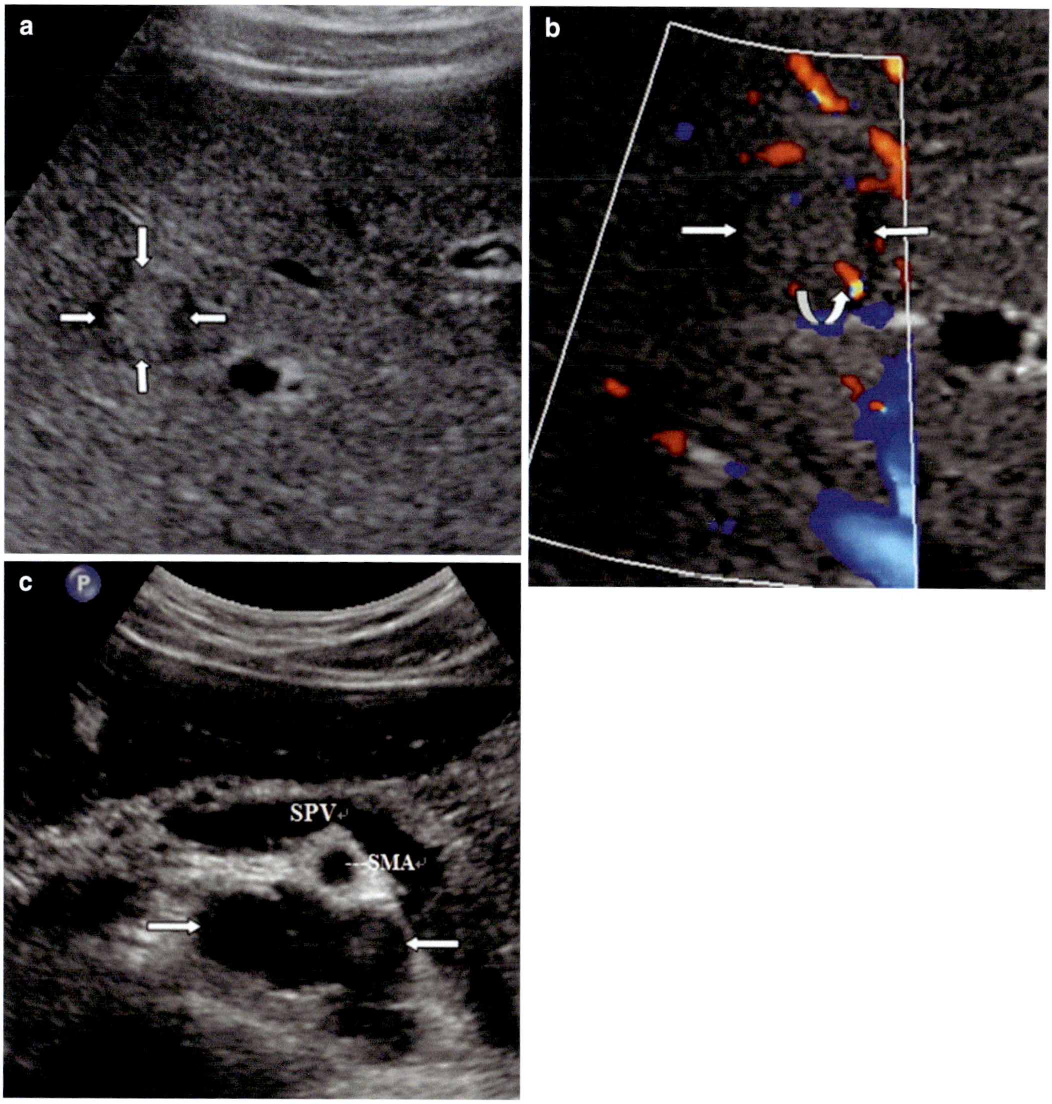

Fig. 7.2 (**a**) Hyperechoic intrahepatic space-occupying lesion with clear boundary and hypoechoic dark rings in surrounding area (*arrow*). (**b**) Liver lesion (*arrow*), observing *dotted color* blood flow signals in surrounding area (*curved arrow*). (**c**) The same patient showing conglomeration of swelling lymph nodes (*arrow*) behind the pancreas (*arrow*). *SPV* splenic vein, *SMA* superior mesenteric artery

manifesting as color blood in the shape of point, linear, or branch. Generally speaking, commonly seen metastatic liver cancer often manifests bypass blood flow in peripheral tumor (Fig. 7.2b), which is then detected by pulsed Doppler as arterial blood flow with often high resistance indexes, in which most of them are above 0.6. As the blood supply of metastatic liver cancer is usually less than that of the primary liver cancer, the color Doppler blood flow detection rate of metastatic liver cancer is usually less than that of the primary liver cancer with the former more abundant than the latter. Based on the blood flow of tumor lesions, color Doppler can often determine whether the lesion is benign or malignant, but, it is difficult to identify a primary lesion from a metastatic one, and the preliminary diagnoses should be made by combining with conventional gray-scale ultrasound.

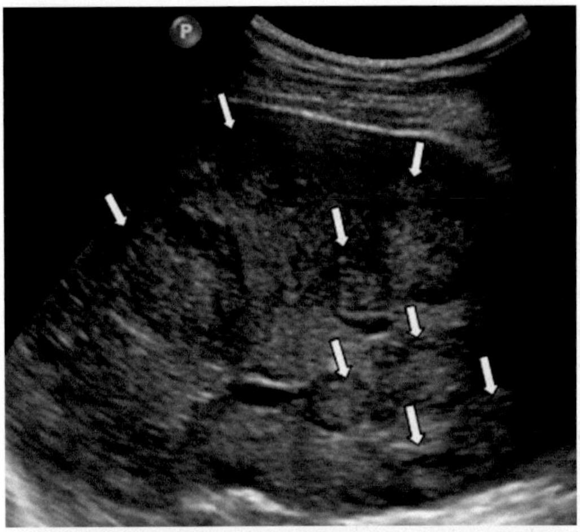

Fig. 7.3 Diffusely distributed hypoechoic intrahepatic space-occupying lesions (*arrow*) of different sizes and bereaving hypoechoic dark rings in surrounding area with some of them being integrated

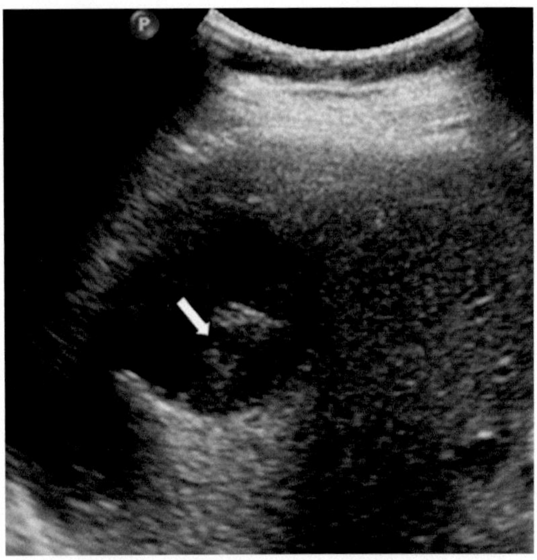

Fig. 7.4 Intrahepatic cystic space-occupying lesion, observing material echo (*arrow*), low-differentiated adenocarcinoma metastasis of ovarian tumor

7.2.3 Contrast-Enhanced Ultrasound

Hepatic malignant tumors often seen in contrast-enhanced ultrasound present rapid enhancement and rapid decline (against liver parenchyma) and are referred to as "rapid in and rapid out." Metastatic liver cancer is also usually manifested in contrast-enhanced ultrasound as "rapid in and rapid out" hepatic malignant tumors characterized by enhancement (Fig. 7.5). Different from primary hepatocellular carcinoma in which the characteristic enhancement way of the former is mostly peripheral enhancement in the manner of ring, and after that the decline often begins from the center toward the around area with hypoechoic change. Sometimes, the center of the lesion begins to decline before completion of the enhancement. Comparing with primary liver cancer, the blood supply to metastatic liver cancer is less, which may contribute to the above situation. In addition, the enhancement way of metastatic liver cancer is different with that of the primary liver cancer.

7.2.4 Interventional Ultrasound

It is a minimally invasive technique often used when the above techniques or other imaging techniques cannot clarify a diagnosis. By using proper puncture needle and automated biopsy gun, this method, under the guidance of conventional two-dimensional ultrasonograph, carries out rapid biopsy of concerned lesions to obtain tissue blocks of 1–2 cm or so for pathological diagnosis. Without doubt, the success of this technique largely depends on the doctors' experiences. For a skilled doctor, the success rate, in theory, is more than 95 %. Therefore, interventional ultrasound has become an indispensable mean in conventional clinical diagnosis.

7.3 Diagnosis and Differential Diagnosis

Ultrasound examination of the patient with a primary malignant tumor indicates that, for single or multiple hypoechoic intrahepatic space-occupying lesions, in particular those with dark rings around and show high-resistant arterial color blood flow, most of them can be preliminarily diagnosed as intrahepatic metastatic tumors. However, for patients with no relevant history, especially physical discoverer, differentiation of it from other diseases such as primary liver cancer and hepatic hemangioma should be the main priority.

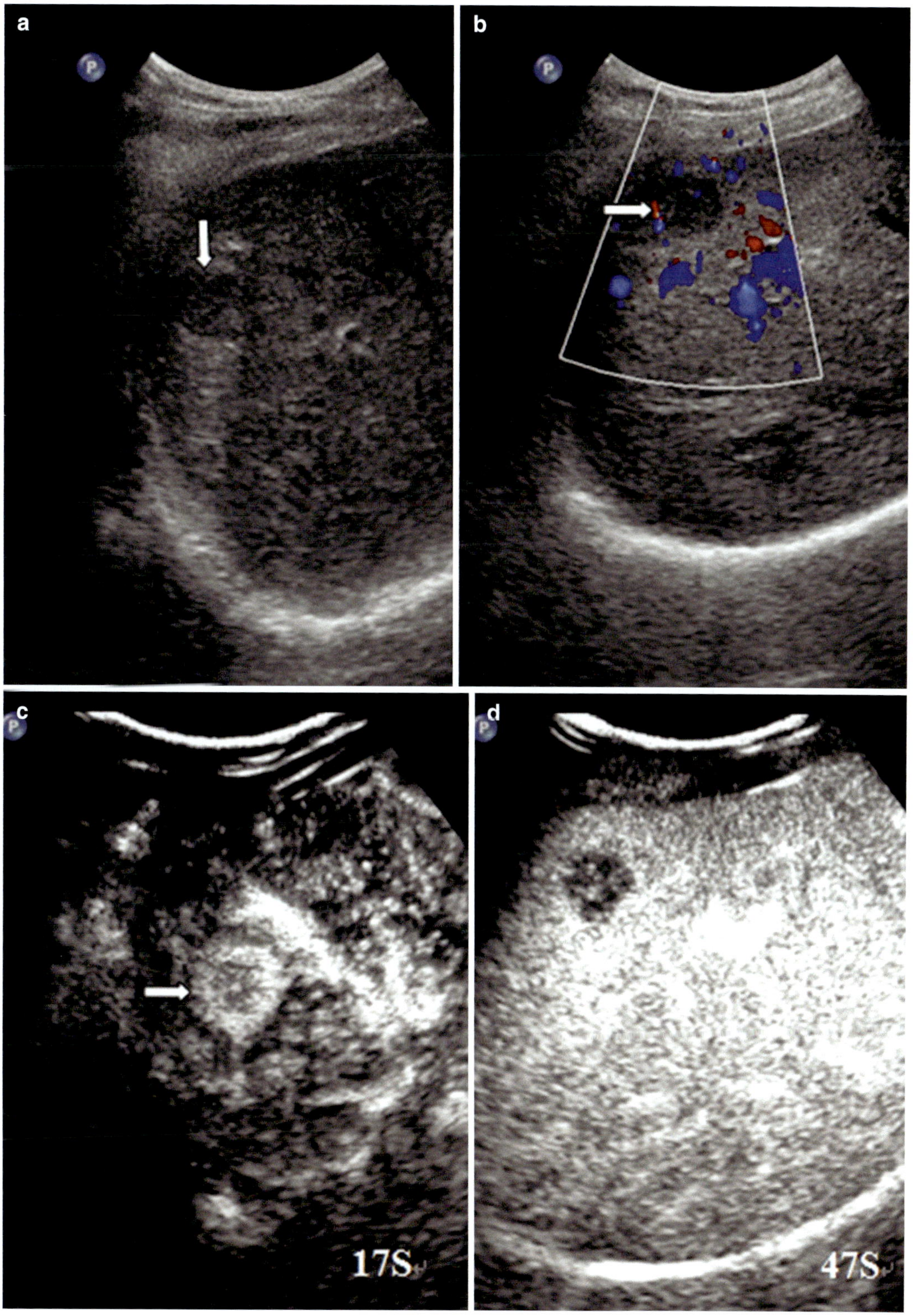

Fig. 7.5 (**a**) Hypoechoic hepatic lesion (*arrow*). (**b**) Color Doppler ultrasound showing linear color blood flow in surrounding area of the lesion (*arrow*). (**c**) Contrast-enhanced ultrasound showing arterial phase of liver lesion (17 s after injection of contrast agent) with obvious enhancement of surrounding area (*arrow*). (**d**) Decrease of portal phase showing obvious hypoechoic change (47 s after injection of contrast agent)

7.3.1 Primary Hepatocellular Carcinoma

It is mainly singly developed with most of them presenting varied degrees of liver cirrhosis. When the tumor is less than 3 cm, it manifests as hypoechoic type with dark ring around, and high-resistant arterial color blood is often found accompanied with symptoms such as portal vein tumor thrombus and portal hypertension, while patients with metastatic liver cancer often have no portal vein tumor thrombus. In addition, contrast-enhanced ultrasounds of the two have obvious differences and can be easily distinguished.

7.3.2 Hepatic Hemangioma

It is the most common benign tumor in the liver. Hyperechoic metastatic cancer is sometimes difficult to be differentiated from hyperechoic hepatic hemangioma. The former has rear sound attenuation, while the latter has no attenuation and no peripheral hypoechoic halo. Hypoechoic hemangiomas often have internal network echo surrounding the peripheral hyperechoic area. Color Doppler ultrasound of most hepatic hemangioma indicates no color blood flow, while small number of it may be detested with arterial blood flow, but the resistance index is often less than 0.6. In addition, hepatic hemangioma manifests itself in contrast-enhanced ultrasound as characteristic of enhancement from peripheral part to the center slowly which is significantly different from metastatic liver cancer.

7.4 Clinical Value

At present, ultrasound has been recognized as the first choice for imaging examination of intrahepatic space-occupying lesions. The accurate examination and diagnosis of intrahepatic space-occupying lesion are of great significance to clarify the stage of and choose treatment for the tumor as well as determine prognosis. Metastatic liver cancer manifests itself varied in ultrasonography. Clinical diagnoses mainly give comprehensive judgments based on conventional gray-scale ultrasound, color Doppler ultrasound, contrast-enhanced ultrasound, etc., and most of them can get diagnoses. But, there are some cases that are difficult to be diagnosed because of their complexity, and in this case, interventional ultrasound biopsy pathological examination may be carried out to further clarify the diagnosis.

In recent years, we have adopted the surgical techniques that cut primary intestinal tract lesions and at the same time primary liver metastases derived originally from intestinal tract and achieved better treatment result. For these cases, accurate diagnosis of liver metastases before surgery is of particularly important. The sensitivity and specificity of conventional gray-scale ultrasound in diagnosing liver metastases are lower than that of enhanced CT and MRI, especially in terms of number detection. According to documents at home and abroad, the sensitivity of conventional gray-scale ultrasound in diagnosing liver metastases is between 40 % and 80 %; the different research results can be varied widely. The reasons might be that detection rate of conventional gray-scale ultrasound in diagnosing small liver metastases is low, especially in diagnosing metastases less than 1 cm; in addition, for diffused liver swelling caused by infiltration of tumors such as leukemia and lymphoma presents no limited space-occupying lesion, it is difficult for ultrasound to detect, thus leading to misdiagnosis (Fig. 7.6a).

The application of contrast-enhanced ultrasound has greatly improved detection rate and accuracy of ultrasound in diagnosing liver metastases (Fig. 7.6b) and greatly enhanced the detection capacity of ultrasound in diagnosing small liver lesions because of its advantages of real time and continuity compared with CT/MRI. According to existing literature reports, the smallest liver metastatic lesion detected by contrast-enhanced ultrasound is between 2 and 4 mm. Meanwhile, the detection rate of metastatic liver cancer is increased by 20–30 % because of contrast-enhanced

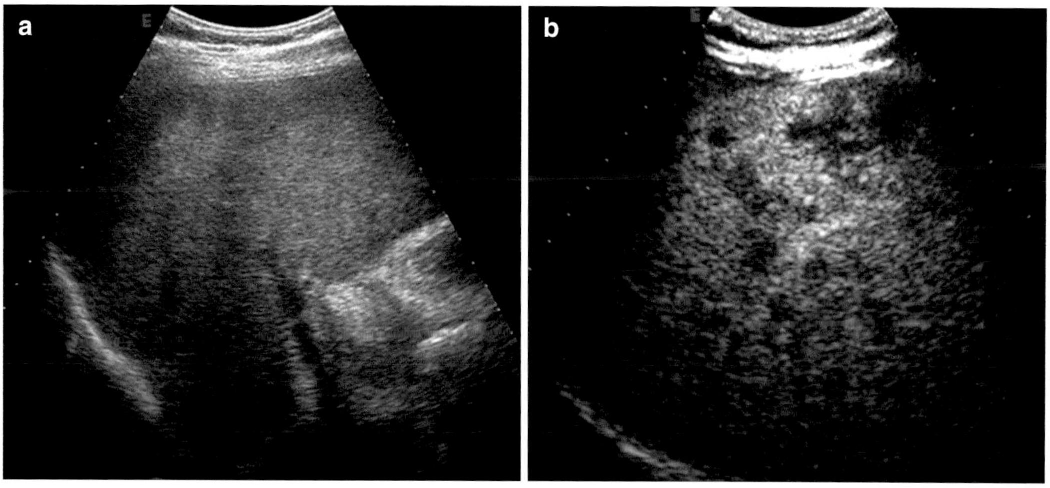

Fig. 7.6 (**a**) Patients with malignant lymphoma. Intrahepatic space-occupying lesion is not found by conventional gray-scale ultrasound. (**b**) Showing diffused distribution of hypoechoic slice shape liver lesions after injection of ultrasound contrast agent

ultrasound application. A number of studies, including studies widely conducted by numerous foreign research centers, also indicate that after the implication of this technique, the sensitivity and specificity of ultrasound in diagnosing metastatic liver cancer have been increased by 94 % and 98 %, respectively, which can achieve equal effects with enhanced CT/MRI and even better than the latter, especially in detecting small liver lesions. In addition, as metastatic liver cancer has a manifestation of enhancement in contrast-enhanced ultrasound different from primary liver cancer, the qualitative diagnosis of ultrasound for this disease is significantly improved, especially in differentiating metastatic liver cancer from primary liver cancer, which were difficult to be differentiated by using conventional ultrasound including color Doppler in the past. Undoubtedly, the application of contrast-enhanced ultrasound is of great significance.

When there are multiple smaller metastatic lesions in the liver, especially for the one that has less than 1 cm, lesions are often difficult to be detected in surgery, during which ultrasound can help to locate small lesions and guide the surgeon remove the lesion precisely. Furthermore, intraoperative ultrasound can help to detect lesions difficult to be identified before the surgery, such as lesions at the top of the liver and diaphragm; those lesions cannot be presented easily by conventional ultrasound due to interference of air in the liver and lead to misdiagnosis, while by using intraoperative ultrasound, this concern will be avoided, as in this technique, the probe will be placed directly on the surface of the liver.

For highly suspected metastatic cancers and/or cases with unknown primary tumors, biopsy guided by ultrasound can help to clarify the nature of lesions while determining sources of primary tumors. For inoperable cases, radio frequency, microwave, and percutaneous ethanol injection therapy guided by ultrasound are the commonly used treatment methods. In addition, radio frequency and microwave can also be used to treat early metastasis. It has been reported that the effectiveness of ultrasound-guided radio frequency or microwave ablation therapy on metastatic liver cancer less than 3 cm is the same with that of surgery.

Certainly, due to the special nature of ultrasound technique, i.e., largely dependent on operation skill and clinical experience of the doctor, the subjectivity of the diagnosis is larger compared with CT and MRI techniques. When the application of ultrasound technique is insufficient to make a determination, it is necessary to carry out comprehensive determination by combining with other imaging techniques and clinical examination.

References

1. Xu Zhi Zhang. Modern abdominal ultrasound diagnostics. Second ed. Beijing: Science Press; 2008. p. 139–40.
2. Cao Haigen, Wang Jinrui. Practical abdominal ultrasound diagnostics. Beijing: People's Medical Publishing House; 1994. p. 179–81.
3. Bates J. Abdominal ultrasound. 2nd ed. London: Elsevier; 2005. p. 93.
4. Jin Wenhao, Li Ruiyong, Jin Zhezhu, et al. B ultrasonographic features of metastatic liver cancer. Mod Oncol. 2005;13(3):365–7.
5. Kamalov IR, Sandrikov VA, Gautier SV, et al. The significance of colour velocity and spectral Doppler ultrasound in the differentiation of liver tumors. Eur J Ultrasound. 1998;7:101–8.
6. Zhao Boshan, Tian Rong, Duan Yunyou, et al. Color Doppler ultrasound Analysis on Primary and Metastatic Liver Cancer. Chinese J Ultrasound Med 2001;17(4):295–8.
7. Srivastava DN, Mahajan A, Berry M, et al. Colour Doppler flow imaging of focal hepatic lesions. Australas Radiol. 2000;44:285–9.
8. Robinson PJA. Imaging liver metastases: current limitations and future prospect. Br J Radiol. 2000;73:234–41.
9. Kopljar M, Brkljacic B, Doko M, et al. Nature of Doppler perfusion index changes in patients with colorectal cancer liver metastases. J Ultrasound Med. 2004;23(10):1295–300.
10. Albrecht T, Blomley MJK, Burns PN, et al. Improved detection of hepatic metastases with pulse-inversion US during the liver-specific phase of SHU 508A: multicenter study. Radiology. 2003;227:361–70.
11. Mann CD, Metcalfe MS, Neal CP, et al. Role of ultrasonography in the detection of resectable recurrence after hepatectomy for colorectal liver metastases. Br J Surg. 2007;94(11):1403–7.
12. Wang Wenping, Li Chaolun, Ding Hong, et al. Real-time contrast-enhanced ultrasound diagnosis for metastatic liver cancer. Chinese J Ultrasound Med. 2008;17(2):127–9.
13. Guo Zhizhong, Liu Zhisu, Huang Jian, et al. Differentiation between colorectal liver metastases and primary liver cancer by contrast-enhanced ultrasound. Med J Wuhan Univ. 2009;30(1):119–26.
14. Hong Ding, WP Wang, BJ Huang, et al. Imaging of focal liver lesions: low-mechanical-index real-time ultrasonography with SonoVue. J Ultrasound Med 2005;24(3):285–97.
15. Chen Xing, Wei Guangyu, Deng Xiaoyun, et al. Value of ultrasonography in diagnosing metastatic liver cancer. J Ultrasound Clin Med. 2006;8(7):409–12.
16. Zhang Huiping, Du Lianfang, He Yingqian, et al. Value of contrast-enhanced ultrasound in diagnosing metastatic liver cancer. J Ultrasound Clin Med. 2009;11(1):24–6.
17. Larsen LPS, Rosenkilde M, Christensen H, et al. Can contrast-enhanced ultrasonography replace multidetector-computed tomography in the detection of liver metastases from colorectal cancer? Eur J Radiol. 2009;69:308–13.
18. Larsen LPS, Rosenkilde M, Christensen H, et al. The value of contrast enhanced ultrasonography in detection of liver metastases from colorectal cancer: a prospective double-blinded study. Eur J Radiol. 2007;62:302–7.
19. Torzillia G, Boteaa F, Procopio F, et al. Use of contrast-enhanced intraoperative ultrasonography during liver surgery for colorectal cancer liver metastases – its impact on operative outcome. Analysis of a prospective cohort study. Eur J Cancer. 2008;6(1):16–23.
20. Liang Ping, Dong Bowei. On the development of ultrasound-guided interventional treatment of liver cancer. Chinese J Ultrasound Med. 2000;16(1):65–8.

The Differential Diagnosis of Hepatic Metastasis by CT and MRI

8

Mengsu Zeng

In addition to ultrasound (US) screening, the current diagnostic imaging techniques of liver lesions are computed tomography (CT) and magnetic resonance imaging (MRI), which are the most commonly used noninvasive techniques. With constantly updated technology, CT and MRI machines have developed into a multispiral CT (320 layers/circle scan) and high-field-strength MRI machines (3 T); the scanning speed, tissue contrast, and spatial resolution have been significantly improved, and so have the diagnostic sensitivity, specificity, and accuracy. It also plays an extremely important role in the metastatic liver cancer detection, differential diagnosis, treatment, and follow-up work [1–3].

8.1 CT and MRI Technology

8.1.1 CT Technology

Patients are required to fast for more than 8 h or at least 4 h before the scan and take 1,000–1,500 ml of water orally half an hour before the scan to fill the gastrointestinal tract, and this can overcome air artifact, so that the gut lumen and wall can be displayed clearly and the relationship between the intestinal tract and its adjacent structures can be known. Normally liver scan includes plain and enhanced scan. Enhanced scan is very important and almost indispensable. Enhanced scanning is performed after the injection of nonionic iodine contrast agent from peripheral vein, which then is mainly distributed in the artery, portal vessels (including vein), and organ parenchyma. Accordingly, the enhanced scan is called the scan of arterial phase, portal venous phase (venous phase), and the substantial balance of the entire liver (layer thickness ≤5 mm, pitch ≤1.5). The following must be emphasized:(1) the total amount of nonionic iodine contrast agent must be calculated at 1.5–2 ml/kg of total body weight, and injection rate should be 3 ml/s; (2) the scan delay time of each phase (calculated when the injection of nonionic iodine contrast agent begins) (arterial phase, 30±5 s; portal venous phase,80±5 s; substantial balance phase, 180 s); (3) iodine contrast agents should be used with caution to patients who have history of drug allergy or severe renal insufficiency; (4) to display the hepatic artery and portal vein and hepatic vein-based CT angiography, the appropriate layer thickness should be ≤1.5 mm; and (5) during the scan, the patient should hold the breath in order to avoid scan plane beating and missing lesions; therefore, the patient's breathing should be trained before the examination. They are required to hold the breath in a calm state in order to maintain the consistency of each breath. This point is very important.

M. Zeng
Department of Radiology, Zhongshan Hospital affiliated to Fudan University, Shanghai, China
e-mail: zeng.mengsu@zs-hospital.sh.cn

X. Qin et al. (eds.), *Multidisciplinary Management of Liver Metastases in Colorectal Cancer*,
DOI 10.1007/978-94-017-7755-1_8

8.1.2 MRI Technology

Patients are only required to fast more than 4 h before the scan. There is no need to make special preparation under normal circumstances, and can also oral negative MRI contrast agent (such as dilute barium, etc.). Spin echo or fast spin echo (SE/FSE) and gradient echo (GRE) techniques are commonly used in liver check with MRI. The following can be used if necessary:

1. Diffusion weighted imaging (DWI): Complimentary to SE, FSE, and GRE sequences; it can improve the sensitivity of lesion detection and differential diagnosis capabilities.
2. Perfusion weighted imaging (PWI): The liver perfusion can be understood with PWI; therefore, doctors can have a quantitative and/or semi-quantitative understanding of liver function and liver blood supply.
3. Magnetic resonance cholangiopancreatography (MRCP): It can display intrahepatic bile duct, common bile duct, cystic duct, hepatic duct, pancreatic duct morphology, and their mutual relations.

SE T1-weighted (T1W) and FSE T2-weighted fat suppression (T2W + FS) axial images (layer thickness ≤5 mm, interval ≤3 mm) are normally used in liver scan. If jointed with real-time navigator and trigger technology, a better image can be collected. Liver examination with MRI focuses more on plain + enhanced scanning with GRE T1-weighted fat suppression sequences. After the injection of magnetic resonance contrast agent (usually gadolinium–diethylenetriamine pentaacetic acid, Gd-DTPA) from peripheral vein, enhanced 2D or 3D fast axial scanning is performed through breath-hold GRE T1-weighted fat suppression (2D layer thickness ≤7 mm, interval of ≤3 mm; 3D layer thickness ≤5 mm), and breath-hold requirements are the same with CT. GRE T1-weighted fat suppression sequence scanning is fast, especially the latest high-strength-field, high-gradient, high-switching-rate, and multi-channel sampling of the aircraft, as with the spiral CT, after injection of Gd-DTPA, and can finish the whole liver scan in artery, portal vein, and substantial balance phase of the liver. Generally, Gd-DTPA total injection is 0.4–0.5 mmol/kg of body weight (in total about 30 ml), 2–3 ml/s of injection rate. At the same time, according to the clinical condition of patients, the coronal enhanced scanning which mainly shows hepatic vessel can be used (using the 3D scan of GRE T1-weighted fat suppression, layer thickness ≤1.5 mm).

In addition to commonly used extracellular Gd-DTPA, the liver-specific contrast agents currently used in clinical area are mainly three types: (1) Mn-DPDP, which is absorbed by the hepatic cells and excreted by biliary, is mainly used to shorten the T1 relaxation; (2) SPIO and USPIO, absorbed by mesh endothelial cells (including macrophages and Kupffer cells), mainly shorten the T2 and T2 * relaxation; and (3) contrast agents of dual functions, absorbed by extra cells and hepatic cells and excreted by biliary, such as Gd-BOPTA (MultiHanceR), Gd-EOB-DTPA (PrimovistR), etc., are used to shorten the T1 relaxation. (1) and (2) liver-specific contrast agents are used mainly as the supplementary to contrast agents in extracellular Gd-DTPA examination, while the contrast agents of dual functions are expected to replace Gd-DTPA and become the common or preferred contrast agents in MR examination.

8.1.3 The Clinical Value of MRI and CT Technology

The liver with CT and MRI examination may help clinicians accurately understand:

1. The location, size, and number of metastatic liver tumors
2. The relationship between foci and the surrounding blood vessels, in particular, with or without the portal vein and hepatic vein involvement, or cancerous thrombi and thrombosis and their identification
3. With or without hilar and retroperitoneal lymph node metastasis

4. Whether there are the cirrhosis, portal hypertension, collateral blood vessel formation, ascites, splenomegaly, etc.
5. Measure the state of liver volume and the blood perfusion and understand liver functions indirectly

8.2 CT and MRI Diagnosis and Differential Diagnosis of Hepatic Livers

The liver is the largest substantial viscera in abdominal organs. Among the noninvasive diagnostic imaging tools, CT and MRI are the most widely used and effective screening tools. It is significant in the diagnosis of liver lesions. The common malignant tumors of livers are HCC, metastatic carcinoma, and cholangiocellular carcinoma; benign tumors include cavernous hemangioma, hepatic adenoma, and angiomyolipoma; tumorlike lesions include focal nodular hyperplasia, inflammatory pseudotumor, cyst-like lesions, focal fatty livers, and so on. Most of these occupying lesions have manifestations on CT and MR and can be identified to help or guide clinical decisions or treatment.

8.2.1 The Features of CT and MRI for Hepatic Metastasis

Hepatic metastasis: Hepatic metastasis can be single or multiple. The most common metastasis is gastrointestinal tumor metastasis, followed by lung cancer, breast cancer, pancreas cancer, gallbladder cancer, ovarian cancer, renal cancer, thyroid cancer, and nasopharyngeal cancer. The features of colorectal liver metastasis are similar to that of other liver metastasis. They display low-density, occasionally slightly calcified, or mucus-like image in the center of lesions through the plain CT scan, which are of great help to the diagnosis of hepatic metastasis. Most hepatic metastasis are lack of blood supply, while a small number of lesions are rich in blood supply. So enhanced scans in arterial phase generally enhance the unobvious or only enhance the edge by rim enhancement, while the typical ring enhancement of the edge of lesions is often visible by the enhanced scans in portal venous phase, in particular, the concentric "bull's-eye sign" or "target sign" is typical in diagnosing hepatic metastasis (see case 1). With MRI, SE sequence, the lesion often shows low signals on T1W image and slightly higher signals onT2W image. If there is clear necrosis or cystic change in tumors, it can show high signals on T2W image clearly. With enhanced scans, it can be presented with edge-enhanced "bull's-eye sign" or "target sign" and sometimes similar to the "petallike" structure (see cases 2 and 3). MRI, in particular DWI, T2W image, and enhanced image, can detect lesions with high sensitivity. Besides, hepatic metastasis is less likely to cause liver subcapsular rupture and portal vein tumor thrombus. In the mean time, the hilar, abdominal, and retroperitoneal enlarged lymph nodes are also found to show ring enhancement, which is helpful for diagnosis.

8.2.2 Differential Diagnosis

8.2.2.1 Hepatocellular Carcinoma (HCC)

Hepatocellular carcinoma (HCC) occurs usually in the "hepatitis B," "hepatitis C," and the high-risk patients with liver cirrhosis. With CT plain scan, liver lesions often show relatively low density, regular or irregular edge, and sometimes even low-density ringlike pseudocapsule in the lesion edge, which is quite characteristic for diagnosing liver cancer. Most of the HCC, particularly small hepatocellular carcinoma lesions, are rich in blood supply - supplied by the main hepatic artery. If with enhanced scan in arterial phase, tumor enhancement is very clear, showing high density, in contrast, in portal phase, it is showing low density (see case 4). This "sped-ascend and sped-descend" enhancement form is the feature of CT in diagnosing hepatocellular carcinoma [4, 5].

With MRI examination SE sequence, HCC often shows low signals on T1W image and slightly higher signals on T2W image. It is more likely to find pseudocapsule of liver cancer on MRI than by CT. There are usually low-signal ringlike images on T1W and T2W images. MRI and enhanced CT findings of liver cancer are similar by dynamic enhanced scanning with GRE sequences, that is to say, the lesion shows significantly higher signals with enhanced scans in arterial phase, while in portal vein phase, it shows low signal (see case 5).

Liver cancers, particularly large hepatocellular carcinoma and invasive liver cancer, easily invade the portal vein and hepatic venous system and can cause the tumor thrombus of portal and hepatic veins as well as the inferior vena cava. Blood metastases of liver cancer are common, such as lung metastasis and bone metastasis; lymph node metastases are rare, only 10–20 %, and are mainly enlarged lymph nodes of liver portal, adjacent structure of the head of pancreas, and posterior peritoneum. The liver capsule indentation, also called "liver capsule contraction," appears after the invasion of liver capsule by liver cancer, which has some value in differential diagnosis [6]; liver tumors, associated with macroscopic tumor thrombus in the bile duct, are rare. According to data of the liver cancer institute in our hospital, only 0.76 %. Besides, the bile duct dilations are relatively rare, caused by the invasion of intrahepatic and hepatic portal bile duct by liver cancer.

8.2.2.2 Cholangiocellular Carcinoma

Cholangiocellular carcinoma: Intrahepatic bile duct carcinomas are rare. According to locations of their occurrence, they can be divided into peripheral cholangiocellular carcinoma and hilar cholangiocellular carcinoma. Peripheral cholangiocellular carcinoma occurs in the left lobe of the liver, especially in the left lateral lobe, which with plain CT scan shows low density and less clear edge and is often accompanied by cystic degeneration, hemorrhage, necrosis, and occasional calcification. There are signs of intrahepatic bile duct dilation in the remote lesions (see case 6). Hilar cholangiocellular carcinomas are generally associated with the extensive and clear dilation of intrahepatic bile duct. Clinically, the patients are often with jaundice. On MRI scan with SE sequence, hilar cholangiocellular carcinomas are often presented with low signal on T1W image. If associated with subacute or chronic hemorrhage, they show high signal zone. They are also presented with high signal on T2W image; if associated with calcification, they show dark zone with signal avoid. The lesion enhancement is not obvious on CT and MR enhanced scan with GRE sequences in arterial phase, and mainly are the edge enhancement. The lesion enhancement continues with enhanced scans in portal venous phase or delayed phase, and the enhancement scope tends to expand. Cholangiocellular carcinoma is characterized by delayed enhancement; with the dilation of the bile duct in delay enhanced zone, the diagnostic value will be greater.

8.2.2.3 Cavernous Hemangioma

Cavernous hemangioma: It is the most common benign tumor of the liver. It can be single or multiple. The size ranges from a few mm to more than ten cm. On CT scan, cavernous hemangioma is presented with low density, no capsule, and often clear edge. It is difficult to distinguish from small hepatocellular carcinoma without capsules only with plain scan. On MRI scan with SE sequence, cavernous hemangioma is presented with low signal on T1W image. On T2W image, the signal becomes higher and higher with the continuous extension of magnetic resonance, as "light bulb" becomes brighter with the improvement of wattage. This is one of the characteristics of cavernous hemangioma differing from other liver tumors.

Cavernous hemangioma has features on enhanced scans of CT and MRI. There are nodular or spotlike, high-density or high-signal enhancement zone on the edge of lesions on enhanced scans in arterial phase, which is similar to aortic enhancement. With time, the range of lesions continues to expand to the center. In the portal venous phase or delayed phase, the lesions continue to be presented with high density or high signal (see case 7).

Individual hemangioma is smaller than 1.0 cm, whose presentation on scan in arterial phase is similar to that of small hepatocellular carcinoma enhancement. The key difference of hemangioma is its homogenous, high-density, and high-signal enhancement in the portal venous phase or delayed phase, while the small liver cell carcinoma often shows low density/low signal, which is the main point for it to be identified [7].

Sometimes in the center of hemangiomas (often more than 5 cm), irregular and more low-density fiber scar zone and calcification are visible on plain CT scan. They are basically presented with low signals on MRI T1W and T2W images or slightly higher enhancement zone on T2W image. The scar tissue zone is not enhanced on enhanced CT and MRI scan.

8.2.2.4 Angiomyolipoma (AML)

Angiomyolipoma (AML): Clinically, angiomyolipoma is not rare. It can occur at any age and is more common in female adults. The histological features are three components, named mature adipose tissue, smooth muscle cells, and tortuous thick-walled blood vessels mixed in different proportions. If with obvious fat tissue, tumors are presented with mixed density, and shapes can be round or oval with clear edge. The diagnosis can be confirmed if the tumors are presented with fat density or signal on CT and MRI scan. The diagnosis can be confirmed even without the enhanced scan.

For adipose tissue or fat tissue less obvious, it is sometimes difficult to diagnose definitely with CT and MRI, which can only provide the possible diagnosis. In general, there is almost no feature on plain CT. The tumor shows apparent heterogeneous enhancement on enhanced CT in arterial phase, and it continues to show a more pronounced delayed enhancement in portal venous phase and delayed phase. It also shows the following features: (a) shows tortuous enhanced vascular in the center of tumor; (b) the edge becomes blurred in portal phase; and (c) there is no tumor capsule, which is the clue to diagnosis. The enhanced pattern of MRI scan is basically the same with that of CT, but with MRI plain scan, the tumor often shows low signal on T1WI. The tumor on T2WI shows slightly higher or high signal. In particular, the diagnosis can be indicated if some signals in tumors are suppressed by using fat suppression, and if there is void vascular image within the tumors, that is more helpful in the diagnosis [8, 9].

8.2.2.5 Hepatocellular Adenoma

Hepatocellular adenoma: It is more reported in foreign literature. It often occurs in middle-aged women taking birth control pills. Hepatocellular adenoma is always associated with bleeding. It is rarely reported in China. In fact, the pathological identification of this tumor and well-differentiated hepatocellular carcinoma tumors is difficult. It is presented on CT scan with low-density and circular image, and the tumor necrosis is rare; therefore, the density of tumor is evenly distributed. If there is bleeding, slightly higher-density image or lower-density image is available depending on the bleeding time. The tumor capsule is usually clear, similar to pseudocapsule of HCC. With enhanced CT scan in arterial phase, the tumor shows a homogeneous enhancement with high density, the degree of whose enhancement is basically similar to aorta enhancement. With scan in portal phase, the tumor lesions are still presented with equal density or slightly higher density, which is different from the HCC. The image findings of MRI are diversified. The tumor is presented with mainly low signals on T1WI, but also with high signals and analogue signals, and slightly higher signals on T2WI, and the minority is with analogue signals and low signals. If accompanied with tumor hemorrhage, regardless of T1WI or T2WI, it often shows mixed signals. The enhanced scan is almost the same like CT manifestation, but MRI is usually more sensitive to display capsule than CT. In addition, some literature reported that patients with glycogen accumulation often were combined with liver adenoma.

8.2.2.6 Focal Nodular Hyperplasia (FNH)

Focal nodular hyperplasia (FNH): FNH often occurs on the liver without cirrhosis. It is more common on the right lobe and has no age and sexual differences. Lesions can be single and multiple. Microscopically, normal liver cells are visible in lesion area. The thick-walled blood vessels and liver tissues separated by scar tissues are visible, between which are lymphocytic infiltration and bile duct hyperplasia but no hepatic lobules and portal area structure.

The typical change is the central starlike scar tissue expanding to the surrounding (liver tissue divided by entity scar tissue type), and individual central starlike scar tissue is replaced by the dilation of blood vessels (dilated capillaries). FNH is now considered to be the reactive hyperplasia of liver parenchyma to preexisting arterial vascular malformation [10].

For typical FNH lesions, both CT and MRI have features to easily confirm the diagnosis. CT plain scan shows low density, with the central starlike and lower-density zone; the form of whole lesions is presented with round or irregular shapes with generally clear edge. With enhanced scan in arterial phase, the lesion enhancement is homogeneous except the central stellate lesion. The degree of enhancement may be similar to that of the aorta, and even the enhanced and distorted vascular image (dilated capillaries) can be often visible in the center; the degree of enhancement in portal phase and delayed phase is reduced slightly, presenting analogue density or low density, and the edge becomes blurred; if capillaries are dilated, the central starlike zone disappears in the delay phase and even changed to spotty enhancement (see case 10), which has special significance for the diagnosis.

On MR T1WI, the lesion often shows low signal, and the central stellate scar shows much lower signal. On T2WI, the enhancement of lesion signal is not obvious and sometimes even showed analogue signals, but the central area of dilated capillaries often shows high signal, which has particular diagnostic value. The changes on enhanced MRI scan are basically the same with that of CT.

For atypical FNH lesions with no stellate scar, their identification through CT and MRI is easily confused with HCC. Generally speaking, in the portal venous phase or delayed phase, HCC is often presented with apparently low density or low signal, while FNH is often presented with analogue density or signal or slightly lower-density or signal. In addition, compared with HCC image on T2WI, the signal of FNH is a little lower and more homogenous, which is helpful for the diagnosis of FNH. In addition, FNH is not coated, which can be used for identification.

If the identification is really difficult, the liver-specific magnetic contrast agent can be added. Because FNH has normal liver cell function and Kupffer cell, therefore, it can intake Mn-DPDP or SPIO and compare it with the signal before the injection so that the diagnosis can be confirmed. In addition, DSA examination is also useful for further identification. With DSA examination, nutrient artery of FNH is colored from the inside to the outward lesions and shows "dendritic" staining, while arterial tumor of HCC is colored from surrounding around tumor and shows "hold ball" staining. This can also be used for differentiation.

8.2.2.7 Hepatic Inflammatory Pseudotumors

Hepatic inflammatory pseudotumors are rare in clinical area. There are less than 1,000 cases reported in the literature so far. Etiology is unclear. They may be related to infection, immune status, and biliary obstruction. The lesions are common on the right lobe. They can be single and multiple, and the divisions between lesions and surrounding tissues are clear. Most lesions have no fibrous capsule. Histology showed fibrosis and myofibroblasts and visible capillaries, among which distribute the histiocytosis, polyclonal plasma cells, and lymphocytes with infiltration. In the mean time, there must be coagulation necrosis.

CT scan often shows homogenous, low-density, and unclear edge, and the shapes can be round, oval, irregular, gourd shaped, and clustered-grape shaped, etc. With enhanced scans in arterial phase, lesions almost have no enhancement; in portal venous phase, lesions show slight enhancement or separate enhancement in the edge. A small number of lesions are without enhancement, but the lesion edge shows more clearly than that with plain CT scan. It often showed low signal on T1WI, and mostly low signal or analogue signal on T2WI, a very small number of lesions can be presented with slightly higher signal, the form of enhanced scan is generally the same with CT, and some lesions can only be usually found on enhanced scans [11].

It is worth mentioning that sometimes it is difficult to differentiate it from HCC which is lack of blood supply, but the lesions with gourd, and clustered-grape shape show low density or low signal in portal phase, in particular on T2WI, they show low or analogue signal and there is no lesion enhancement in arterial phase, which support the diagnosis of inflammatory pseudotumor. In addition, chronic inflammation or chronic abscesses are often considered as inflammatory pseudotumor; in fact, the writer thinks that pathological lesions of inflammatory pseudotumor should be massive, besides the existent of fibrous tissue and inflammatory cells; there also should be coagulative necrosis. This point should be noticed.

8.2.2.8 Hepatic Cyst

Hepatic cyst: Hepatic cyst is the common congenital lesion, single or multiple, or part of multiple cystic lesions. With CT scan, the lesion is presented with round or oval, low-density, and water-like image, and the edge is clear, wall is thin as paper, and CT value is close to zero (see case 8). It shows homogenous low signal on T1W image with SE sequences, and it shows high signal like water on T2W image. There is no lesion enhancement after the injection of contrast medium. Complicated hepatic cyst such as infective hepatic cysts and hemorrhagic cysts sometimes are required to be distinguished from malignant liver cancer. The manifestations of hydatid disease of liver and hepatic cyst are similar. The asci are in mother cyst. The location and calcification are their characteristics.

8.2.2.9 Focal Fatty Change Is Common in the Normal Liver

Focal fatty change is common in the normal liver. It can be single or multiple with diameter of a few cm. Pathological features are liver steatosis with vesicular shape, distributing diffusely in the hepatic lobule, and the lobule structure exists. CT scan showed a homogenous, slightly low-density image, and the edge is clear. It shows no enhancement and low signal in arterial phase and portal venous phase, slightly higher signal on T1WI, and high or slightly higher signal on T2WI. With fat-suppressed T1WI and T2WI, the lesions are presented with low signal, which is helpful in the diagnosis. The manifestations of enhanced scans of MRI are the same with that of CT.

8.2.2.10 Liver Abscess

Liver abscess: Liver abscess in early period is sometimes difficult to distinguish with hepatocellular carcinoma. The comprehensive judgments must be made by combining clinical presentation with laboratory findings. For difficult cases, if necessary, doctors can have short-time follow-up after biopsy or positive anti-inflammatory. In abscess formation period, with CT scanning, the lesions show mixed low density with blurred edge; the lesion center shows low signal on T1W with SE sequences, the wall of the abscess shows low signal on T2W image, central liquefaction necrosis shows high signal, and peripheral edema regions show flap-like and slightly higher signal. With enhanced scanning of CT and MRI, the lesions are more typical. The abscess shows concentric circles like a "target sign," which consists of unenhanced liquefaction necrosis, enhanced wall, and band edema in the center, or the lesion image shows "honeycomb-like" shape on enhanced scan, which is also quite typical (see case 9). On CT image, the gaseous image, in particular, the gas-fluid levels are occasionally visible in the lesions, which is helpful for diagnosis of liver abscess. In addition, liver abscess is often accompanied by a small amount of ipsilateral pleural fluid.

8.2.2.11 Fatty Liver

Fatty liver: The place involved with fatty liver shows lower density using CT plain scan, and in the place with lower density, normal liver blood vessel image is clearly visible with relatively low density. The enhancement of fatty liver is the same with normal liver but still remains of relatively low density. Fatty liver on MRI scan with SE sequences, T1W and T2W images, can show relatively high signal. If the fat suppression technique is increased, the affected liver shows low signal, which is more conducive to the diagnosis of fatty liver. It should be noted that when part of the normal liver tissue present with ball shape in the fatty liver, it is called "liver island" in the radiography, which is often mistaken as a space-occupying lesion by ultrasound, while it cannot be misdiagnosed by CT and MRI, the key performances are: with enhanced scan, its change rule is consistent with that of the already enhanced fatty liver.

8.3 Optimization of Imaging Procedures

Ultrasound, DSA, and PET can be also used in imaging diagnosis of hepatocellular carcinoma. In addition to B-mode ultrasound, there are also Doppler ultrasound, CO2 contrast ultrasound, and intraoperative ultrasound. Therefore, in clinical practice, it is required to understand and know how to use the diagnostic imaging technology correctly, reasonably, and orderly. Based on our current experience, B-mode ultrasound or Doppler ultrasound (which may include ultrasound imaging) is generally preferred. If there are some problems, it is recommended to use enhanced spiral CT scan. If the diagnosis still cannot be confirmed, we can use MRI, and if necessary, we can use liver-specific MR contrast agent for further examination, and the ultrasound-guided needle biopsy is the last choice. DSA is usually only used in the process of TACE. At present, the sensitivity of PET in diagnosing liver cancer is low, and specificity is relatively high, which remains to be further studied.

References

1. Zeng MS. CT and MRI manifestations of hepatocellular carcinoma with portal hypertension. Chin J Pract Surg. 2002;22(9):517–9.
2. Zeng MS, Wang WP. The status and process of imaging diagnosis of small hepatocellular carcinoma. Chin Med J (Engl). 2003;38(9):13–6.
3. Zeng MS, Yan FH, Zhou KR, et al. The significance of liver capsule indentation in CT diagnosis of hepatocellular carcinoma. J Pract Radiol. 1996;12(6): 327–30.
4. Yan FH, Zeng MS, Zhou KR, et al. Helical dual-phase dynamic scanning in the diagnosis of small hepatocellular carcinoma. Chin J Radiol. 1996;30:829.
5. Yan FH, Zhou KR, Shen JZ, et al. A comparative study of the enhancement features of small hepatocellular carcinoma with MR and CT dynamic scan. Chin J Radiol. 2001;23:413.
6. Zeng MS, Yan FH, Zhou KR, et al. The study on hepatic enhancement with spiral CT in displaying hepatic and portal vein. Chin J Radiol. 2000;34(5): 345–9.
7. Yan FH. Imaging diagnosis of liver hemangioma. Chin J Pract Surg. 2003;23:324.
8. Yan F, Zeng M, Zhou K, et al. Hepatic angiomyolipoma: variable appearances on two-phase contrast scanning of spiral CT. EJR. 2002;41:12.
9. Yan FH, Zeng MS, Zhou KR, et al. The analysis of CT and MR images of angiomyolipoma of the liver. Chin J Pract Surg. 2001;35:821.
10. Yan FH, Zhou KR. Focal nodular hyperplasia (FNH): the manifestations with multiphase spiral CT scanning. Chin J Radiol. 1999;18:468.
11. Yan F, Zhou K, Jiang Y. Inflammatory pseudotumor of the liver: MRI findings. WJG. 2001;7:422.

Diagnostic Value of PET/CT in Metastatic Liver Cancer

9

Haibo Tan and Yihui Guan

There are many diagnostic imaging methods applicable to metastatic liver cancer, including CT, MRI, ultrasound, etc. In some cases, the specificity and sensitivity of these methods are limited, because of the influence of anatomical structures and the lack of blood supply to lesions, making early diagnosis difficult and delaying early treatment. Improving the early diagnosis of metastatic liver cancer and providing a theoretical basis for early treatment are ongoing focuses of medical and clinical medicine research. Positron emission tomography (PET) uses the distribution of positron radiopharmaceuticals in the body to reflect the metabolism of physiological and biochemical features. Fluoro-deoxy-glucose positron emission tomography (FDG PET) uses the increased glucose metabolism in tumor tissue to identify benign or malignant lesions and diagnose them in the early stage as a complement to other imaging technology. The basic principles and application of PET imaging for metastatic liver cancer are briefly discussed in this paper.

H. Tan (✉) • Y. Guan
Department of Radiology, Zhongshan Hospital, Fudan University, Shanghai, China
e-mail: tan.haibo@zs-hospital.sh.cn; guan.yihui@zs-hospital.sh.cn

9.1 Principles of PET Imaging and Common Tracers

9.1.1 Principles of PET Imaging

The physics principle behind positron emission tomography (PET) imaging is the use of a cyclotron to accelerate charged particles (protons, deuterons) to bombard target nuclei. Positron radionuclides (such as 11C, 13N, 15O, 18F, etc.) are produced by nuclear reactions; the appropriate imaging agent is introduced and observed in the target organs after the patient is placed in a thermal chamber. During the decay process, these nuclides emit positrons, which move short distances in the tissue (<1 mm). These positrons interact with the surrounding materials, causing annihilation radiation that emits two photons with equivalent energy (511 kev) in opposite directions. PET imaging uses a series of detectors paired with each other at 180° angles and connected with DHC to detect the annihilation photons; thus, the tomography of the body's positron radionuclides is formed. This method shows the metabolism, function, blood flow, cell proliferation, and receptor distribution of organ and lesion cells at the molecular level to provide clinicians with detailed diagnostic information about physiological and pathological aspects. Such methods are known as molecular imaging or biochemical imaging. The application of PET imaging has introduced a new era of molecular nuclear medicine [1].

X. Qin et al. (eds.), *Multidisciplinary Management of Liver Metastases in Colorectal Cancer*, DOI 10.1007/978-94-017-7755-1_9

9.1.2 The Common Tumor Metabolic Tracers Used in PET Imaging

9.1.2.1 18F-FDG

18F-FDG (2-fluorine-18-fluoro-2-deeoxy-d-glucose) is a glucose analogue. It is the most commonly used imaging agent in clinical settings. 18F-FDG is intravenously injected and then transported into the cell through the cell membrane with the help of the glucose transporter. The 18F-FDG in the cell is phosphorylased under the action of hexokinase, generating 6-PO4-18F-FDG, which differs structurally from glucose (the hydroxyl groups of the 2-position carbon atom are replaced by 18F) and cannot be further metabolized. Because it cannot pass through the cell membrane, 6-PO4-18F-FDG remains in the cells for several hours. Its retention is almost equivalent to the glucose consumption of tissue cells; therefore, 18F-FDG can reflect glucose utilization in vivo.

Most cancer cells have a high metabolism. In particular, malignant cells proliferate faster than normal cells, and their energy consumption is correspondingly higher. As one of the main energy sources of cells, glucose becomes overused as a result of the abnormal proliferation of malignant cells; consequently, the cell aims to increase the capacity of its membrane to transport glucose and the activities of key regulatory enzymes in the glucose metabolism channel. The increased glycolysis of malignant cells is related to the increase in the activity of glycolytic enzymes, including hexose kinase, 6-phosphofructokinase, and pyruvate dehydrogenase. At present, it is clear that the increased mRNA expression of glucose transporters in malignant tumors leads to an increase in glucose transporters. Therefore, a large amount of 18F-FDG is accumulated in tumor cells. PET imaging can display the tumor location, shape, size, and number and the distribution of radioactivity within the tumor. Primary and metastatic lesions of tumor cells have similar metabolic characteristics. Whole-body imaging can be easily performed with one injection of 18F-FDG. 18F-FDG PET whole-body imaging has a unique value for revealing the extent of tumor involvement throughout the body. Clinically, for tumors, 18F-FDG is mainly used for diagnosing benign or malignant tumors, determining clinical staging, evaluating efficacy, and monitoring recurrence.

9.1.2.2 Amino Acids

Amino acids are essential nutrients for the human body. They are mainly metabolized via protein synthesis, which changes them into enzymes and hormones with important biological activity. Amino acids are transformed into carbon dioxide, urea, and other substances and used by tissues or excreted after transportation, deamination, and decarboxylation, in which protein synthesis is the major metabolism. Abnormal protein synthesis can result from diseases and physiological or biochemical changes. Labeled amino acids can display abnormal changes.

Currently, the labeled amino acids used in human PET imaging are L-methyl-11C-methionine (11C-MET), L-1-11C-leucine, L-11C-tyrosine, L-11C-Phe acid, L-1-11C-methionine, L-2-18F-tyrosine, O-(2-18F-fluoroethyl)-L-tyrosine(FET), L-6-18F-fluorination dopa (18F-FDOPA), L-4-18F-phenylalanine, and 11C-and 13N-glutamic acid. In 11C- and 18F-labeled amino acid imaging, the ratio of radioactivity between tumor tissue and normal tissue is high, and the image is clear, which is useful for identifying tumor tissue and inflammation or lesions with strong glucose metabolism. Combining these amino acids with 18F-FDG can make up for the deficiencies of 18F-FDG alone, and they can also be used to identify tumor recurrence after radiotherapy changes.

9.1.2.3 Nucleotides

11C-thymidine (11C-TdR) and 5-18F-fluorouracil (5-18F-FU) are commonly used nucleic acid imaging agents. These agents are involved in nucleic acid synthesis and reflect the speed of cell division and propagation. 11C-TdR is mainly used for tumor imaging. The results show that 11C-TdR has a rapid clearance in blood. A clear image of a brain tumor can be obtained 20 min after administration. 5-18F-FU can be used to evaluate the treatment effects of chemotherapy. In addition, 5-18F-deoxyuridine and 11C-thymidine can also be used for tumor imaging.

9.1.2.4 Choline

Methyl-11C-choline is the most commonly used choline metabolic imaging agent. It is mainly used for prostate cancer, bladder cancer, brain tumors, lung cancer, esophageal cancer, and colon cancer imaging. We also use 18F-labeled choline, such as 18F-methyl choline, 18F-fluoroethyl choline, and 18F-fluoro-propyl choline; the imaging effects of 18F-fluoro-methyl choline and methyl-11C choline are similar. The advantage of using a choline metabolic imaging agent is the high ratio of radioactivity between tumors and non-tumors and the clarity of tumor imaging. Imaging can be performed a short time after intravenous administration.

9.1.2.5 11C-Acetate

11C-acetate can be absorbed by myocardial cell and then transformed into the 11C-acetyl coenzyme A, which is oxidized to carbon dioxide and water after it enters citric acid circulation. It can reflect citric acid in the myocardial flow and is proportional to the myocardial oxygen consumption. It can also be used to estimate myocardial viability and for tumor imaging. It has particularly important diagnostic value for more highly differentiated HCC.

9.2 Applications of PET/CT in the Diagnosis of Liver Metastases

9.2.1 Diagnosing the Primary Tumor

Colonoscopy is the first clinical choice for diagnosing primary colon cancer tumors. Lesions can be observed with direct vision, and pathological findings can be confirmed by biopsy. The primary tumor of colorectal cancer can also be detected with 18F-FDG PET imaging. While this method has high sensitivity for detecting colorectal cancer, its main clinical application is the simultaneous detection of metastases; specifically, it is used to gain comprehensive understanding of the extent of disease involvement and accurate clinical staging for clinical use to provide a reasonable scientific basis for treatment. PET shows images of radioactive accumulations because colorectal tumors have a high uptake of 18F-FDG. Abdel-Nabi et al. studied 48 cases of colorectal cancer and reported that the sensitivity of 18F-FDG PET imaging for detecting primary colorectal cancer was 100 %, and its specificity, positive predictive value, and negative predictive value were 43 %, 90 %, and 100 %, respectively. Thirty-five patients with colorectal polyposis showed no 18F-FDG accumulations.

9.2.2 Finding Metastases in the Liver and Other Remote Organs

More lymph node and remote organ metastases appear in intermediate and advanced colorectal cancer. Before and after surgical treatment, it is important to clarify the presence or absence of metastases, have a comprehensive understanding of the area of disease involved, and accurately determine clinical staging to clarify treatment options; 18F-FDG PET offers considerable advantages, particularly for patients with increased serum CEA and those whose lesions cannot be found using clinical fiber-optic colonoscopy, B-ultrasound, CT, MRI, and other tests. The metastases and primary lesions of malignant tumors have the same metabolic characteristics, and systemic imaging can be performed with one injection of 18F-FDG; therefore, systemic PET imaging can not only detect the primary tumor in an early stage but also can provide a comprehensive view of the area of disease throughout the body to provide an objective basis for clinical staging and choosing appropriate treatments [2].

Compared with CT, MRI, and other anatomical imaging methods, PET has the following advantages: (1) hole-body imaging, in which a comprehensive assessment of the metabolism of various tissues throughout the body can reveal metastasis beyond the target organs, and (2) enhanced ability to identify benign and malignant lesions, in which CT and other anatomic imaging techniques can clearly show obvious changes in the tissue structure, but sometimes it is difficult to determine the

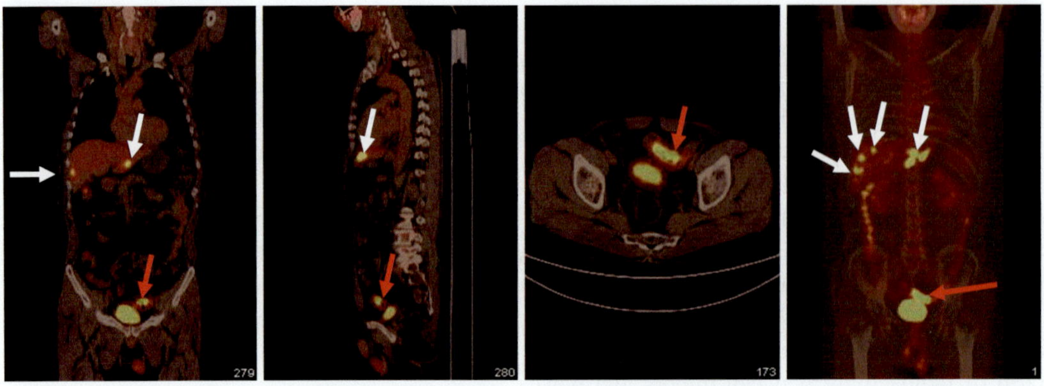

Coronal plane Sagittal plane Cross section Planar section

Fig. 9.1 The PET/CT image of colorectal cancer liver metastases (colonic lesions, *red arrows*; liver metastases, *white arrows*). Coronal plane, sagittal plane, cross section, planar section

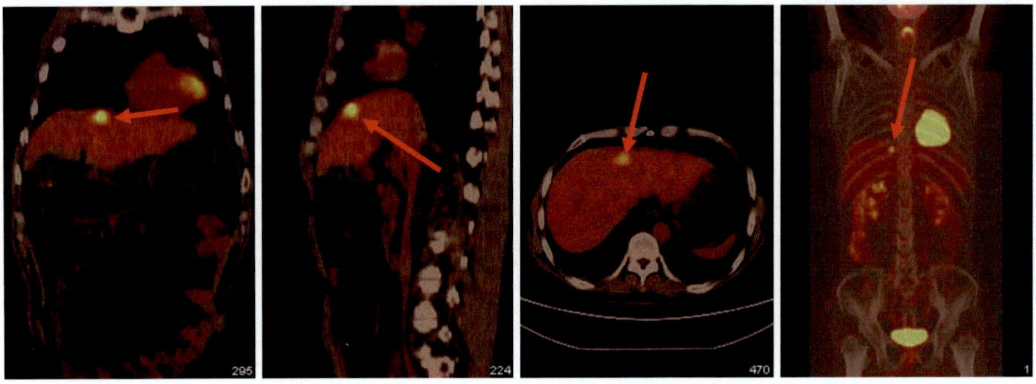

Coronal plane Sagittal plane Cross section Planar section

Fig. 9.2 Male patient, age 43. Liver metastases were detected 3 months after colorectal cancer surgery (liver metastases: *red arrows*). Coronal plane, sagittal plane, cross section, planar section

nature of these changes' pathology. PET, which is based on metabolism, provides CT images of tissue metabolism, which makes it better able to identify pathological characteristics that change the nature of the structure. Therefore, PET is a noninvasive imaging technique that can indicate the metabolism of the normal and abnormal tissue via quantitative detection.

Whiteford et al. reported that the sensitivity of PET for detecting liver metastases was 89 %, while the sensitivity of CT was 71 %. The specificity of PET and CT was similar: 98 % and 92 %, respectively. Among patients believed to have only extrahepatic metastasis, PET found liver metastasis in 20 %. Ogunbiyi et al. reported that the sensitivity of PET for diagnosing intrahepatic multiple metastases was also superior to that of CT (Figs. 9.1, 9.2, and 9.3). Some studies also compared PET with MRI (Table 9.1). FDG PET/CT is not only used for diagnosing liver metastases, but it is also better than other anatomical imaging methods for monitoring therapeutic effects after treatment (Fig. 9.2) [3].

The overall diagnosis of extrahepatic metastases of colorectal cancer remains unresolved. The sensitivity and accuracy of CT for diagnosing liver metastases are high, but CT is not ideal for diagnosing extrahepatic metastasis, especially abdominal lymph node metastases, which can usually only be diagnosed according to the size of the lymph nodes: Enlarged lymph nodes (larger than

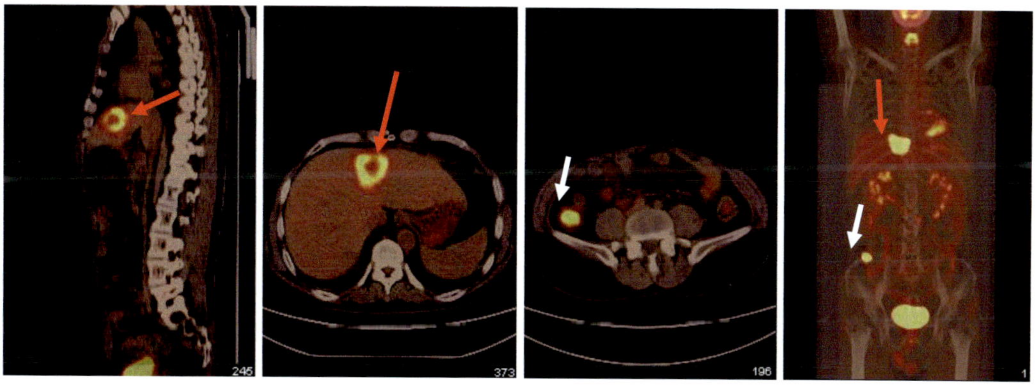

Fig. 9.3 Recurrent lesions were detected 6 months after colorectal cancer surgery, and the liver metastases had grown bigger (recurrent lesions, *white arrows*; liver metastases, *red arrows*). Sagittal plane, cross section, cross section, planar section

Table 9.1 Comparisons of the diagnostic value of PET, PET/CT, and MRI for colon cancer liver metastases

	PET	PET/CT	MRI
Accuracy (in %)	79	92	91
Sensitivity (in %)	61	84	73
Specificity (in %)	98	100	100
PPV (in %)	98	100	100
NPV (in %)	70	86	88

1 cm) are considered to be metastases; however, many are enlarged because of chronic inflammation. Furthermore, metastases of smaller lymph nodes are mistaken for normal lymph nodes. PET identifies metastases according to the metabolic activity of the lymph nodes, which is a more accurate indicator than size. Research has shown that the sensitivity of PET for detecting nonlocal recurrence of extrahepatic metastases is 94 %, while that of CT is only 67 %; PET and CT have similar specificity of 98 % and 96 %, respectively [4].

In addition, although the surgical removal of liver metastasis of colorectal cancer is still the most effective treatment, if the cancer is associated with extrahepatic metastases, liver surgery alone cannot benefit patients and may aggravate their condition. Therefore, PET is more helpful than CT in identifying the overall situation of patients. It can be combined with CT to select more appropriate patients for the radical resection of tumor recurrence or metastases and to avoid unnecessary extended resection.

Although PET has the advantages of high sensitivity, good resolution, and high accuracy for diagnosing liver and other metastasis of colorectal cancer, it should be used with anatomical imaging methods such as CT and MRI and serum markers to improve cancer diagnosis because of its low spatial resolution and less clear display of anatomical structures. Currently, different types of imaging devices can be used together because of improvements in medical imaging equipment; for example, the image fusion method can be used to join the anatomical image and the PET CT image, which can then be analyzed simultaneously to provide more accurate information for clinical diagnosis [5].

With the development of image fusion technology, PET/CT has been widely used in clinical areas. PET/CT provides the advantages of both the PET image and CT anatomical image. The information from PET and CT and the joined information from both are available in one image. This method has significant value for tumor diagnosis, staging, restaging, and efficacy monitoring [6]. Compared with conventional PET, PET/CT has the following advantages:

- Significantly reduced image acquisition time and increased patient turnover
- Improved accuracy of lesion orientation, which is beneficial for improving the interpretation of PET images and reducing the false-positive and false-negative rates of PET

- Diagnostic accuracy superior to that of PET or CT alone combined with the joint view of PET and CT
- CT can promote the detection of FDG uptake-negative tumors
- PET/CT can orient the biological target volume (BTV) of tumors to guide the precise formulation of a radiotherapy plan

The value of CT in PET/CT is greater than its ability to correct attenuation and its ability to precisely orient PET to the radioactive uptake-abnormal lesions.

References

1. Whiteford MH, Whiteford HM, Yee LF, et al. Usefulness of FDG-PET scan in the assessment of suspected metastatic or recurrent adenocarcinoma of the colon and rectum. Dis Colon Rectum. 2000;43: 759–67.
2. Ogunbiyi OA, Flanagan FL, Dehdashti F, et al. Detection of recurrent and metastatic colorectal cancer:comparison of positron emission tomography and computed tomography. Ann Surg Oncol. 1997;4:613–20.
3. Torizuka T, Tamaki N, Inokuma T, et al. Value of 18F-FDG-PET to monitor hepatocellular carcinoma after interventional therapy. J Nucl Med. 1994;35: 1965–9.
4. Donckier V, Van-Laethem JL, Goldman S, et al. 18F-FDG PET as a tool for early recognition of incomplete tumor destruction after radiofrequency ablation for liver metastases. J Surg Oncol. 2003; 84:215–23.
5. Vikram R, Iyer RB. PET/CT imaging in the diagnosis, staging, and follow-up of colorectal cancer. Cancer Imaging. 2008;4(8 S):46–51.
6. Cantwell CP, Setty BN, Holalkere N, et al. Liver lesion detection and characterization in patients with colorectal cancer: a comparison of low radiation dose non-enhanced PET/CT, contrast-enhanced PET/CT, and liver MRI. J Comput Assist Tomogr. 2008; 32(5):738–44.

10 Surgical Treatment of Rectal Cancer

Jin Gu

Rectal cancer operation is commonest in clinic, especially in colorectal surgery. Usually, the radical resection of rectal cancer includes abdominoperineal resection (APR); Chinese surgeons often use Miles operation, low anterior resection (LAR), and Hartmann's operation. So far, the minimally invasive surgery under laparoscope for middle or lower rectal cancer and the transanal endoscopic microsurgery (TEM) for early rectal cancer have developed rapidly. However, due to the limitation of devices or technical condition, they cannot be popularized in a short time. The anatomical background and the steps of transabdominal APR, LAR, and Hartmann's operations are introduced in this chapter.

10.1 Practical Anatomy Relevant to Radical Resection of Rectal Cancer

10.1.1 Anatomical Segment of the Rectum

According to the classical anatomy, the rectum usually consists of three parts [1]: the lower segment usually indicates the area 3–6 cm to the anus, the middle segment is 6–10 cm to the anus, and the upper segment is 10–15 cm to the anus. The upper one third of the rectum is usually coated with the peritoneum, which is named as intraperitoneal viscera; only a part of the middle one third is coated with the peritoneum, named as interperitoneal viscera; the lower one third of the rectum is completely outside of the peritoneum, named as extraperitoneal viscera. According to the National Comprehensive Cancer Network (NCCN) Guide of the United States, it is defined as "the intestinal tube within 12 cm from anus after measurement by proctoscope" [2].

10.1.1.1 Clinical Significance

Usually, in clinic, rectal cancer can be classified as the upper rectal cancer and the middle or lower rectal cancer according to the distance between the tumor and anus. In China, 70 % of rectal cancers are middle or lower rectal cancer [3]. The therapy for middle and lower rectal cancer is much different from that for upper rectal cancer. For cancers in middle and lower segments of the rectum, standard total mesorectal excision (TME) is usually adopted in clinic, while the therapy for upper rectal cancer is usually the same as that for carcinoma of the sigmoid. Moreover, for middle and lower rectal cancer, if the tumor is in T3 stage according to preoperative evaluation, or lymphatic metastasis occurs, preoperative neoadjuvant chemoradiotherapy should be applied, while upper rectal cancer can directly receive operation [2]. It must be pointed out that, after thorough dissociation of the rectum in operation, the distance

J. Gu
Department of Surgery, School of Oncology, Peking University, Beijing, People's Republic of China
e-mail: zlguj@bjmu.edu.cn

X. Qin et al. (eds.), *Multidisciplinary Management of Liver Metastases in Colorectal Cancer*,
DOI 10.1007/978-94-017-7755-1_10

between tumor and the anus is usually extended to 5 cm [4]; therefore, for a part of low rectal cancer, after dissociation, enough distance can be obtained so that the sphincter preservation operation can be carried out.

10.1.2 Concept of the Mesorectum

The middle and lower segments of the rectum are extraperitoneal viscera. Actually, in terms of histology, there is no mesorectum. The so-called mesorectum was described by Maunsell first, and RJ Heald stressed this concept in TME recommended in 1982 [5]. According to RJ Heald, "this is an exclusive conception of surgery, a descriptive noun irreplaceable" [6], of which the nature is the connective tissues such as fat and vessels around the rectum; the posterior border of it is the fascia pelvis visceralis, and there are collateral ligament and Denonvilliers' fascia at the side and front. In TME, it should be ensured that all mesorecta or that over 5 cm from the far end of tumors should be resected. There are several hypotheses about the structure of mesorectum; most of the scholars agree that the mesorectum has a closed structure; i.e., the pelvic fascia is around the whole rectum, while Denonvilliers' fascia is isolated from the visceral fascia [7, 8].

10.1.2.1 Clinical Significance

The key points of TME operation is to ensure the whole resection of the mesorectum and ensure the completeness of peripheral incisal margin. In terms of the complexity of operation, the posterior gap, or the "holy plane" [9] described by Heald, is usually easy to find out and separate, but the finding and separation of anterior and lateral gaps are relatively difficult. Therefore, during the operation, a proper reversed traction to the rectum should be maintained to reveal these gaps sufficiently, and then accurate sharp separation should be carried out by electric coagulation; thus, hemorrhage during operation can be decreased significantly, and a good separation result can be achieved. As worrying about the injury of the ureter, some surgeons would rather not to operate along the plane of gap close to pelvic wall; instead, they operate in the mesorectum, which could lead to hemorrhage and make the visual field unclear.

10.1.3 Concept of Denonvilliers' and Waldeyer's Fascia

Denonvilliers' fascia and Waldeyer's fascia are two critical structures at the anterior and posterior boundaries of the mesorectum. The former is a fibrous tissue extending vertically in front of the mesorectum, starting from the peritoneal reflection and ending at the perineal body; for male, there are seminal vesicle and prostate in front, while for female, there is posterior vaginal wall (Fig. 10.1). Waldeyer's fascia is a tougher fibrous tissue at the level of fourth sacral vertebra, connecting posterior fascia pelvis visceralis and presacral fascia; therefore, it is also called as rectosacral fascia.

10.1.3.1 Clinical Significance

As mentioned above, Denonvilliers' fascia is the front boundary of the mesorectum; therefore, sometimes, it is recommended to resect it completely in TME operation [10]. Some researches indicated that there are an amount of metastatic lymph nodes with small diameters in anterior mesorectum; it was necessary to ensure the complete resection of the mesorectum. Some researches indicated that pelvic nerve was adjacent to the sides of Denonvilliers' fascia; if the sides of Denonvilliers' fascia were to be separated, injury should be avoided [11, 12] (Fig. 10.2). Our experience is that, under the condition that the front seminal vesicle or posterior vaginal wall is not injured, fibrous tissues of Denonvilliers' fascia should be resected as much as possible; occasionally, capillary hemorrhage may occur from posterior vaginal wall, which could be controlled rapidly by surface coagulation with electric knife under argon mode.

The significance of Waldeyer's fascia is that if the tough layer of the fascia is not disconnected, it is difficult to reach the bottom of the pelvis, and the coccyx cannot be revealed. As shown in

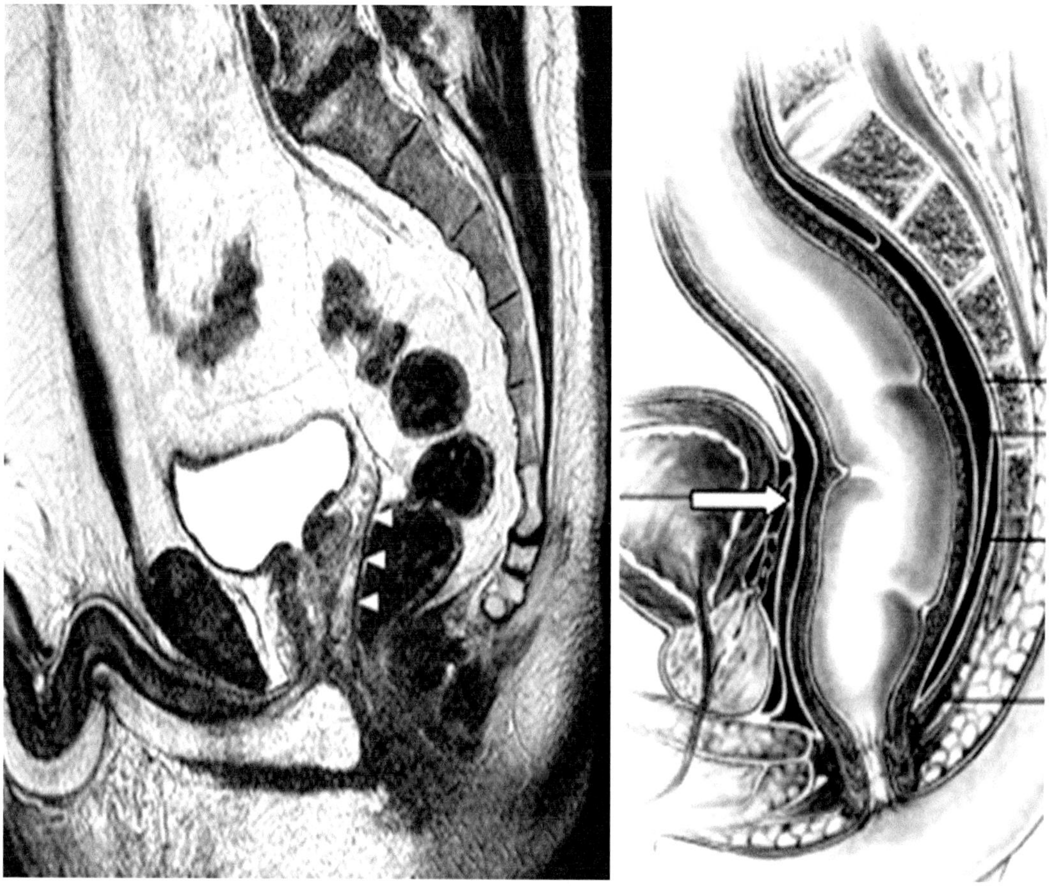

Fig. 10.1 Image and schematic diagram of Denonvilliers' fascia in MRI (*white arrow*)

Fig. 10.3, after entering the surgical plane between the fascia pelvis parietalis and fascia pelvis visceralis, this fascia must be sharply disconnected and separated to the upper level of coccyx. Thus, for both low-position anastomosis and APR operation, the most sufficient dissociation of the rectum can be achieved [13].

10.1.4 Concept of Lateral Ligament of the Rectum

It is disputed whether or not there is an anatomic structure named lateral ligament of the rectum. According to histological research, the so-called lateral ligament is actually located between the middle and lower segments of the rectum and the lateral pelvic wall, which may include histological bundle consisting of nerve fibers, fat, and arteriae rectalis caudalis; however, the structure may vary. In the operation, during separation of lateral sides of the rectum, fibrous bundle structure was also found. Anatomical researches on lateral ligament lead to various results. Sato et al. believed that there was a lateral ligament, consisting of arteria rectalis media and branches of pelvic plexus nerve [14]. Nano et al. also agreed that there was a lateral ligament structure; however, it consisted of only fibrous tissues, and the rectal arteries and branches of pelvic plexus nerve are located under the ligament structure [14] (Figs. 10.4 and 10.5).

10.1.4.1 Clinical Significance

Although there is controversy on the existence of lateral ligament, the lateral bundle structure

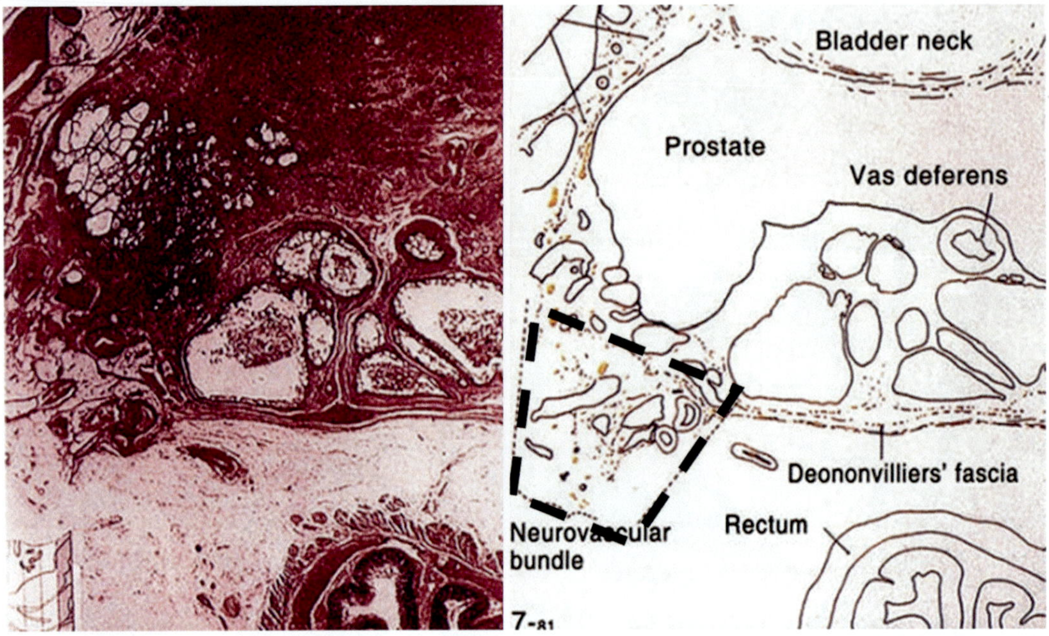

Fig. 10.2 Correlation between sides of Denonvilliers' fascia and the pelvic plexus (male)/branches of pelvic plexus are in the trapezoidal area

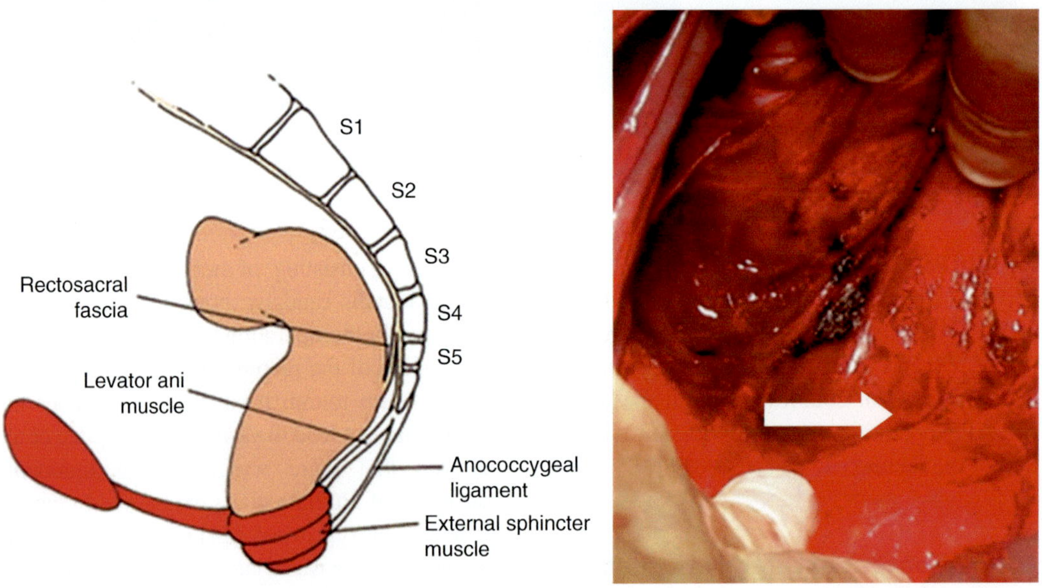

Fig. 10.3 In the operation, after disconnection of Waldeyer's fascia (*white arrow*), posterior rectal wall can be dissociated completely, and anococcygeal ligament can be revealed

must be treated in the operation of rectectomy. In order to avoid injuring of the lateral pelvic plexus, sharp disconnection should be carried out by electric knife, and disconnection should be achieved near the rectum under the condition that the structure is maintained. There may be arteriae rectalis caudalis in the lateral ligament, but ultrasonic knife or electric coagulation can usually seal them, and clamping or ligation is not necessary; this is very important to maintain

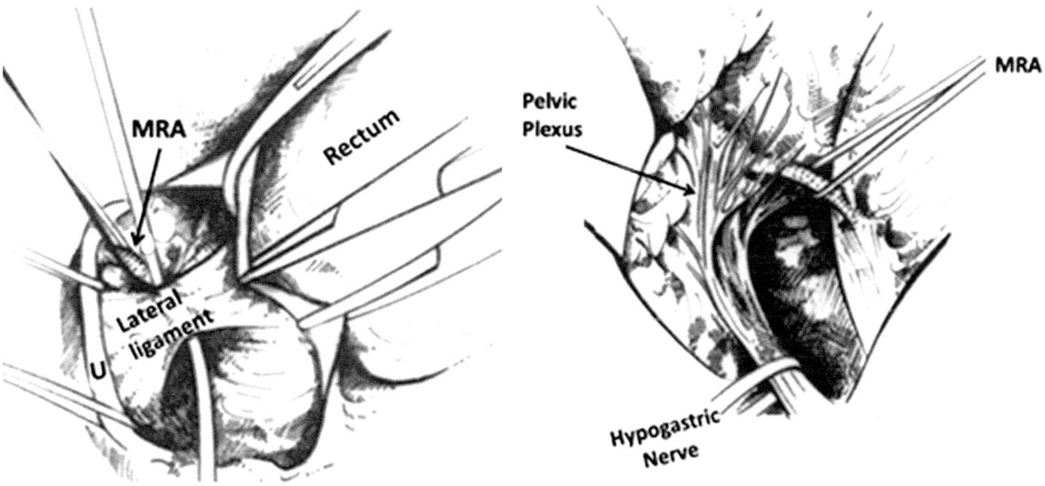

Fig. 10.4 Correlation of the lateral ligament, arteriae rectalis caudalis (*MRA*), hypogastric nerve, ureter (*U*), and pelvic plexus (the lateral ligament in the right diagram has been cut)

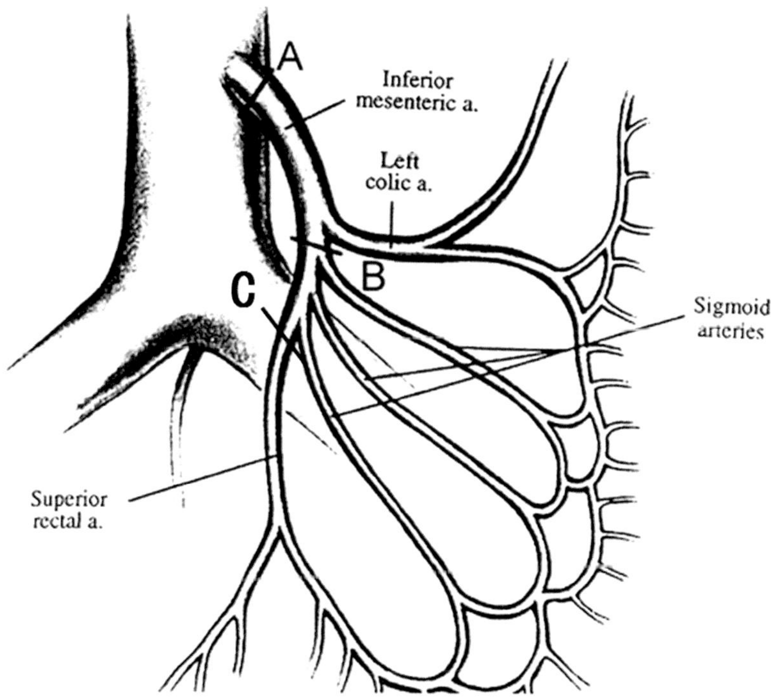

Fig. 10.5 Ligation level of blood vessels in radical resection of rectal cancer. (**a**) Classical high ligation at the root of the inferior mesenteric artery. (**b**) Low ligation involving sigmoid arteries. (**c**) Low ligation only involving superior rectal artery

the completeness of the lateral side of the mesorectum.

10.1.5 Blood Supply to the Rectum

Blood vessels feeding the rectum are mainly from inferior mesenteric artery that comes from aorta abdominalis and then branches into the left colic artery, arteriae sigmoideae, and superior rectal artery. Arteriae rectalis caudalis from the internal iliac artery or internal pudendal artery also supplies blood to the rectum. Another important content of anatomy of rectum-related blood vessels is presacral venous plexus.

10.1.5.1 Clinical Significance

In traditional opinion of therapy against colon cancer, high ligation should be carried out to the inferior mesenteric artery. Classical high ligation means that the main trunk of the inferior mesenteric artery should be ligated and disconnected 2 cm away from aorta abdominalis at the root of the inferior mesenteric artery. However, in recent years, more and more findings of evidence-based medicine indicated that high ligation does not improve the prognosis of patients; instead, it may lead to complications such as ischemic necrosis [15]. Therefore, NCCN guide recommends that, if intraoperative exploration finds there is no swollen lymph node at the root of the mesentery, routine high cleaning and ligation are not necessary; instead, ligation of the root of the superior rectal artery is enough; a part of branches of blood vessels in the sigmoid colon may be ligated selectively according to the intraoperative colon tension.

Arteriae rectalis caudalis, coming from the internal pudendal artery or internal iliac artery, is a small artery distributed at the lateral side of middle and lower segments of the rectum, of which the diameter is about 1–2 mm with a big anatomic variation. It is reported that the possibility of occurrence of arteriae rectalis caudalis is 22–100 % [14, 16, 17]. If it is found in operation, this blood vessel can be disconnected and coagulated with electric knife, while clamping and ligation are not necessary.

Presacral venous plexus is a structure of blood vessels in front of the sacral periosteum, consisting of two big lateral sacral veins and one median sacral vein. Presacral venous hemorrhage is a severe and dangerous intraoperative event during separation of posterior of the rectum, especially Waldeyer's fascia, of which the anatomic background is that the presacral venous plexus will retract to sacral foramen after breakage [18]. Therefore, during presacral venous hemorrhage, clamping and ligation cannot stop hemorrhage; moreover, it may tear presacral vein and aggravate hemorrhage. At present, there are two hemostatic methods in clinic: (1) Resect a piece of rectus abdominis, of which the diameter is 2 cm, press it on the bleeding point, and carry out electric coagulation (recommended electric coagulation value >100); then the charring of muscle will coagulate the contacted venous plexus [19] (Fig. 10.6); (2) press a tailor-made thumb pin on the bleeding point, penetrate the venous plexus, and stabilize it in the sacrum; with the help of local pressing, the purpose of hemostasis is achieved; it should be noted that the distance between the midline of the sacrum and the point where the thumb pin is pressing in should be less than 2 cm at S1 level, while at S5 level, it should

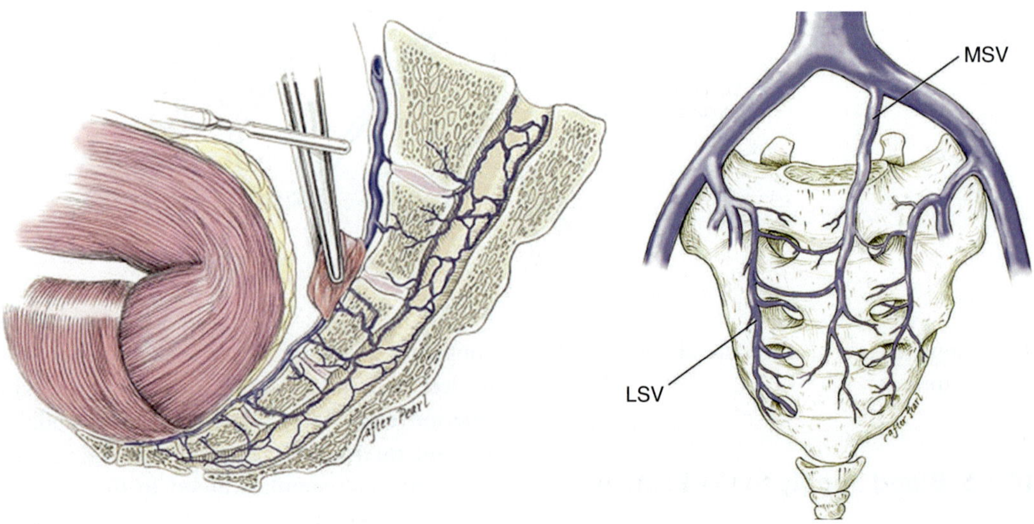

Fig. 10.6 Presacral venous plexus and treatment of presacral hemorrhage (rectus abdominis electric coagulation method)

be less than 1 cm, in order to avoid damaging the lateral sacral nervous plexus [20].

10.1.6 Pelvic Autonomic Nerve Preservation (PANP)

As the nerve controlling the rectum is usually resected along with the rectum in operation, what we stressed here is the pelvic autonomic nerve to be protected and preserved in the rectal operation. The critical nerve adjacent to the rectum usually has the following anatomical structure:

1. Hypogastric plexus: a nerve plexus resulted from confluence of the sympathetic nerve coming from thoracic vertebra 11 and lumbar vertebrae 2 and the lumbar splanchnic nerves coming from lumbar ganglia 3–4, formed in front of aorta abdominalis, at the branch of common iliac artery, also named as presacral nerve or nervi praesacralis.
2. Hypogastric nerve: two branches of nerve fascicles, of which the diameter is about 3 mm, starting from hypogastric plexus, going down with iliac vessels, bringing the adrenergic nerve into the pelvic organ, and controlling the function of ejaculation in male; hypogastric nerve is easy to identify in clinic, because it consists of thick yellowish fibers.
3. Pelvic splanchnic nerves: parasympathetic nerve fibers started from sacral nerve 2–4 and entered the right bottom corner of the pelvic plexus, which controls the function of erection in male.
4. Pelvic plexus: also named as hypogastric plexus. Pelvic plexus results from the confluence of hypogastric nerve, sacral splanchnic nerves, and pelvic splanchnic nerves and is located at the outer side of arteriae rectalis caudalis and lateral ligament of the rectum. Usually, the pelvic plexus is difficult to identify in a living body (Figs. 10.7 and 10.8).

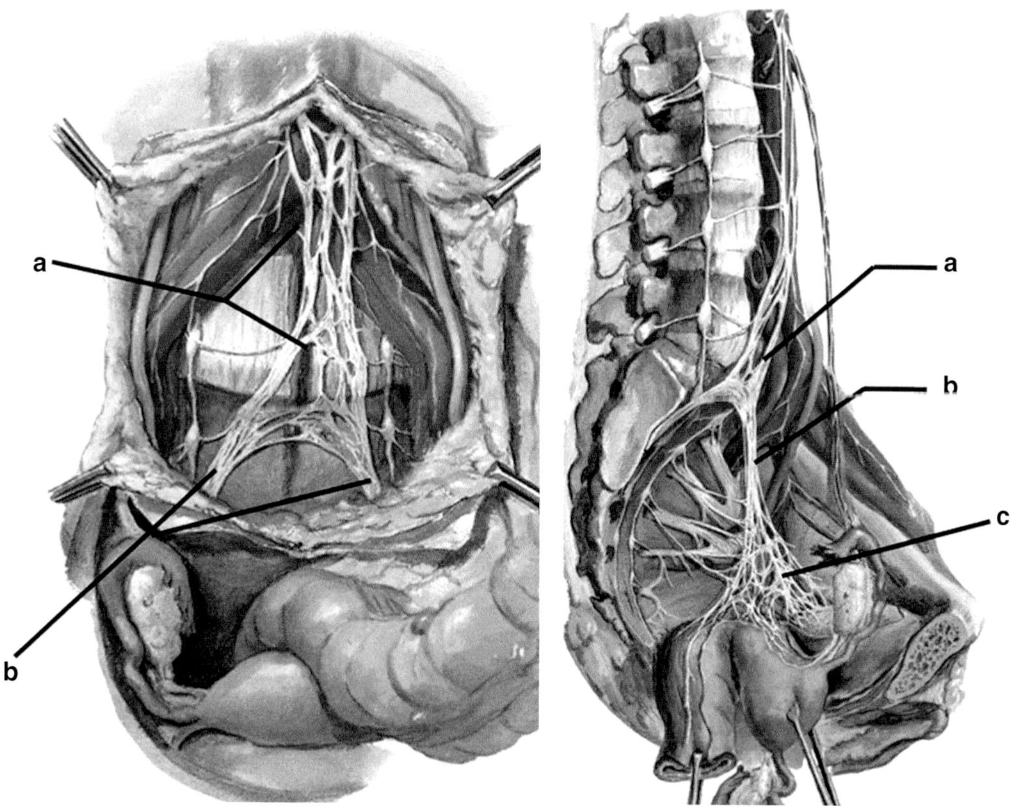

Fig. 10.7 (**a**) Hypogastric plexus. (**b**) Hypogastric nerve. (**c**) Pelvic plexus

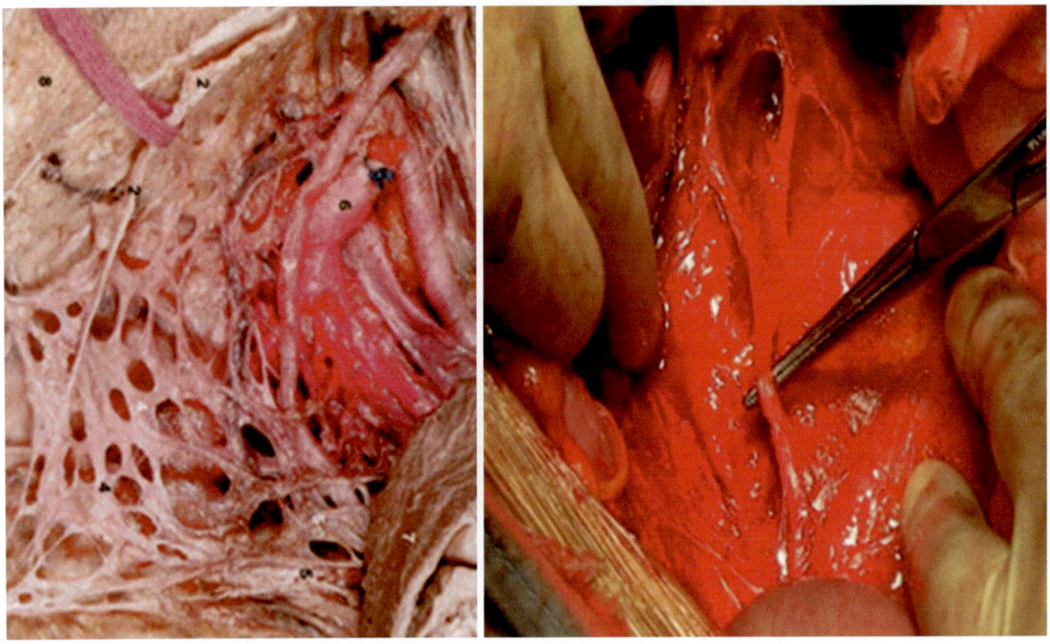

Fig. 10.8 The pelvic plexus (necrotomy) and trunk of hypogastric nerve (observed during operation)

10.1.6.1 Clinical Significance

In rectal surgery, especially radical resection of rectal cancer, the pelvic nerve structure should be protected as much as possible, in order to ensure that the patient can get good urinary and sexual function. In TME surgery, attention should be paid to the following: (1) After opening the lateral peritoneum at the inner side of the ureter, before entering the "holy plane," attention must be paid to the dissociation and protection of hypogastric nerve at both sides. If dissociation is carried out directly along the loose gap that appears first, the hypogastric nerve would usually be disconnected at the posterior-lateral side of the rectum. Therefore, after the appearance of the gap, one should find the starting site of two hypogastric nerves from superior hypogastric nerve in front of sacropromontory (note the nerve trunk at this part is usually thick), sharply dissociate the main trunk of hypogastric nerve from the back of the mesorectum until the place where it enters the lateral pelvic wall to form the pelvic plexus, and then carry out the successive operation of TME. (2) Disconnection of the lateral ligament should be carried out adjacent to the rectum, in order to avoid injuring the pelvic plexus. (3) During the traction and dissociation of the sigmoid mesocolon to the branch of aorta abdominalis, the starting part of the hypogastric nerve at the left side is usually tracked together; at this time, the hypogastric nerve at the left side should not be injured [21].

10.1.7 Conception of Lateral Lymph Node Dissection (LLND)

Lateral lymph node metastasis usually occurs in advanced lower rectal cancer. Lateral lymph nodes mainly include the common iliac and internal iliac lymph nodes distributed along the direction of iliac vessels and the obturator lymph nodes distributed along the obturator vessels/nerve. The lateral dissection of rectal cancer should start from the branch of aorta abdominalis, and clean the fat/lymph tissues adhered to the front of the aorta and inferior vena cava; open the lateral peritoneum, clean the fat tissues on the surface of common iliac blood vessels and at the corner of common iliac blood vessels and iliopsoas muscle, and reveal the obturator nerve and blood vessels; further bare the obturator nerve and clean the obturator lymph nodes.

10.1.7.1 Clinical Significance

In recent years, according to the finding of evidence-based medicine, lateral lymph node metastasis indicated a worse prognosis, while lateral lymph node dissection increased the postoperative injury to urinary and sexual function significantly and could not improve the survival rate of patients [22]. Especially, as application of neoadjuvant preoperative radiotherapy can lower the local incidence after operation, some researches indicate that lateral dissection after preoperative radiotherapy has no significant meaning [23]. Therefore, lateral disconnection can act as optional operation at present; during the operation, if lateral swollen lymph nodes are contacted, they should be disconnected.

10.1.8 Concept of Anal Tube

The explanation of anal tube is different in anatomists, embryologists, pathologists, and surgeons. Usually, the following two classes of definitions are given for anal tube: the concept of anatomical, histological, embryological, and pathological anal tube is identical, while that closely related to surgeon is called as surgical or clinical anal tube. Usually, the length of surgical anal tube is about 4 cm, of which the range is from the upper edge of sphincter ani internus to the edge of the anus, while the length of anatomical anal tube is about 2 cm, of which the range is from the upper edge of dentate line (the upper edge of anal transitional zone) to the edge of the anus. The two concepts are not conflicted, and the former includes the latter. The horizontal tissues above and below the dentate line have completely different epithelial structure and nerve control, which have been described in detail in many textbooks. Perianal means the range 5 cm around the anus.

10.1.8.1 Clinical Significance

In order to judge the possibility of anus-preserving operation, surgeons usually carry out digital examination of the rectum to explore the position of tumor; the distance between the lower margin of tumor and the surgical anal tube is a factor to decide whether or not the anus can be preserved. If this distance is less than 1 cm, a distal margin with pathological negative is hard to obtain during operation; thus, the risk of local recurrence after anus preservation is increased significantly. The distance between the tumor and the dentate line (or the anatomical anal tube) has a less important meaning in guiding surgery operation.

10.1.9 Construction of Levator Ani Muscle

Levator ani muscle consists mainly of puborectal muscle, pubococcygeus muscle, and iliococcygeal muscle (Fig. 10.9). The iliococcygeal muscle, whose distal ends are located at the lateral pelvic wall and coccyx, respectively, is the main muscle to be treated during dissociation of posterior levator ani muscle.

10.2 Abdominoperineal Resection (APR)

10.2.1 Development of APR

In 1908, Miles brought forward the conception of APR according to the achievements of study on lymph drainage of rectal cancer, which lowered the postoperative local recurrence rate of middle or lower rectal cancer significantly. In recent 70 years, APR operation was always the standard operation for lower rectal cancer [24]. With the development of concept and skill of TME, more and more colorectal surgeons care about the whole dissociation of the mesorectum, other than stress on the resection range of levator ani muscle and fat tissues in ischiorectal fossa. With the development of pathology of rectal cancer and image technology, more and more attention have been paid to the question how to ensure to get a negative circumferential resection margin (CRM) after radical resection of rectal cancer [25]. The study of evidence-based medicine

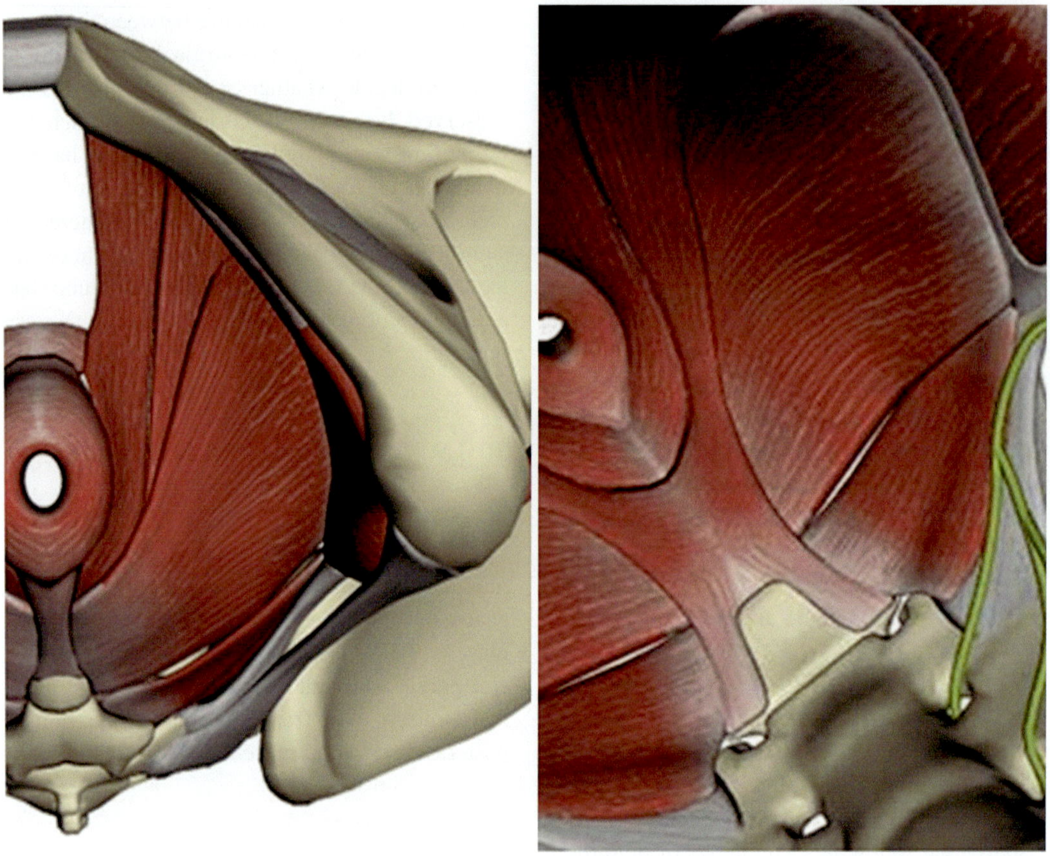

Fig. 10.9 Construction of levator ani muscle (outside and inside): from left to right, external rectal sphincter, puborectal muscle, pubococcygeus muscle, iliococcygeal muscle, and coccygeal muscle; the levator ani muscle is usually the generic term of the former three muscles

also indicated that APR operation has a worse prognosis than the anus-preserving LAR operation, because of the higher rate of positive CRM after APR operation, which may lead to local recurrence [26]. Therefore, on the basis of TME, the cylindrical APR operation, in which the resection range of levator ani muscle is extended, has attracted attention of colorectal surgeons gradually [27].

10.2.2 Indications of APR Operation

Because of the development of lower stapling technique, a distance <6 cm from the lower margin of tumor to the edge of the anus is no longer the absolute indication of APR operation. We suggest that the common indication is the rectal cancer, of which the distance between tumor and the anus is less than 5 cm. Application of APR needs correct preoperative staging, good operation, and cautious intraoperative decision.

The following conditions were often met: (1) Preoperative MRI judged that the tumor had invaded levator ani muscle, or digital examination of the anus indicated that the distance between tumor and upper edge of surgical anal tube was less than 1 cm. (2) During operation, pelvic canal stenosis or giant tumor was founded; thus, the lower rectum was difficult to be dissociated and stapled. (3) After sufficient dissociation of the rectum, satisfactory distal incisal margin (>1 cm) was not yet obtained, or rapid pathological examination indicated a positive recisal margin. (4) After local resection of early lower rectal cancer, pathological examination indicated a positive incisal margin or a lesion over T2 stage.

10.2.3 Preoperative Preparation for APR Operation

10.2.3.1 Routine Preoperative Preparation

Preoperative evaluation of physical state and nutrition support; preparation of blood and blood transfusion (when necessary); cleaning the vagina for female patients; skin preparation of the perineum and abdomen.

10.2.3.2 Preoperative Intestinal Tract Preparation: Insertion of Gastrointestinal Decompression Tube and Urine Drainage Tube

In classical surgery, a routine 3-day intestinal tract preparation should be carried out before operation for rectal cancer, including oral intake of antibiotics, mechanical lavage of intestinal tract, preoperative gastrointestinal decompression, and urine drainage tube insertion. However, researches of evidence-based medicine in recent years indicated that preoperative oral intake of antibiotics and mechanical lavage of intestinal tract could not decrease the incidence of postoperative complications such as anastomotic leakage and infection [28, 29]. After routine intestinal tract lavage, the patients may suffer a higher incidence of postoperative anastomotic leakage and infection [30]. In addition, according to the rapid recovery opinion advocated at present, preoperative intestinal tract preparation, gastrointestinal decompression, and urine drainage tube insertion may be carried out to some patients with rectal cancer but not routinely [31].

10.2.3.3 Permanent Colostomy and Marking

Please refer to Sect. "10.5.10.1 Colostomy."

10.3 Steps of APR Operation

10.3.1 Selection of Anesthesia, Position, and Incision

As APR operation has a large resection range and will take a long time, general anesthesia should be used. Lithotomy position should be adopted to reveal perineum. It should be noted that (1) after anesthesia, the operation table can be adjusted so that the head is in a lower position and the feet are in a higher position; thus, the small intestine will be set at the front of surgery field; (2) the coccyx of patients should be extruded, and the angle between thighs and trunk should be less than 90°, so that the perineal region can be revealed enough to facilitate operation; (3) during the setting of lithotomy position, the position of patient's leg should be adjusted to avoid pressing the common peroneal nerve. The incision is usually selected at the center of the abdomen around the navel, of which the bottom should reach the pubic symphysis and the top boundary depends on the condition of the patient. During the incision of abdominal wall to the lower part, avoid injure bladder. For female patients, womb can be suspended to facilitate revealing.

10.3.2 Exploration of Abdominal Cavity and Pelvic Cavity

After entry of the abdomen, explore whether or not there is ascites, hepatic metastasis, or peritoneal metastasis and collect information of abdominal visceral organ such as the colon and stomach; explore whether or not there are swollen lymph nodes at the root of the inferior mesenteric artery, in front of aorta abdominalis, or at the area of iliac vessels; for female, attention should be paid to the bilateral ovary. Finally, explore the tumor and pay attention to the dissociation degree of the tumor and the relation of the tumor to adjacent organs and pelvic wall; during operation, preoperative pelvic MRI image should be combined to identify the local condition of tumor.

10.3.3 Preligation of Rectal Vessels and Intestinal Canal

After complete exploration, the operation table can be adjusted so that the head is in a lower position and the feet are in a higher position; push the small intestine to the side of the head. Ligate the intestinal canal with tape at the boundary of the rectum and sigmoid colon above the tumor. Tract the tape so that the sigmoid mesocolon has a certain stress, touch to identify the direction of superior rectal artery and sigmoid arteries, open the peritoneum at the surface of the mesentery, and preligate at the root of superior rectal artery. For patient who has a shorter length of sigmoid colon, a narrow pelvic cavity, or an overweight body, under the precondition that the proximal end of the rectum is long enough to be brought out of abdominal wall, the rectum-sigmoid colon can be disconnected with an occluder; thus, traction and dissociation of proximal end of the rectum are helpful for revealing the posterior rectal wall.

10.3.4 Dissociation of the Sigmoid Colon

First of all, disconnect the physiological adhesion between the left side of the sigmoid colon and lateral pelvic wall, and open the peritoneum with electric knife at the inner side of the ureter; then the loose gap at the starting part of mesorectum will appear; this plane is also a critical plane for fulfilling the TME operation. Disconnect upward along the abovementioned loose gap, and the sigmoid colon at left side can be dissociated completely to the end of descending colon. Then the dissociation of the sigmoid colon can be paused.

10.3.5 Protection of Hypogastric Nerve and Dissociation of Posterior Rectal Wall

After dissociation of the sigmoid colon, find out the hypogastric plexus at the branch of aorta abdominalis, and identify the starting point of the trunk of the hypogastric nerve at both sides in front of the sacral promontory. Then track the rectum fore-upward to reveal the loose gap between the fascia pelvis visceralis and the fascia pelvis parietalis at the posterior rectal wall, which is the operation plane of TME; at this plane, carry out sharp disconnection carefully with electric knife, and a precise operation will not lead to hemorrhage. During sharp disconnection, the following details should be noted: (1) The trunk of hypogastric nerve acts as the boundary of this plane; this plane consists of an anterior gap and a posterior gap (Fig. 10.10); although the gap between the trunk of the hypogastric nerve and the fascia pelvis parietalis is looser, dissociation along this plane will disconnect the trunk of hypogastric nerve, resulting in failure of nerve protection. The correct operation should be that as follows: after entering the starting part of the loose gap, dissociate and protect the trunks at both sides, and then dissociate along the relatively dense gap between the trunk of the hypogastric nerve and fascia pelvis parietalis (i.e., the fascia on the surface of posterior mesorectum). (2) After entering the right place, the electric

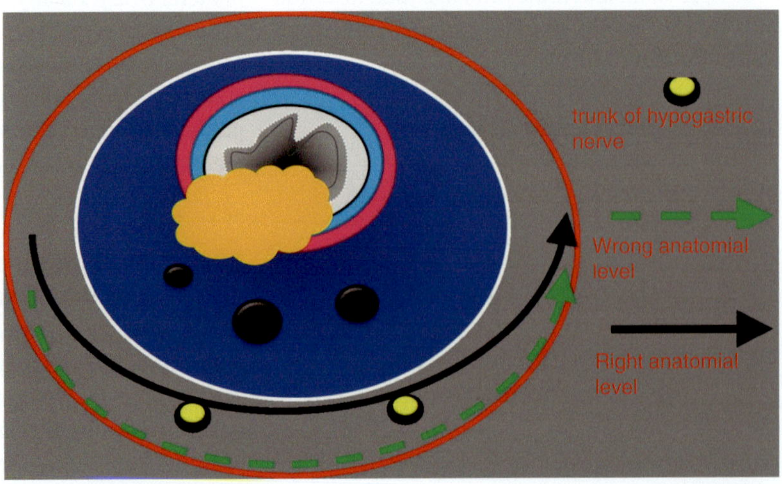

Fig. 10.10 Schematic diagram of dissociation of posterior rectal wall: the trunk of the hypogastric nerve often adheres to the fascia pelvis visceralis (the fascia at posterior wall of the mesorectum); the correct place is not the looser gap

knife should deflect to the mesorectum in order to avoid injuring anterior sacral veins. (3) As the place where the trunk of hypogastric nerve enters lateral pelvic wall is most brittle and thin, after successful dissociation of posterior rectal wall, the main trunk of hypogastric nerve should still be protected until the complete dissociation of lateral rectal wall.

10.3.6 Dissociation of Lateral Rectal Wall and Protection of the Pelvic Plexus

After dissociation of the posterior wall, extend to both sides along the gap of dissociation and continue the protection of the trunk of the hypogastric nerve until it enters into the lateral pelvic wall. Dissociate to the directions of 3 o'clock and 9 o'clock; then the gap usually gets unclear; instead, connective tissues with unclear boundaries, or the so-called lateral ligament of the rectum, will appear. Then the surgery field should be revealed enough; by assistant's dragging hook and operator's pushing rectal tube reversely, the lateral ligament structure will be stretched. Sharp disconnection should be carried out near the rectum; thus, injury of the pelvic plexus can be avoided. According to our experience, increase of the power of electric knife (electric coagulation value, 60–80) can ensure a satisfactory electric coagulation to the median artery; usually, the dissociation of the lateral rectal wall can be fulfilled without the ligation of the median artery.

10.3.7 Dissociation of Front Rectal Wall

After the dissociation of frontal and lateral wall, drag the rectum toward the posterior interior direction, and open the peritoneum with electric knife at the lowest point near the front of folding of the peritoneum. The assistant can push the frontal tissues toward pubis with dragging hook; then a layer of tough fascia consisting of longitudinal fibrous structure will appear; this is the Denonvilliers' fascia (Fig. 10.11); dissociation in front of this fascia can maintain the completeness of anterior mesorectum. For male patients, if there is no tumor invasion or adhesion, hemorrhage will hardly occur between the Denonvilliers' fascia and the seminal vesicle; for female patients, as there are much blood vessels at the posterior vaginal wall, the electric knife with argon spray mode should be used to achieve good hemostasis on the surface without burning the posterior vaginal wall.

10.3.8 The Level of Rectum Dissociation During Abdominal Operation

In traditional APR operation, dissociation of the rectum should be carried out downward as much as possible during abdominal operations. For male patients, the dissociation of frontal wall should be over the level of seminal vesicle; for female patients, most of posterior vaginal wall

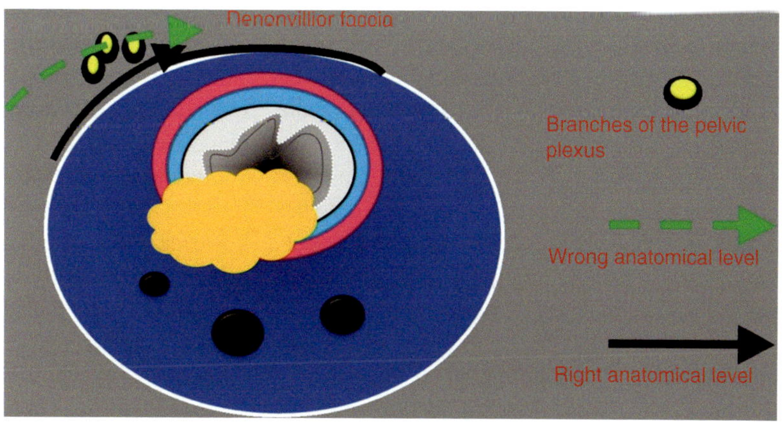

Fig. 10.11 Schematic diagram of dissociation of frontal-lateral wall of the rectum: dissociation should be carried out near the mesorectum, and the Denonvilliers' fascia should be resected to ensure the completeness of the mesorectum

should be dissociated until the perineal bodies. The dissociation of posterior wall should reveal the coccyx to reach the level of levator ani muscle.

However, at present, it is recommended to carry out cylindrical APR resection for patients with late T stage and invasion of levator ani muscle. At frontal wall, dissociation is enough to the level of seminal vesicle or the middle segment of posterior vaginal wall; at the posterior wall, dissociation is enough to the starting part of the coccyx (the boundary of the coccyx and sacrum). Successive dissociation will be carried out at perineal region.

10.3.9 Permanent Colostomy at Abdominal Wall

Please refer to Sect. " 10.5.10.1 Colostomy."

10.3.10 Operation at the Perineal Region

Traditional APR operation: after suture of the anus, make a fusiform incision around the anus, of which the frontal edge is the projection of the perineal conjoined tendon on the skin, the back edge should reach the tip of coccyx, and the lateral edge should reach the exterior side of the middle point of anus-tuber ischiadicum. Incise the skin and subcutaneous adipose tissue until the levator ani muscle plane. Then, find out the bony marker of the coccyx and disconnect the anococcygeal ligament. Levator ani muscle appears mainly as iliococcygeal muscle at the back; combination of electric knife and clamping should be used to treat the fascicle. After treatment of the second half ring of levator ani muscle, the surgeon's operation for the perineum and those for the abdomen can meet at the coccyx, and drag the closed proximal end of the rectum out of the pelvic cavity. Thereafter, drag the specimen to reveal the left and right lateral anterior walls, respectively, and continue the ligation of levator ani muscle fascicle. Once the specimen adheres only to frontal wall, incise the conjoined tendon and puborectal muscle at the perineum. Then, the deep area of anterior rectal wall to be treated is the place where effusion of blood occurs most frequently in APR operation. Here, for male patients, there is prostate in front; for female patients, there is the lower segment of posterior vaginal wall; for both and male and female, there is the vascular plexus between this place and anterior rectal wall. Experiences for treatment of this place include: (1) After dissociation to some extent, it is recommended to stanch first before recovering the dissociation; otherwise, the unclear surgery field is easy to lead to wrong dissociation. (2) Here hemostasis can be carried out with ultrasonic knife or suture, while electric knife or electric coagulation often gets an unsatisfactory result. (3) For female patients, the assistant can help to guide in the vagina to avoid injury; for male patients, during dissociation, the surgeon can keep feeling the position of the ureter and prostate to get a right position. After complete dissociation of anterior wall, the specimen can be removed completely; attention should be paid to the examination of the prostate and vagina to detect whether or not they are injured; if so, repairing is necessary. If hemostasis occurs to anterior wall, posterior wall, or lateral wall, suture to staunch.

Cylindrical APR operation: It can be subdivided as standard cylindrical APR and cylindrical APR combined with coccyx resection. In this operation, during abdominal operation, the mesorectum cannot be dissociated completely; at the posterior wall, it is enough to reach the joint of the coccyx-sacrum; at the anterior wall, it is enough to reach the seminal vesicle/middle segment level of posterior vaginal wall (Fig. 10.12). The incision at perineal region and the resection range of perianal tissues under levator ani muscle plane are identical.

Standard cylindrical APR requires a body position identical to that for traditional APR; however, after entering the level of levator ani muscle, one should open surgery field further toward the lateral and posterior walls and find the end point of fascicle on the pelvic wall and disconnect it (Fig. 10.13). As the operation position is deep there, it is difficult to treat the fascicle

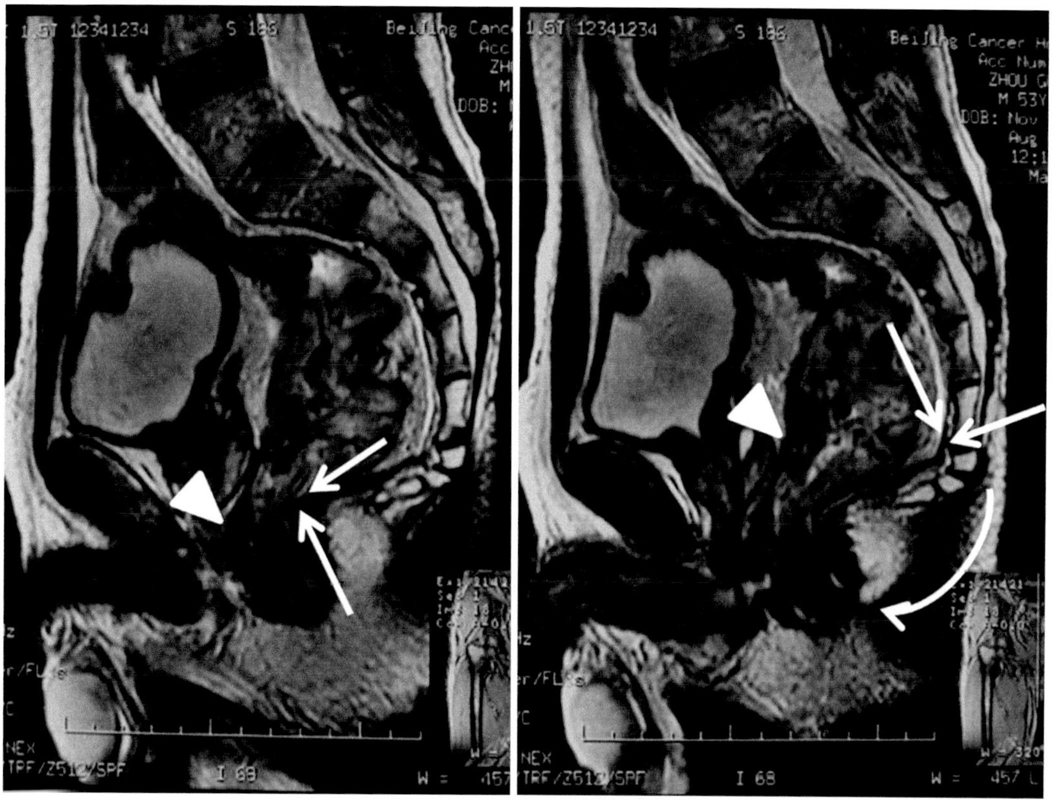

Fig. 10.12 Comparison of cylindrical APR and traditional APR: the *thicker arrow* indicates the end point of anterior wall disconnection; in cylindrical resection, it is at the seminal vesicle level, while in traditional resection, it is adjacent to levator ani muscle. The *thin arrow* indicates the meeting point of abdominal operation and perineal region operation; in cylindrical APR, it is at the border of the coccyx and sacrum, while in traditional APR, it is at the border of anal tube and levator ani muscle. The *curved thin arrow* indicates the range of posterior resection of cylindrical APR combined with coccyx resection

with ligation by clamping; the author is accustomed to dragging the fascicle with left hand and coagulating and disconnecting the fascicle with right hand by ultrasonic knife at a slow speed. The treatment of anterior wall is not significantly different from that in traditional APR. The advantage of this operation is that the patient does not have to change position, and the operation technique is easy to grasp. However, the disadvantage is that the poor revealing of APR operation is not resolved yet; as the dissociation range is narrow in epigastrium, the operation in deep perineal region is difficult. For patients with invasion at levator ani muscle level but the anterior wall is not involved, standard cylindrical resection at lithotomy position can increase the rate of radical cure and is very safe.

Cylindrical resection combined with coccyx resection: After the dissociation of the sigmoid colon and mesorectum through the abdomen and the construction of artificial stoma, place the upper segment of the rectum into the pelvic cavity and rebuild the peritoneum at the pelvic floor and then close the abdomen gradually and routinely. Change the body position of the patient from lithotomy position to jackknife position, re-sterilize, and prepare drape. The incision range should include the range along the direction of the coccyx besides fusiform incision around the anus (Fig. 10.14). After incision of the fascia of the skin covering the coccyx, disconnect the tendon of the gluteus maximus adhered to the coccyx-sacrum and reveal the posterior gap of the coccyx. Bluntly disconnect the border of the

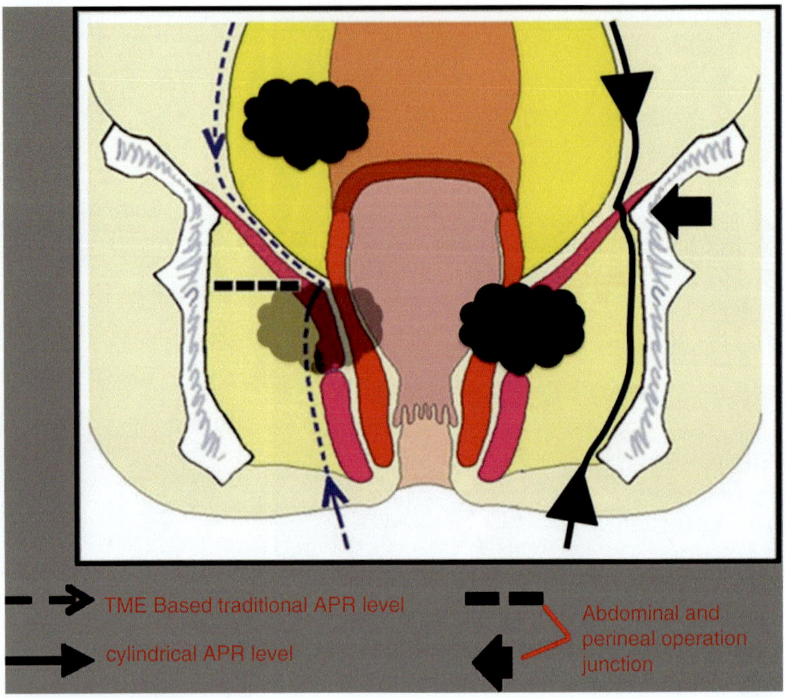

Fig. 10.13 Schematic diagram of traditional APR and cylindrical APR for rectal cancer: for rectal cancer at very low position combined with levator ani muscle invasion, cylindrical APR can achieve a better resection range than traditional APR to ensure a negative incisal margin

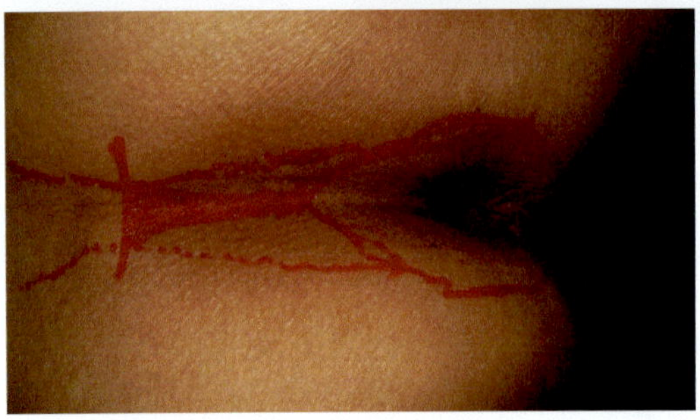

Fig. 10.14 Cylindrical APR combined with coccyx resection: jackknife position, the incision should include the range along the direction of the coccyx; the deep conical area is the projection of the coccyx on the body surface

coccyx-sacrum with periosteum detacher and incise the posterior fascia of the coccyx with electric knife to enter the pelvic cavity. Thereafter, the assistant can clamp and drag the coccyx to guide the following operation: as iliococcygeus adheres to the coccyx, dragging the coccyx leftward can reveal the end point of iliococcygeus at the pelvic wall very well; the operator should insert the left index finger and middle finger into the pelvic cavity through the coccyx, and put them behind iliococcygeus; meet thumb with the index and middle fingers, and touch iliococcygeus to identify the end position of fascicle on the pelvic wall. Then, coagulate with clamping ligation or ultrasonic knife at a low rate, and disconnect the right lateral iliococcygeus gradually from the pelvic wall. After disconnection of left lateral iliococcygeus by the same method, the posterior and lateral walls of levator ani muscle can be dissociated completely, and the rectum can be dragged out of the pelvic cavity. As the patient is set at a jackknife position, after disconnection of the coccyx and all posterior and lateral levator ani muscle, the anterior rectal wall can be revealed very well, and the operator can achieve precise dissociation and hemostasis to anterior wall under direct observation. For patients with partial invasion to anterior wall, partial resection of prostate or resection/repairing of posterior vaginal wall can be carried out under direct observation. According to the photo of image, for cylindrical APR, there isn't a "middle" part at levator ani muscle level, which existed in traditional APR operation; as the dissociation of

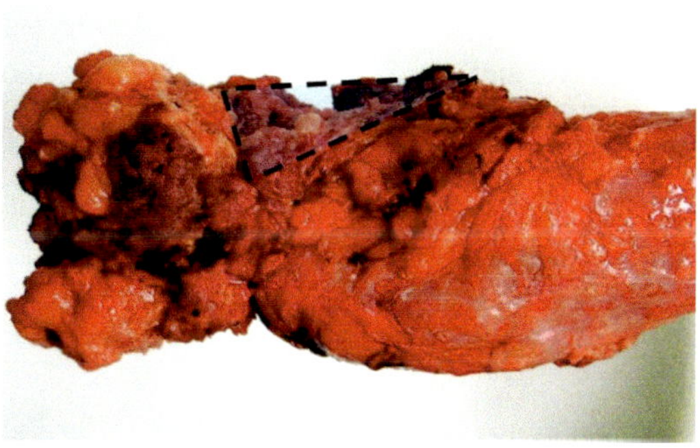

Fig. 10.15 Photo of cylindrical APR specimen (lateral posterior): the triangular area is the levator ani muscle resected more than traditional APR

mesentery is carried out only to the levator ani muscle level, mesentery and levator ani muscle are resected together, just like a cylinder (Fig. 10.15). The author recommends that, for patients with anterior wall invasion but critical cure can be achieved by extended resection, cylindrical APR combined with coccyx resection should be adopted; according to the experience of the author, by changing the body position, resection of coccyx can lead to a good surgery field, which can result in a precise intraoperative hemostasis; even the prostate or vagina is resected, operation in perineal region still leads to little hemorrhage. The disadvantage of this operation is that the change of body position during operation will elongate the duration of operation; thus, the risk of anesthesia is higher.

10.3.11 Rebuilding of the Pelvic Floor and Occlusion of Abdominal Wall and Perineal Incision

Rebuilding of pelvic floor: Lateral peritoneum should be interruptedly suture to prevent small intestine from dropping into the pelvic cavity. The stitch should be dense here, and ureter should not be injured.

Abdominal wall incision: Use Vicryl suture to close the peritoneum, and use polydioxanone synthetic (PDS II) absorbable suture to close protheca; alternatively, one may use PDS II suture to carry out continuous suture of the peritoneum and protheca. After routine interrupted suture of the skin and subcutaneous tissue, close the abdominal incision.

Closure of perineal incision: After presacral drainage, close the subcutaneous tissue with interrupted or continuous suture and then suture or staple the skin interruptedly. For patients with large surface of wound, unsatisfactory hemostasis, or large incisal tension, gauze can be used to fill the incision, which will be removed in 2–3 days after operation; the perineal incision can be cured gradually by hip bath.

10.4 LAR Operation

10.4.1 Development of LAR Operation and Indications

With the common application of double stapling technique, anus-preserving surgery for low-positioned rectal cancer has become a well-accepted operation [32]. At present, the argument about LAR operation is focused on the length of distal incisal margin of intestinal canal. NCCN guide recommended that the distal incisal margin should reach 2 cm. In some researches, for tumors at very low positions, a distal incisal margin of 1 cm is also acceptable, but rapid intraoperative pathological analysis should be carried out to ensure the distal incisal margin negative [33]. Moreover, on the basis of LAR, inter-sphincter resection is derived to treat the tumors at very low position, by which satisfactory long-term therapeutic effect has been achieved in some researches [34]. With the development of technique mentioned above, indications of LAR operation are more flexible. Under the precondition that the radical resection is ensured and the function of external sphincter is preserved, if the low-positioned stapling can be fulfilled, LAR operation should be tried positively. However, whether or not LAR operation can be applied depends mainly on the position of tumor and the condition of the pelvis; if the condition of the pelvis is unsatisfactory, the anus may not be preserved even the tumor is at a higher position [35].

10.4.2 Preoperative Preparation of LAR Operation

Identical to the preoperative preparation of APR operation.

10.5 Steps for LAR Operation

10.5.1 Selection of Anesthesia, Body Position, and Incision

Identical to the preoperative preparation of APR operation.

10.5.2 Exploration of Abdominal and Pelvic Cavities

Identical to the preoperative preparation of APR operation.

10.5.3 Preligation of Rectal Vessels and Intestinal Canal

Identical to that of APR operation.

10.5.4 Dissociation of the Sigmoid Colon

The basic principle is the same as that of APR operation. During treatment of the rectum at proximal end, in order to ensure the low-position stapling without tension, the sigmoid colon should be dissociated sufficiently; when necessary, splenic flexure should be loosened. Disconnect the sigmoid mesocolon at the ligated part. (Note: the edge of mesocolon should be protected to prevent ischemia of the stapled site.)

10.5.5 Protection of Hypogastric Nerve and Dissociation of Posterior Rectal Wall

Identical to that of APR operation basically. However, in LAR operation, Waldeyer's fascia at posterior rectal wall should be resected to reveal the coccyx and make the incision reaching the pelvic floor directly.

10.5.6 Dissociation of Lateral Rectal Wall and Protection of the Pelvic Plexus

Identical to that of APR operation.

10.5.7 Dissociation of Anterior Rectal Wall

Identical to that of APR operation basically. For female patients, the vagina should be dissociated sufficiently at the distal end of the rectum to be resected, in order to avoid rectovaginal fistula resulted from triggering of stapler.

10.5.8 Resection of Distal Mesorectum and Exposure of Myotube

After sufficient dissociation of the mesorectum, incise the mesorectum at distal end and expose the myotube for stapling. At that time, arteriae rectalis caudalis has usually been disconnected, and the blood supply to the rectum comes from superior rectal artery; the latter branches in posterior mesorectum at the top segment of the rectum, and surround the anterior mesorectum. Therefore, during the process that the mesorectum is incised to reach myotube, hemorrhage occurs easily at the anterior lateral side of the mesorectum at low segment, while it occurs hardly at the posterior side. On the other hand, for middle and high-position rectal cancer, if only 5 cm of the mesorectum is resected at the distal end, during the process of incision through which operation approaches myotube from the mesorectum, hemorrhage is easy to occur at the anterior lateral side of the mesorectum. Incision of the mesorectum at the end segment usually leads to little hemorrhage, and electric knife can usually be used for coagulation; hemorrhage is more severe at the middle segment of the mesorectum, and suture is necessary sometimes for hemostasis. The readers can get more experience on this in clinical practice. With the development of medical devices, application of ultrasonic knife can get a satisfactory result during treatment of the mesorectum.

10.5.9 Low-Position Anastomosis by Double Stapler Method

After closing the rectum at distal end with stapler, perfect hemostasis should be carried out to the residual end. Before insertion of tubular stapler through the anus, sufficient expansion of anal sphincter should be carried out; if necessary, paraffin oil can be used to lubricate anal tube. Before triggering stapler, the assistant should drag the anterior viscera with hook; especially, for female patients, the posterior vaginal wall should be separated from the stapling site to avoid injury. After anastomosis, the completeness of anastomosis ring should be examined; if the anastomosis is not satisfactory, air test should be carried out to exclude anastomotic leakage; when necessary, protective ileostomy can be carried out. After anastomosis, insert a pelvic drainage tube through the sacrum or abdomen.

10.5.10 Rebuilding of the Pelvic Floor and Closing of Abdominal Wall Incision

Identical to that of APR operation

10.5.10.1 Colostomy

Colostomy consists of temporary colostomy and permanent colostomy; in the former, transverse colon is usually used, while the sigmoid colon or descending colon is used in the latter.

Indications of transverse colostomy include the ileus, perforation, trauma, and congenital abnormality of distal rectum, the encopresis, and the protection of anastomosis; the stoma should be one stage opened. The character of transverse colostomy is that ileus can be released rapidly, and the operation is not difficult, which can save time for successive therapy. Transverse colostomy is seldom to be used in protective colostomy after low-position rectal cancer operation, because in transverse colon, there is more formed stool than in the ileum, which is inconvenient for nursing. On the other hand, as the blood transport in the colon is much less than that in small intestine, after stoma apothesis, the possibility of anastomotic leakage increases significantly; therefore, protective transverse colostomy is usually replaced by ileostomy. For patients to whom protective colostomy is not carried out but anastomotic leakage occurs or ileus occurs due to severe anastomotic stenosis, as the transverse colostomy leads to small wound and takes effect rapidly, it is usually used for salvage bypass operation.

The selection of surgical opportunity for transverse colostomy is very important; it may not always be so that all postoperative anastomotic leakages need anastomosis, and all anastomotic leakages can be resolved by anastomosis. For the leakage with little syndrome and drainage and without complication, surgical treatment is not necessary; after insertion of drainage tube, parenteral nutrition, and reasonable application of antibiotics, most leakage can cure. As for those with much drainage, general peritonitis, or significant systemic toxic symptoms and those whose drainage tube has been pulled out and local treatment is difficult, surgical treatment should be adopted immediately. Transverse colostomy is the most common operative technique; usually, the intestinal segment with large activity should be chosen for loop double-barrel anastomosis; the stool should be transported away to decrease the stimuli of intestinal juice and stool to downstream anastomosis, which will benefit the growth and cure of anastomosis. The time for stoma apothesis is usually 3–5 months after operation [36]. For anastomotic leakage with bad anastomosis and severe pelvic infection, which cannot be resolved by pure anastomosis, Hartmann's operation should be carried out [37].

The site of colostomy is usually chosen at the part with much straight muscle, skin wrinkle, navel, and operative incision, or bony bulge should be avoided to prevent complications such as stoma retraction, artificial fistula-induced hernia, and infection of incision. The stoma should be observed by the patient, and it should not affect daily cloth wearing; thus, the self-nursing of stoma can be achieved, and the life quality can be improved [38].

Attention should be paid to the permanent colostomy after abdominoperineal resection: the pore size of the stoma on the skin should be somewhat less than that of the intestinal tube to be dragging out of the stoma; a crucial incision can be used to incise the anterior rectus sheath; bluntly drag away the muscle along the direction of the rectus abdominis muscle; incise the posterior rectus sheath, and drag out of the intestinal tube. The length of intestinal tube dragged out of the abdomen should not be excessively long; after dragging out, the mesentery should be trimmed to some extent; usually, the height of the stoma should be 2 cm after eversion of mucosa. Interruptedly suture the peritoneum, serous layer of intestinal wall, anterior rectus sheath and seromuscular layer, and intracutaneous tissue and margin of the stoma.

After colostomy, common complications include stoma retraction, anastomotic stenosis, stoma side hernia, stoma-peripheral inflammation, stoma hemorrhage, stoma necrosis, and stoma prolapse, of which the total incidence is about 25 %, among which 40 % occur within 1 month after operation [39]. The occurrence of stoma complication is related to various factors, including the self-physical condition of patients, the operation, and the postoperative nursing. The postoperative nursing of the stoma is very important; good nursing and education of health can lower the incidence of complications and improve the life quality of patients [40, 41].

References

1. Rosenberg SA. Cancer: principles and practice of oncology, 6th edition. Netherlands: Lippincott Williams & Wilkins; 2001. p. 1271.
2. Engstrom PF, Arnoletti JP, Benson 3rd AB, Chen YJ, Choti MA, Cooper HS, Covey A, Dilawari RA, Early DS, Enzinger PC, et al. NCCN clinical practice guidelines in oncology: rectal cancer. J Natl Compr Canc Netw. 2009;7(8):838–81.
3. Li M, Gu J. Changing patterns of colorectal cancer in China over a period of 20 years. World J Gastroenterol. 2005;11(30):4685–8.
4. Wolff BG, Fleshman JW, Beck DE, Pemberton JH, Wexner SD. The ASCRS textbook of colon and rectal surgery. Germany: Springer; 2007. p. 4.
5. Chapuis P, Bokey L, Fahrer M, Sinclair G, Bogduk N. Mobilization of the rectum: anatomic concepts and the bookshelf revisited. Dis Colon Rectum. 2002;45(1):1–8. discussion 8–9.
6. Morgado PJ. Total mesorectal excision: a misnomer for a sound surgical approach. Dis Colon Rectum. 1998;41(1):120–1.
7. Lindsey I, Warren BF, Mortensen NJ. Denonvilliers' fascia lies anterior to the fascia propria and rectal dissection plane in total mesorectal excision. Dis Colon Rectum. 2005;48(1):37–42.
8. Bisset IP, Chau KY, Hill GL. Extrafascial excision of the rectum: surgical anatomy of the fascia propria. Dis Colon Rectum. 2000;43(7):903–10.
9. Heald RJ, Moran BJ. Embryology and anatomy of the rectum. Semin Surg Oncol. 1998;15(2):66–71.
10. Heald RJ, Moran BJ, Brown G, Daniels IR. Optimal total mesorectal excision for rectal cancer is by dissection in front of Denonvilliers' fascia. Br J Surg. 2004;91(1):121–3.
11. Lepor H, Gregerman M, Crosby R, Mostofi FK, Walsh PC. Precise localization of the autonomic nerves from the pelvic plexus to the corpora cavernosa: a detailed anatomical study of the adult male pelvis. J Urol. 1985;133(2):207–12.
12. Kinugasa Y, Murakami G, Uchimoto K, Takenaka A, Yajima T, Sugihara K. Operating behind Denonvilliers' fascia for reliable preservation of urogenital autonomic nerves in total mesorectal excision: a histologic study using cadaveric specimens, including a surgical experiment using fresh cadaveric models. Dis Colon Rectum. 2006;49(7):1024–32.
13. Gordon PH. Principles and practice of surgery for the colon, rectum, and anus. 3rd ed. London: Informa Healthcare; 2007. p. 5.
14. Sato K, Sato T. The vascular and neuronal composition of the lateral ligament of the rectum and the rectosacral fascia. Surg Radiol Anat. 1991;13(1):17–22.
15. Lange MM, Buunen M, van de Velde CJ, Lange JF. Level of arterial ligation in rectal cancer surgery: low tie preferred over high tie. A review. Dis Colon Rectum. 2008;51(7):1139–45.
16. DiDio LJ, Diaz-Franco C, Schemainda R, Bezerra AJ. Morphology of the middle rectal arteries. A study of 30 cadaveric dissections. Surg Radiol Anat. 1986;8(4):229–36.
17. Havenga K, DeRuiter MC, Enker WE, Welvaart K. Anatomical basis of autonomic nerve-preserving total mesorectal excision for rectal cancer. Br J Surg. 1996;83(3):384–8.
18. Wang QY, Shi WJ, Zhao YR, Zhou WQ, He ZR. New concepts in severe presacral hemorrhage during proctectomy. Arch Surg. 1985;120(9):1013–20.

19. Harrison JL, Hooks VH, Pearl RK, Cheape JD, Lawrence MA, Orsay CP, Abcarian H. Muscle fragment welding for control of massive presacral bleeding during rectal mobilization: a review of eight cases. Dis Colon Rectum. 2003;46(8):1115–7.
20. Nivatvongs S, Fang DT. The use of thumbtacks to stop massive presacral hemorrhage. Dis Colon Rectum. 1986;29(9):589–90.
21. Gu J. Malignant tumor of rectum and anus. Beijing: Peking University Medical Press; 2007. p. 138–40.
22. Hida J, Yasutomi M, Fujimoto K, Maruyama T, Okuno K, Shindo K. Does lateral lymph node dissection improve survival in rectal cancer? Examination of node metastases by the clearing method. J Am Coll Surg. 1997;184(5):475–80.
23. Nagawa H, Muto T, Sunouchi K, Higuchi Y, Tsurita G, Watanabe T, Sawada T. Randomized, controlled trial of lateral node dissection vs. nerve-preserving resection in patients with rectal cancer after preoperative radiotherapy. Dis Colon Rectum. 2001; 44(9):1274–80.
24. Corman ML. Classic articles in colonic and rectal surgery. A method of performing abdominoperineal excision for carcinoma of the rectum and of the terminal portion of the pelvic colon: by W. Ernest Miles, 1869–1947. Dis Colon Rectum. 1980;23(3):202–5.
25. Nagtegaal ID, Quirke P. What is the role for the circumferential margin in the modern treatment of rectal cancer? J Clin Oncol. 2008;26(2):303–12.
26. den Dulk M, Marijnen CA, Putter H, Rutten HJ, Beets GL, Wiggers T, Nagtegaal ID, van de Velde CJ. Risk factors for adverse outcome in patients with rectal cancer treated with an abdominoperineal resection in the total mesorectal excision trial. Ann Surg. 2007;246(1):83–90.
27. West NP, Finan PJ, Anderin C, Lindholm J, Holm T, Quirke P. Evidence of the oncologic superiority of cylindrical abdominoperineal excision for low rectal cancer. J Clin Oncol. 2008;26(21):3517–22.
28. Miettinen RP, Laitinen ST, Makela JT, Paakkonen ME. Bowel preparation with oral polyethylene glycol electrolyte solution vs. no preparation in elective open colorectal surgery: prospective, randomized study. Dis Colon Rectum. 2000;43(5):669–75; discussion 675–7.
29. Slim K, Vicaut E, Launay-Savary MV, Contant C, Chipponi J. Updated systematic review and meta-analysis of randomized clinical trials on the role of mechanical bowel preparation before colorectal surgery. Ann Surg. 2009;249(2):203–9.
30. Wille-Jorgensen P, Guenaga KF, Matos D, Castro AA. Pre-operative mechanical bowel cleansing or not? an updated meta-analysis. Colorectal Dis. 2005;7(4):304–10.
31. Nehlet H. Fast-track colorectal surgery. Lancet. 2008;371(9615):791–3.
32. Moran BJ, Blenkinsop J, Finnis D. Local recurrence after anterior resection for rectal cancer using a double stapling technique. Br J Surg. 1992;79(8):836–8.
33. Rutkowski A, Bujko K, Nowacki MP, Chmielik E, Nasierowska-Guttmejer A, Wojnar A. Distal bowel surgical margin shorter than 1 cm after preoperative radiation for rectal cancer: is it safe? Ann Surg Oncol. 2008;15(11):3124–31.
34. Chamlou R, Parc Y, Simon T, Bennis M, Dehni N, Parc R, Tiret E. Long-term results of intersphincteric resection for low rectal cancer. Ann Surg. 2007;246(6):916–21. discussion 921–912.
35. Gu J, Bo XF, Xiong CY, Wu AW, Zhang XP, Li M, An Q, Fang J, Li J, Zhang X, et al. Defining pelvic factors in sphincter-preservation of low rectal cancer with a three-dimensional digital model of pelvis. Dis Colon Rectum. 2006;49(10):1517–26.

Colostomy

36. Eckmann C, Kujath P, Schiedeck TH, Shekarriz H, Bruch HP. Anastomotic leakage following low anterior resection: results of a standardized diagnostic and therapeutic approach. Int J Colorectal Dis. 2004;19(2):128–33.
37. Kanellos I, Vasiliadis K, Angelopoulos S, Tsachalis T, Pramateftakis MG, Mantzoros I, Betsis D. Anastomotic leakage following anterior resection for rectal cancer. Tech Coloproctol. 2004;8 Suppl 1:s79–81.
38. Xu HL, Yu DH, Lu MF, Shen YF, Yang R, Zhang NJ, Lu S. Preoperative nursing of enterostomy. Chin J Nurs. 2001;10:S10-2–4-5.
39. Duchesne JC, Wang YZ, Weintraub SL, Boyle M, Hunt JP. Stoma complications: a multivariate analysis. Am Surg. 2002;68(11):961–6.
40. Burch J. The pre- and postoperative nursing care for patients with a stoma. Br J Nurs. 2005;14(6):310–8.
41. Bradshaw E, Collins B. Managing a colostomy or ileostomy in community nursing practice. Br J Community Nurs. 2008;13(11):514–8.

11 Laparoscopic Resection for Colorectal Cancer

Zhen Fan and Conor Delaney

11.1 Introduction

Colorectal carcinoma is a very common malignancy in most western countries. Based on data from National Cancer Institute in 2008, it is estimated that 148,810 new cases would be diagnosed (108,070 colon, 40,740 rectal) in the United States. The combined mortality is estimated to be 49,960, making colorectal carcinoma the second most common cause of combined male and female mortality after lung cancer and the most common solid tumor after skin malignancies.

While the incidence of colorectal cancer had been relatively stable in the USA, it is rising in China. Based on a cancer registry in Shanghai, China, the overall colorectal cancer incidence rates increased more than 50 % between 1972–1977 and 1990–1994. This represents approximately a 2 % increase per year [1].

Z. Fan, MD
Spring Branch Medical Center, Memorial Hermann Memorial City Medical Center, Houston, TX, USA

Cleveland Clinic, Cleveland, OH, USA

C. Delaney, MD (✉)
Colon and Rectal Surgery,
University Hospital Case Medical Center,
Cleveland, OH, USA

Cleveland Clinic, Cleveland, OH, USA
e-mail: delanec@ccf.org

11.2 Laparoscopic Surgery in the Treatment of Colon Cancer

Only recently has laparoscopic gastrointestinal surgery been accepted among general surgeons. In 1983, the first laparoscopic gastrointestinal surgery, laparoscopic appendectomy, was performed. Subsequently, in 1987, the first laparoscopic cholecystectomy was performed [2, 3]. Over the last 20 years, laparoscopic surgery has had a tremendous impact on gastrointestinal surgery. The technique of laparoscopy is considered the standard care for the treatment of gallbladder disease, obesity, gastroesophageal reflux, and many others.

The first laparoscopic colonic resection was performed in 1991. Unlike laparoscopic biliary surgery, this technique was not adopted as quickly. Initially, there were concerns that laparoscopic resection of colorectal carcinoma might cause higher recurrence and inferior long-term survival rates compared to the open technique. We now know that based on the current evidences, laparoscopic surgery for malignancy has equivocal rates of recurrence and survival compared to the open technique.

In particular, there were significant concerns over port site metastasis when early reports revealed unusually high incidence of local wound recurrence, in some reports as high as 21 %. This observation was made even in some patients with

X. Qin et al. (eds.), *Multidisciplinary Management of Liver Metastases in Colorectal Cancer*,
DOI 10.1007/978-94-017-7755-1_11

very early stage colorectal cancer. Most of the recurrences occurred within the first year of surgical resection. Concerns about port site metastases soon limited the introduction of laparoscopic surgery for colorectal malignancies. Subsequently, multiple studies had addressed the issue of port site metastases. Several multicenter randomized controlled studies have revealed no difference in wound or port site recurrence rate between the open and laparoscopic approaches. A recent MEDLINE review of >100 articles concluded that the incidence of port site metastases, generally <1 %, was similar to that of wound recurrence rate in open surgery. It appears that poor surgical technique and failure to follow oncologic principles in the early development of the laparoscopic technique were the causes of this problem [4, 5].

Another explanation for the slow acceptance of laparoscopic approach for colorectal malignancy was the concern for overall recurrence and long-term survival. This has only been recently resolved by the publication of the survival results of the Clinical Outcomes of Surgical Therapy (COST) trial in the USA and similar trials from Europe and Australia.

Cancer-free survival is, by definition, a long-term outcome. Therefore initial studies could only focus on potential surrogate markers between the laparoscopic and open approach. Both Milsom and Lacy have reported equivalence in resection margin and lymph node yielded between open and laparoscopic approaches. Before multicenter randomized trials were completed, there were already several single-center studies (shown in Table 11.1) showing that the long-term results were similar between laparoscopic and open approaches [6–8].

In 2004, the results of the Clinical Outcomes of Surgical Therapy (COST) trial were published in *The New England Journal of Medicine*. Eight hundred and seventy-two patients in 48 institutions were randomly assigned to open and laparoscopic approach for cancer. 3 years later, there were no difference in tumor recurrence (16 % LC vs. 18 % OC), wound recurrence (<1 % in both LC and OC), or overall survival (86 % LC vs. 85 % OC). The rates of intraoperative and overall complications were similar between the laparoscopic and open group, but perioperative recovery was faster in the laparoscopic surgery group. Another large randomized trial, the Conventional versus Laparoscopic-Assisted Surgery in Colorectal Cancer (CLASICC), was conducted in the UK. The results of this study were published in 2007. Seven hundred and ninety-four patients in 27 UK medical centers were randomly assigned to laparoscopic (526) and open (268) approach for cancer, in a 2:1 fashion. 3 years later, there was no difference in OS (68.4 % LC vs. 66.7 % OC), DFS (66.3 % LC vs. 67.7 % OC), local recurrence, distant recurrence, or port site/wound recurrence. This trial again confirmed that in terms of recurrence and long-term survival, a laparoscopic

Table 11.1 Single-center studies showing that the long-term results were similar between laparoscopic and open approaches

Author	Method	Tumor recurrence	Cancer-related death
Fleshman (1996)	Retrospective review, 372 patients	Local implantation 3.6 % (3 years), distant implantation 1.1 % (3 years)	Survival similar to those reported in OC (3 years)
			4 % – stage I
			17 % – stage II
			31 % – stage III
			70 % – stage IV
Hartley (2000)	Prospective comparative trial, 114 patients	Similar between OC and LC 25 % in OC, 28 % in LC (>2 years)	Similar between OC and LC 46 % in OC and LC (>2 years)
Lacy (2002)	Randomized trial, 219 patients	Reduced in LC (95 %CI 0.19–0.82)	Improved in LC (95 % CI 0.16–0.91)

OC open colectomy, *LC* laparoscopic colectomy

approach for colon carcinoma is at least as good as the open approach. In addition, a subset of patients was used to demonstrate that OS, DFS, and local recurrence after laparoscopic rectal resection for rectal cancer were comparable with those of the open approach. The third largest randomized trial, the Colon cancer Laparoscopic or Open Resection (COLOR) trial in Europe, showed similar results, and several meta-analyses have been published from these data, confirming the results. Based on the outcomes of the COST study and other trials, the American Society of Colon and Rectal Surgeons (ASCRS) and Society of American Gastrointestinal Surgeons (SAGES) released the following statement: "Laparoscopic colectomy for curable cancer results in equivalent cancer-related survival to open colectomy when performed by experienced surgeons…" [9–11].

Technical difficulty also contributed to the slow adoption of the laparoscopic approach to colorectal cancer. Unlike other laparoscopic procedures such as Nissen fundoplication or cholecystectomy, laparoscopic colorectal resection requires multiple steps, including significant dissection in multiple abdominal quadrants, division of large vessels, removal of a specimen, and reanastomosis. There is a significant learning curve associated with laparoscopic colorectal surgery. It was recommended that a surgeon should have at least 20 laparoscopic colorectal resections to be considered sufficient and probably much more to be considered experienced. Fortunately, developments in video imaging, energy delivery, and stapling technology in the past decades have made it easier for more surgeons to adopt the laparoscopic technique. In addition, some have modified the technique. Surgeons have utilized the insertion of a handport into a small 7–9 cm incision to perform hand-assisted laparoscopic colorectal surgery. Proponents claim that this technique allows tactile and depth sensation and therefore shortens the learning curve. However, to date, there is no convincing evidence supporting clinical or training benefits of this technique over the standard laparoscopic approach.

While initial concerns about poor oncological outcomes associated with laparoscopic colon resection have been put to rest by the mountain of evidence presented, substantial data also demonstrated significant benefits associated with laparoscopic approach. Most of these studies have revealed that laparoscopic approach is linked with decreased hospital stay, less pain, less bleeding, earlier recovery of gastrointestinal function, shorter recovery, and a reduction in wound and other complication rates compared to the open approach [8, 9, 12–14]. Some meta-analyses also showed reduction in perioperative mortality [15].

A final concern with laparoscopic colectomy is that it may end up being much more expensive than open colectomy. This is particularly noted when length of hospital stay is not reduced or minimally reduced. Many single-center reports that have been published showing improvements or worsening of hospital costs. Most recently, some reports have suggested that in a multicenter approach the procedure can be completed with modest increase in costs of approximately $400 [14, 16–20].

Compared to segmental laparoscopic colon resection, laparoscopic rectal resection is technically more challenging. In the pelvis, manipulation of the bowel and its mesentery are limited by the narrow, long pelvis, particularly in males, tall patients, and in the obese. While avoiding injury to important structures such as the ureters, pelvic autonomic nerves, and the presacral veins, one must perform an oncologically sound total mesorectal excision. Despite these limitations, laparoscopic surgery can potentially enhance pelvic dissection in experienced hands by offering a view with higher magnification. In our opinion, using laparoscopic visualization, the correct anatomical planes can be identified and followed at least as well as in open surgery. Although this could potentially result in improved oncological outcomes and reduction in local recurrence rates, this is unlikely to ever be shown in randomized trials because of variability between patients, surgeons, and techniques, and the fact that the most difficult patients are likely to be performed open because of complicating factors such as prior surgery, obesity, and male gender.

For laparoscopic rectal cancer surgery, there are fewer studies to evaluate the oncological outcomes. However, several series have shown prominent results with laparoscopic approach. Morino et al. reported a prospective series of 100 consecutive laparoscopic TME for middle and low position rectal tumors. The conversion rate was 12 %, anastomotic leak rate was 17 %, and overall postoperative morbidity was 36 %. With a median follow-up of 46 months, the port site metastasis rate was 1.4 % and the overall local recurrence rate was 4.2 %. Five-year survival rates for stage I, II, and III disease were 92 %, 79 %, and 67 %, respectively. This series reveals that the oncological outcomes are equivalent to open published series [21].

Dulucq et al. reported their 12-year experience of 218 patients with a mean follow-up of 57 months. Seventy six patients underwent laparoscopic anterior resection and 142 patients underwent laparoscopic TME. Their conversion rate was 12 % and anastomotic leak rate was 10.5 %, and no port site metastases occurred. The local recurrence rate was 6.8 %. Overall survival rate was 67 % at 5 years and 53 % at 10 years. The short-term complication rate and the long-term oncological outcome in this series are comparable with their prior open reports. Although a case series, this study also forcefully reveals that laparoscopic anterior resection and TME with anal sphincter preservation of rectal cancer can be safe and effectively performed by experts [22].

Kim et al. conducted a series of 312 patients who underwent laparoscopic rectal cancer resection performed by a single surgeon. The conversion rate was 2.6 %, anastomotic leak rate was 6.4 %, and overall morbidity rate was 21 %. Sphincter-preserving surgery was performed in 86 %. The circumferential resection margin positivity rate was 4.2 %. Even though only six patients received preoperative radiotherapy, the recurrence rate was 2.9 % at a mean follow-up of 30 months. No port site recurrence was observed. This report demonstrated that laparoscopic rectal cancer resection can achieve remarkable short- and long-term outcomes in highly skilled surgeon [23].

A meta-analysis carried by Heriot et al. was recently published. The data of all the studies between 1993 and 2004 which compared open and laparoscopic surgery for rectal cancer were pooled and analyzed. Overall, 2,071 patients in 20 studies matched the selection criteria. 990 (44 %) patients underwent laparoscopic surgery and 1,162 (56 %) patients underwent open surgery for rectal cancer. This study showed that there was equivalent in oncologic clearance between laparoscopic and open surgery. However, there were some short-term benefits linked with laparoscopic surgery. It was found that time to first bowel movement, feeding solids, and lengths of hospital stay remarkably reduced after laparoscopic surgery. In abdominoperineal resections patients, wound infection and requirement for postoperative analgesia were also prominently reduced in the laparoscopic group. This study demonstrated that laparoscopic rectal cancer surgery results in a resected specimen that is oncologically equivalent to open surgery and a shorter postoperative recovery [24].

The largest comparative randomized trial thus far accruing patients with rectal cancer is the CLASSIC trial (shown in Table 11.2). Unlike the COST study, rectal cancers were included in CLASSIC trial. Seven hundred and ninety-four patients with colon and rectal carcinoma were randomly assigned to laparoscopic and open surgery in a 2:1 fashion. Approximately 50 % of the patients had rectal cancer. The conversion rate for the rectal cancer patient was high at 34 %. The circumferential resection margin positivity rates were higher in patients undergoing laparoscopic anterior resection (12 % vs. 6 %). However, the

Table 11.2 CLASSIC trial

CLASSIC rectal cancer			
	Laparoscopy	Open	*P*
Number of patients	253	128	
Conversion	34 %	N/A	
APR/AR	63/196	34/96	ns
Positive CRM (APR)	20 %	26 %	ns
Positive CRM (AR)	12 %	6 %	ns
Number of lymph nodes examined	12	13.5	ns
Anastomotic leak	10 %	7 %	ns
Perioperative morbidity	13 %	11 %	ns
Hospital stay	11	13	ns

CRM circumferential resection margin

difference was not statistically significant ($P = 0.19$). At 3-year follow-up, there were undifferentiated in terms of OS, DFS, or local recurrence between laparoscopic AR and open AR patients. Longer follow-up was recommended but not available to date [10].

Although many reports showed promising outcomes for laparoscopic rectal resection, one has to note that most of these surgeons have surpassed their learning curves and have considerable expertise in laparoscopic surgery. It is difficult to generalize these results. More prospective, randomized studies are recommended for accurate comparison between laparoscopic and open approach for rectal cancer. Several other groups have published similarly excellent results, pending the completion of prospective randomized trials addressing laparoscopy for rectal cancer [25–28].

11.3 Surgical Procedures

11.3.1 Preoperative Planning

Preoperative preparation of the patient for laparoscopic colorectal surgery depends on the urgency and magnitude of the procedure, the medical condition of the patient, and the underlying tumor pathology. The surgeon must grasp the exact general medical condition of patient, including any comorbidities that may predispose the patient to cardiopulmonary, cerebrovascular, or musculoskeletal complications. These comorbidities should be corrected or optimized prior to operation. Fluid and electrolyte disorders should be corrected and nutritional states should be optimized. All patients should have bowel preparation to facilitate laparoscopic bowel manipulation. Prophylaxis for deep venous thrombosis shoul be carried out for every patient in the form of heparin and SCDs (brand of antithrombus stretch socks). In the case of rectal cancer, it is important for the surgeon to have all the information regarding tumor location, preoperative tumor stage, and tumor response to preoperative chemoradiotherapy (CRT). Only then can the surgeon decide an operation that will offer patient the best chance for cure, with minimal morbidity and optimal functional results.

11.3.2 Positioning

In our practice, patients are positioned in a standard way regardless of the type of resection. The patient is positioned and secured on a bean bag which will allow angulation of the OR table intraoperatively, to use gravity as an assistant in holding structures in position. The arms are tucked at the patient's side. The legs are placed in stirrups, with the knee slightly flexed and the hips straight. The perineum is positioned at the break of the table, which is especially important for left-sided lesions. An orogastric tube and a Foley catheter are inserted. The abdomen is then prepared and draped routinely. The surgeon and assistant usually stand at either side of the patient, while the scrub nurse with the instrument table stand between the patient's legs.

11.3.3 Surgical Instruments

As laparoscopic surgery continues to advance, the instrumentation also continues to improve with time. It should be noted that all the instruments described below are currently available, both in reusable and disposable format.

11.3.3.1 Laparoscopic Ports

The laparoscopic ports consist of an outer cannula and an inner introducer trocar. The trocar may be sharp or blunt tipped. The ports should be comfortable to use, not easily dislodged during operation, and allow for exchange of surgical instruments efficiently. The port size required reflects the largest instrument that will be introduced through the working port. In most cases, this reflects the stapling devices such as endoscopic GIA, which requires a port size of 12–15 mm diameter.

11.3.3.2 Graspers and Retractors

Bowel graspers are used to hold and manipulate the bowel without tearing it. Therefore, use only atraumatic graspers for this purpose. They should be nonconductive to avoid conduction thermal injury. The coating on the instruments should not be highly reflective in order to avoid impairment of the laparoscopic light detecting system.

There are certain situations that require the use of traumatic graspers. A Maryland grasping forceps has serrated edges and can be useful in grasping small bleeding vessels for coagulation and hemostasis. The laparoscopic Allis forcep is particularly useful for left-sided colectomy. This instrument is used to grasp the anvil of a circular stapler for approximating a left-sided or low rectal anastomosis.

There are several types of retractors, such as the fan retractor, the paddle retractor, or the "snake" retractor, that one can use for retraction of the bowel. However, these retractors are designed for retraction of a solid organ, such as the liver, and they do not work as well for small bowel. In colorectal surgery, we depend on gravity heavily by tilting the table in severe angles to aid in the displacement of the bowel. Most often, this type of maneuver is adequate for the operation. The fan retractor may also be used in the pelvis for retraction of the mesorectum.

11.3.3.3 Energy-Based Dissecting Instrumentation

There are two major types of energy-based dissecting instruments – the Harmonic and the LigaSure. The Harmonic is an ultrasonic-based dissector. The generator generates high-frequency ultrasound waves, which are converted to mechanical vibrations in the functional operating blade. This instrument can be used through the 5 mm ports. The maximum size of the vessels that can be safely divided by the Harmonic is about 5 mm in diameter.

The LigaSure works through a different mechanism by applying pressure and bipolar cautery, generating heat to seal the vessels. This instrument comes in 5 mm and 10 mm diameter. The maximum size of the vessels that can be safely divided by LigaSure is about 7 mm in diameter. The thermal injury to the surrounding tissue is limited to only about 2 mm. In our practice, the LigaSure is routinely used to seal large vessels such as the ileocolic, middle colic, and left colic arteries. We apply double-firing technique to assure hemostasis before division of these large vessels. Although both of these energy sources are effective, we perform most dissection using scissors and monopolar cautery, as we feel this is the most expedient technique for dissection.

11.4 Operative Procedures

11.4.1 Laparoscopic Right Hemicolectomy

11.4.1.1 Step 1. Position and Equipment (Fig. 11.1)

The patient is positioned on a bean bag and secured to the table. After induction of general anesthesia, an orogastric tube and Foley catheter are inserted. The legs are placed in stirrups and the arms are tucked at the patient's side. We use the atraumatic 5 mm bowel graspers for manipulation of the bowel and use the cautery scissors for dissection. An Endo GIA with vascular load or LigaSure is used for division of the ileocolic artery.

11.4.1.2 Step 2. Port Placement (Fig. 11.2)

A 10 mm subumbilical incision is made. The fascia is opened and the abdomen entered using Hasson technique. A purse-string stitch on the fascia and a Rommel tourniquet is used to pre-

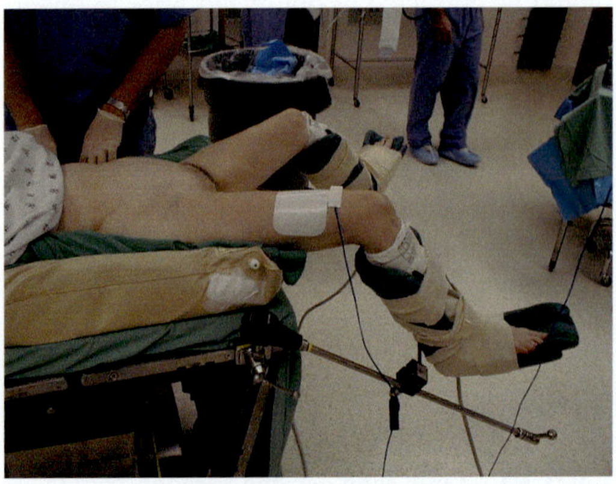

Fig. 11.1 Position (R hemi)

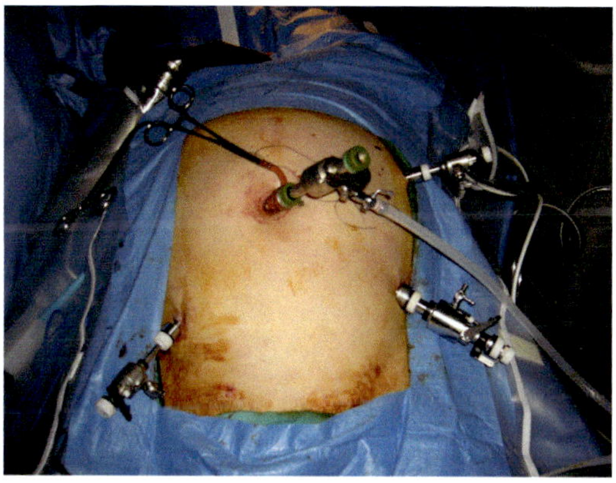

Fig. 11.2 Port placement (R hemi)

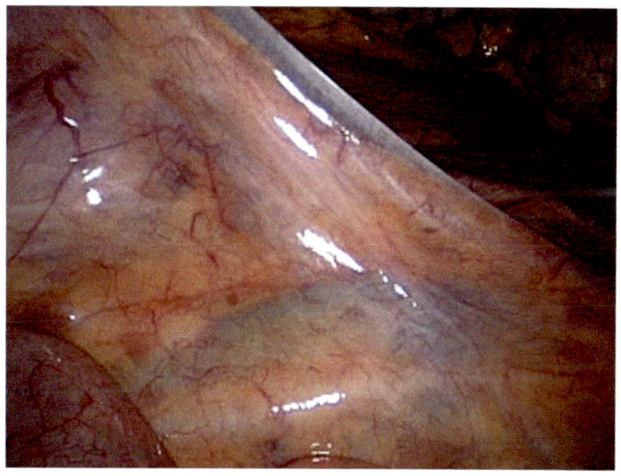

Fig. 11.3 Exposure of operating field (R hemi)

vent air leak. A 10 mm port is inserted. The abdomen is insufflated with CO_2 to pressure of 15 mmHg. Under direct vision, a 12 mm port is inserted in the left lower quadrant (10 mm if planning to use LigaSure for vessel division). Its location is approximately 3 cm medial and superior to the anterior superior iliac spine. Further 5 mm ports are placed in the left upper, right lower, and sometimes right upper quadrant. For obese patients, one may move the left-sided ports more medially. Make sure at least a hand's breadth is present between all ports.

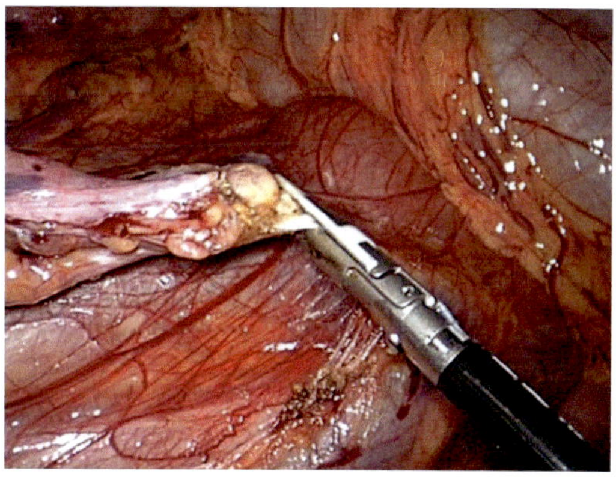

Fig. 11.4 Division ileocolic artery (R hemi)

11.4.1.3 Step 3. Exposure of the Operating Field (Fig. 11.3)

The assistant now moves to the left side of the patient, standing caudad to the surgeon. The patient is placed in slight Trendelenburg position and rotated to the left. The greater omentum is lifted over the stomach, above the transverse colon. The small bowel is grasped and moved medially so that the cecum, terminal ileum, and the ileocolic pedicle are exposed. Gravitational force alone is often adequate for displacement of the small bowel.

11.4.1.4 Step 4. Identification and Division of the Ileocolic Artery (Fig. 11.4)

The mesentery of the terminal ileum is grasped and lifted up. This will expose and stretch the ileocolic artery. The peritoneum is opened with cautery scissors along a line between the ileocolic artery and the superior mesenteric artery. Using blunt dissection, the ileocolic pedicle is lifted up. An opening is made with cautery scissors just lateral to the ileocolic artery. Thus a window is created around the ileocolic artery for vessel division. It is important for the dissection to be carried just anterior to the congenital peritoneum, so that the retroperitoneal structures such as the ureter will not be injured and need not be displayed. The vascular division may be done with stapler, energy source, or clips. High ligation of the ileocolic artery is performed for cancer cases.

11.4.1.5 Step 5. Mobilization of the Hepatic Flexure (Fig. 11.5)

After ligation of the ileocolic artery, the plane between the ascending colon mesentery and the

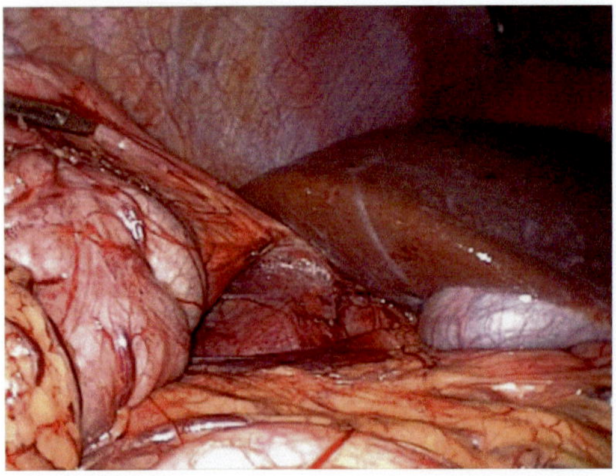

Fig. 11.5 Mobilization of hepatic flexure (R hemi)

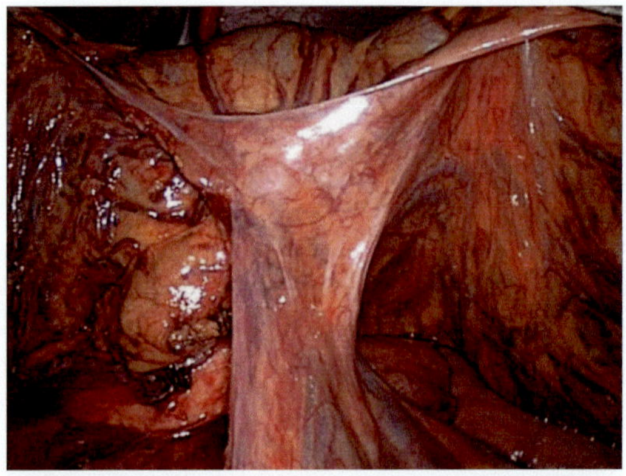

Fig. 11.6 Division of right branch of middle colic artery (R hemi)

retroperitoneum is developed with blunt dissection. Laterally the dissection reaches the congenital white line of Toldt. Superiorly the dissection reaches the transverse colon, separating the mesentery off the anterior surface of the duodenum and the pancreas. The patient is then put in reverse Trendelenburg position. The transverse colon is grasped and pulled inferiorly exposing the gastrocolic ligament. Using cautery scissors or other energy-based dissection device, the gastrocolic ligament is divided. Dissection continues laterally and inferiorly. This dissection will connect to the prior retroperitoneal dissection. Laterally, the white line of Toldt is then completely divided right down to the base of the cecum.

11.4.1.6 Step 6. Identification and Division of the Right Branch of the Middle Colic Vessels (Fig. 11.6)

In order to easily exteriorize the right colon and tension-free anastomosis, the middle colic artery's right branch is identified and divided.

11.4.1.7 Step 7. Mobilization of the Ileocecal Junction (Fig. 11.7)

The patient is now positioned in Trendelenburg position. The small bowel is placed superiorly and medially. The plane between the mesentery of the terminal ileum and the retroperitoneum is

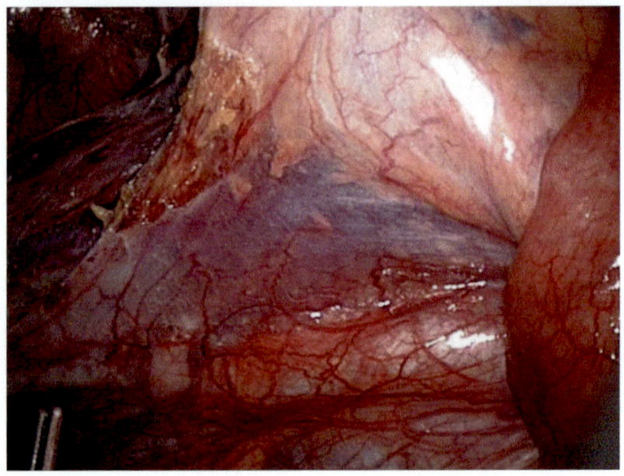

Fig. 11.7 Mobilization of ileocecal junction (R hemi)

developed with sharp dissection. The dissection is carried medially to the third portion of duodenum. The colon is now completely mobile to the midline.

11.4.1.8 Step 8. Exteriorization of the Specimen (Fig. 11.8)

Before extraction of the specimen, the right colon is grasped and tested for its mobility. Hemostasis is assured. All trocar incisions larger than 5 mm (except the subumbilical incision) are closed with a Carter-Thompson suture passer and an 0 Polysorb tie. The cecum is grasped with an atraumatic bowel clamp. Pneumoperitoneum is deflated and subumbilical incision is extended to 3–4 cm. For colon carcinoma, exteriorizing the specimen should always be got through a wound protector (protractor, medium or small) to reduce the risk of port site metastasis. The small bowel, colon, and the mesentery are divided. Specimen is removed to a nearby table and opened to confirm pathology and margin.

11.4.1.9 Step 9. Creation of Anastomosis

An ileocolic anastomosis is fashioned. The mesenteric window does not require closure. It is necessary to check for hemostasis and integrity of the anastomosis and then returned it to abdomen.

11.4.1.10 Step 10. Wound Closure

The midline incision fascia is closed in the standard fashion. The subcutaneous spaces are irrigated, and wounds are sutured with subcuticular 4-0 absorbable sutures.

Hints

- Use a Rommel tourniquet for the umbilical port.
- Use Carter-Thompson with 0 Polysorb tie to close any port >5 mm.
- Have endoclip in room.
- Use Endo GIA or LigaSure for division of the ileocolic artery.
- Use a wound protector for cancer cases. (Protractor, small or medium)

11.4.2 Laparoscopic Sigmoid Hemicolectomy

11.4.2.1 Step 1. Position and Equipment

The patient is positioned on a bean bag and secured to table. After induction of general anesthesia, an orogastric tube and Foley catheter are inserted. The legs are placed in stirrups and the arms are tucked at the patient's side. The perineum should be at or below the break of the table (Fig. 11.1). Atraumatic 5 mm bowel graspers are used for manipulation of the bowel, and cautery scissors for dissection. An Endo GIA with vascular load or LigaSure is used for division of the inferior mesenteric artery. The laparoscopic Allis forceps is used for firm holding of the anvil of a circular stapler.

11.4.2.2 Step 2. Port Placement (Fig. 11.9)

A 10 mm subumbilical incision is made. The fascia is opened and the abdomen entered using Hasson technique. A purse-string stitch on the fascia and a Rommel tourniquet is used to prevent air leak. A 10 mm port is inserted. The abdomen is insufflated with CO_2 to pressure of 15 mmHg. Under direct vision, a 12 mm port is inserted in the right lower quadrant. Its location is approximately 3 cm medial and superior to the anterior superior iliac spine. Further 5 mm ports are placed in the right upper and left lower quadrant. A left

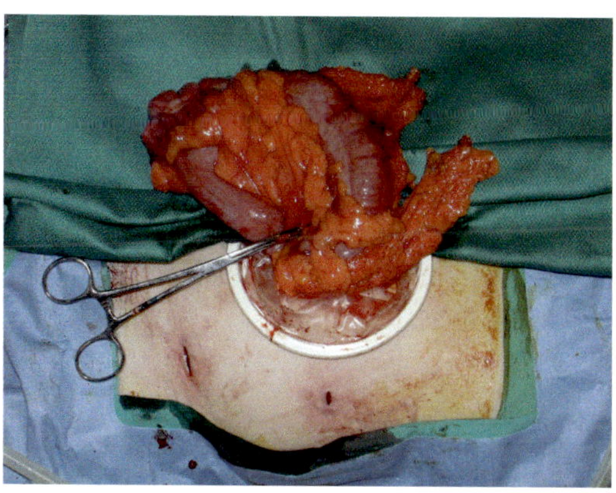

Fig. 11.8 Exteriorization of specimen (R hemi)

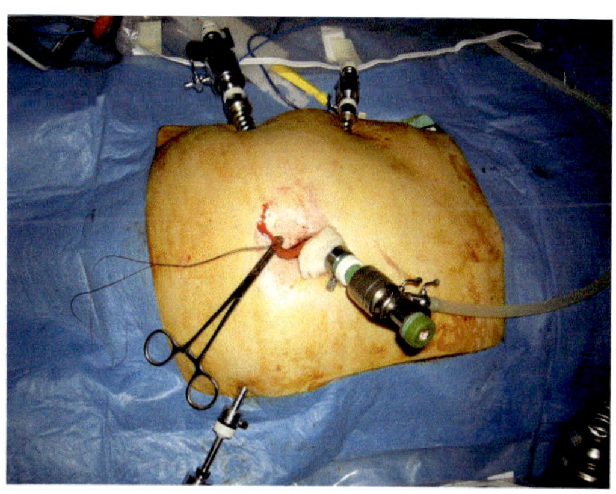

Fig. 11.9 Port placement (sigmoid colectomy)

upper quadrant port is selectively inserted to assist splenic flexure mobilization. For obese patients, one may move the right-sided ports more medially. Make sure there is at least a hand's breadth distance between all ports.

11.4.2.3 Step 3. Exposure of the Operating Field (Fig. 11.10)

The assistant now moves to the right side of the patient, standing cephalad to the surgeon. The patient is placed in Trendelenburg position and rotated to the right. The greater omentum is lifted superiorly to above the transverse colon. The small bowel is grasped and moved to the right side so that the medial aspect of the rectosigmoid mesentery is exposed. Gravitational force alone is often adequate for displacement of the small bowel.

11.4.2.4 Step 4. Identification of Inferior Mesenteric Vessels and Left Ureter (Fig. 11.11)

The rectosigmoid mesentery at the level of the sacral promontory is grasped and lifted anteriorly and superiorly. The contour of the inferior mesenteric artery (IMA) pedicle at the level of the pelvic brim is demonstrated. The peritoneum beneath the IMA groove is opened with cautery scissors. This opening is extended to the origin of the inferior mesenteric artery cranially and to the sacral promontory caudally. Using a blunt instrument, the inferior mesenteric artery is lifted. A dissection plane is developed to reveal the posterior surface of the capsule of the IMA. This keeps the hypogastric nerves posteriorly and ureter posterolaterally safe from injury. Unlike laparoscopic right hemicolectomy, it is necessary to identify the ureter before proceeding with the rest of the operation. If the left ureter cannot be discovered, the anatomy may be too deep in the retroperitoneum. In this situation, the ureter has often been elevated on the back of the inferior mesenteric pedicle. The surgeon should try to perform the dissection close to the vessel to discover the ureter and to protect the autonomic nerves. If the surgeon still can't find the ureter, then a lateral to medial approach often helps. Starting just distal to the sacral promontory is usually an easy way to discover the correct plane. Rarely the left ureter might not be identified, or else the options are either insertion of ureteric stents or conversion to open surgery.

11.4.2.5 Step 5. Division of the Inferior Mesenteric Artery (Fig. 11.12)

An opening is made with cautery scissors lateral to the inferior mesenteric artery to create a window in the peritoneum. The vascular division may be got with an energy source, stapler, or clips. High ligation (division above the left colic artery) of the vessel is performed. There

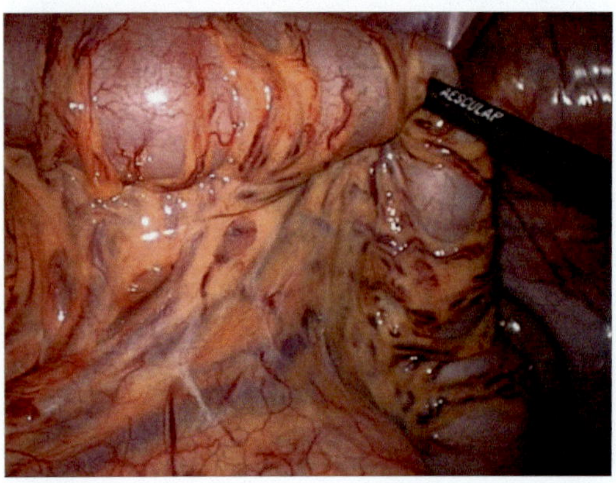

Fig. 11.10 Exposure of operating field (sigmoid colectomy)

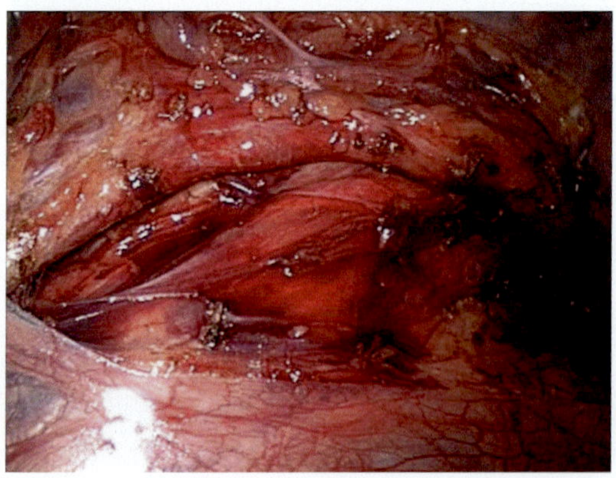

Fig. 11.11 Identification of IMA and left ureter (sigmoid colectomy)

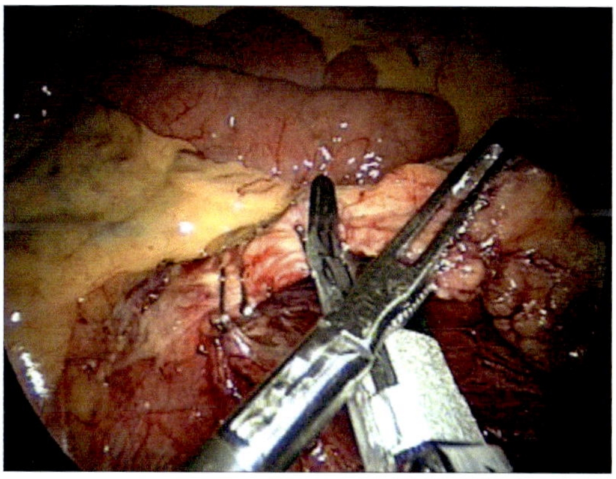

Fig. 11.12 Division of IMA (sigmoid colectomy)

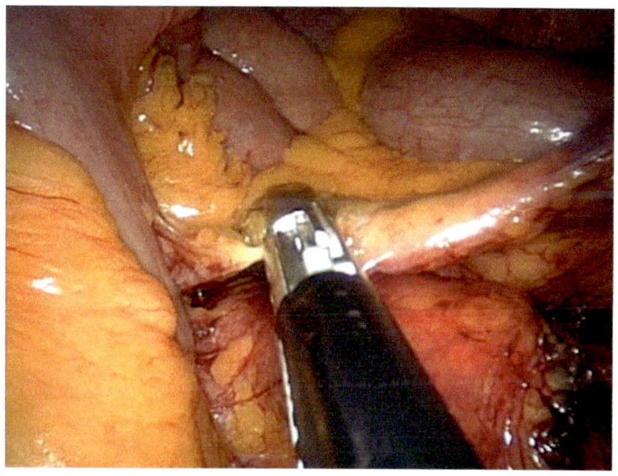

Fig. 11.13 Division of IMV (sigmoid colectomy)

are several advantages in performing high ligation of the IMA. This removes the apical lymphatic nodes along with the resected surgical specimen. It maintains collateral supply to the left colon by preserving the bifurcation of the ascending and descending branches of the left colic artery. A high ligation of the IMA also assists in attaining a tension-free colorectal anastomosis; this is especially true for low rectal carcinomas.

11.4.2.6 Step 6. Division of the Inferior Mesenteric Vein (IMV) (Fig. 11.13)

The peritoneum is dissected along the lower border of the IMV from the IMA up to the ligament of Treitz. Division of the IMV at this level assists in mobilization of the left colon and attaining a tension-free colorectal anastomosis. The vascular division is performed with an energy course, stapler, or clips.

11.4.2.7 Step 7. Mobilization of the Left Colon (Fig. 11.14)

After division of the inferior mesenteric vessels, the plane between the left mesocolon and the retroperitoneum is developed. By gentle dissection, the left mesocolon can lightly be lifted off the retroperitoneum from a medial approach. This plane is developed laterally to the white line of Toldt (lateral attachment of the colon). Superiorly the dissection is carried toward the splenic flexure, dissecting the bowel off the anterior surface

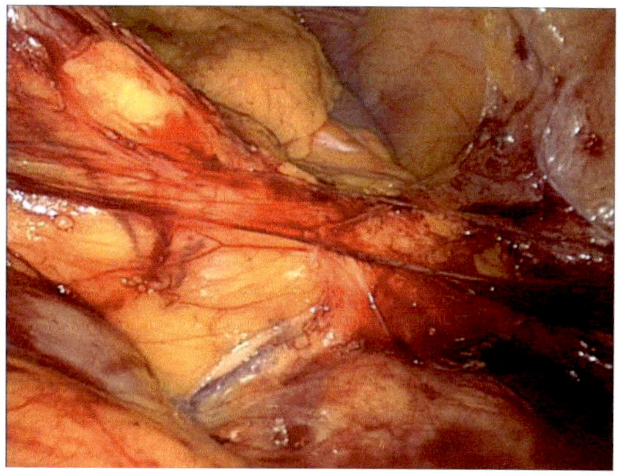

Fig. 11.14 Mobilization of left colon (sigmoid colectomy)

of the Gerota's fascia. Dissection is then carried inferiorly to mobilize the right side of the mesorectum.

After completing the medial dissection, a lateral dissection is carried out. The rectosigmoid junction is grasped and drawn to the right side of the patient. The lateral attachments of the sigmoid colon and the descending colon are divided using cautery scissors. Once this is done, the left and sigmoid colon are completely free and become a midline structure.

11.4.2.8 Step 8. Division of the Upper Rectum and Mesorectum (Fig. 11.15)

The rectosigmoid junction is grasped and drawn out of the pelvis. This reveals the

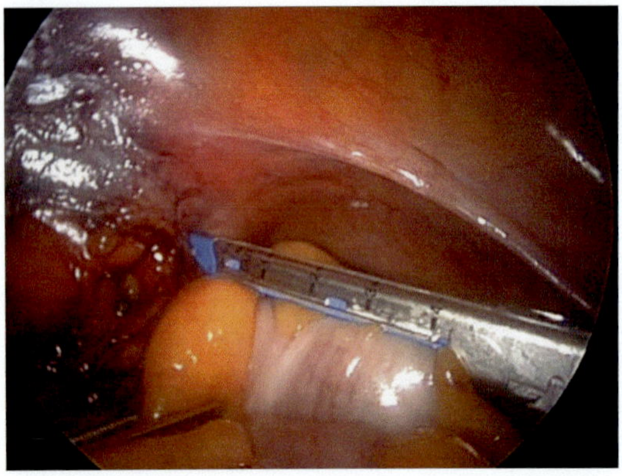

Fig. 11.15 Division of upper rectum (sigmoid colectomy)

posterior surface of the mesorectum and the presacral space. A decision is made about the distal margin of resection (a flexible endoscope may be inserted to identify for position of the carcinoma). The peritoneum is opened with cautery scissors perpendicular to the colon. A tunnel between the rectum and the mesorectum is then developed using atraumatic bowel graspers. This step is carried out very carefully to prevent perforation of the rectum or avulsion of small vessels off the back of the mesorectum. A laparoscopic linear stapler, such as Endo GIA stapler, is inserted through the 12 mm port in the right lower quadrant to divide the rectum.

11.4.2.9 Step 9. Division of the Upper Rectum and Mesorectum (Fig. 11.16)

The left lower quadrant port site incision is enlarged to 3–4 cm. For colon carcinoma, exteriorizing the specimen should always be got through a wound protector (protractor, medium or small) to reduce the risk of port site metastasis. The specimen is then exteriorized. The descending colon mesentery and the bowel are divided. A Babcock clamp is placed on the proximal end of the colon to prevent it from slipping back inside the abdomen. The specimen is examined to confirm adequacy of margins.

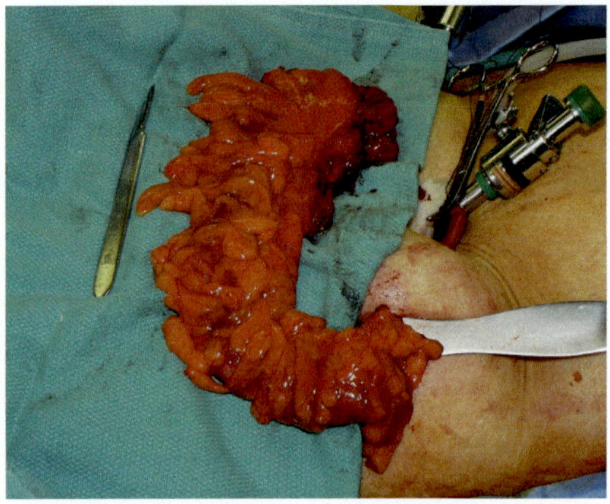

Fig. 11.16 Exteriorization of specimen (sigmoid colectomy)

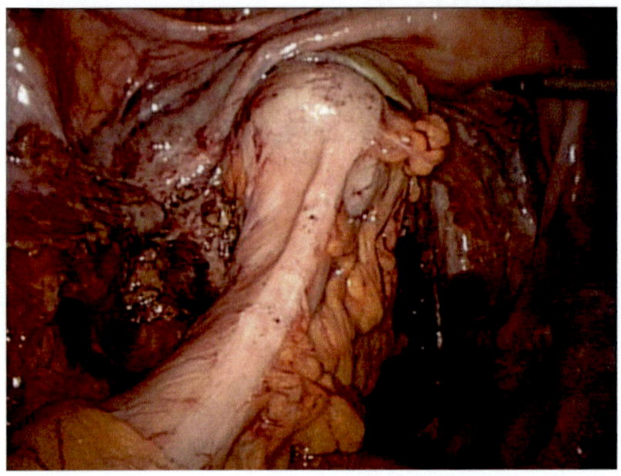

Fig. 11.17 Colorectal anastomosis (sigmoid colectomy)

11.4.2.10 Step 10. Creation of the Anastomosis (Fig. 11.17)

A purse-string suture is placed on the proximal end of the colon. The anvil of a circular stapler is inserted (normally size 28 in our practice) and the purse-string suture tied. The colon end with the anvil is returned to the abdomen and the fascia is closed. The abdomen is then insufflated again. It is important to make sure that there is adequate reach so that there is no tension on the anastomosis. It is also important to check the colonic mesentery orientation to avoid torsion of the anastomosis. If reach is not adequate, then further mobilization of the splenic flexure is necessary. The circular stapler is inserted through the anus and discreetly advanced up to the rectal remnant resection line. Then the anastomosis is made under direct vision.

The anastomosis is checked with the following steps. First the doughnuts are examined to be sure that they are completely intact with all layers. Then the rectum is insufflated with air with the pelvic cavity filled with water. If during these steps the anastomosis was found to be inadequate, then it should either be redone or strengthened with sutures.

11.4.2.11 Step 11. Wound Closure

All trocar incisions larger than 5 mm are sutured. The subcutaneous spaces are irrigated, and wounds are sutured with subcuticular 4-0 absorbable sutures.

Hints

- Use a Rommel tourniquet for the umbilical port.
- Use Carter-Thompson with 0 Polysorb tie to close any port >5 mm.
- Have endoclip in room.
- Use Endo GIA or LigaSure for division of the inferior mesenteric vessels.
- For division of the rectum, two firings are usually required with the Endo GIA.
- To check for reach (for anastomosis), place the colon with anvil into the pelvis. If it lies there without falling back into abdomen, then reach is adequate.
- Use a wound protector for cancer cases (protractor, small or medium).

11.4.3 Laparoscopic Low Anterior Resection

The decision for abdominoperineal resection with colostomy or a low anterior resection is based on oncological principles, patient preference, and the experience of the surgeon. Abdominoperineal resection is normally reserved for patients with tumors abutting the sphincter complex or those patients with anal incontinence.

11.4.3.1 Step 1. Position and Equipment

As per description of laparoscopic sigmoid hemicolectomy.

11.4.3.2 Step 2. Port Placement

As per description of laparoscopic sigmoid hemicolectomy.

11.4.3.3 Step 3. Exposure of the Operating Field

As per description of laparoscopic sigmoid hemicolectomy.

11.4.3.4 Step 4. Identification of Inferior Mesenteric Vessels and Left Ureter

As per description of laparoscopic sigmoid hemicolectomy.

11.4.3.5 Step 5. Division of the Inferior Mesenteric Artery

As per description of laparoscopic sigmoid hemicolectomy.

11.4.3.6 Step 6. Division of the Inferior Mesenteric Vein

As per description of laparoscopic sigmoid hemicolectomy.

11.4.3.7 Step 7. Mobilization of the Left Colon

As per description of laparoscopic sigmoid hemicolectomy

Complete mobilization of the left colon is not necessary. The left colon is only mobilized enough to give adequate length for the colostomy.

11.4.3.8 Step 8. Proximal Division of the Left Colon

The division level of the left colon is selected to secure a healthy and well-functioning stoma. The left colon mesentery is divided at the preferred level. The marginal artery can be clipped and divided. The surgeon can also use an energy source to divide the mesentery up to the bowel edge. The colon is then divided with a laparoscopic linear stapler.

11.4.3.9 Step 9. Mobilization of the Rectum

As per description of laparoscopic sigmoid hemicolectomy.

To perform a total mesorectal excision is necessary; however, the pelvic dissection does not go to the anal canal but rather stops at the tip of the coccyx posteriorly and below the prostate anteriorly. A sponge is placed posteriorly at this site, which will be removed during the perineal dissection. The levator ani muscles are usually divided from below after making the perineal incision.

11.4.3.10 Step 10. Creation of Left Iliac Fossa Colostomy

A skin disk is excised at the left iliac fossa colostomy site. The anterior rectus fascia is opened longitudinally with cautery. The rectus muscle is then split with a long Kelly. The peritoneum is grasped and opened. The distal end of the left colon is delivered through the ostomy site and grasped by a Babcock forceps. The colostomy is then matured with absorbable sutures in the standard fashion.

11.4.3.11 Step 11. Perineal Dissection

The anus is closed with a 2-0 nylon suture, and the perineum usually requires to be re-prepared and draped. An elliptical skin incision is made around the anus. Laterally, the dissection plane is outside the external anal sphincter muscle. The incision continues deeply to enter the ischiorectal fossae bilaterally. The tip of the coccyx is the posterior landmark of the dissection. However, in some posterior rectal cancer, the coccyx may be resected with the specimen to ensure a safe resection margin. The dissection continues laterally and posteriorly to expose the levator ani muscles. The levator ani muscles are then divided posteriorly, entering the pelvis at the distal margin of the abdominal dissection and removing the sponge that had been placed laparoscopically. The remaining lateral and anterior attachments are then divided. Technically the anterior dissection is often the most challenging. The urethra in men and the posterior vaginal wall in women must not be injured during anterior dissection. Once the perineal dissection is completed, the specimen can be delivered through the perineal opening. The perineal wound is then thoroughly irrigated to wash out blood and debris. Pelvic and perineal hemostasis is secured and the wound closed in layers.

11.4.3.12 Step 12. Wound Closure

All trocar incisions larger than 5 mm are sutured. The subcutaneous spaces are irrigated, and wounds are sutured with subcuticular 4-0 absorbable sutures.

Hints

- Use a Rommel tourniquet for the umbilical port.
- Use Carter-Thompson with 0 Polysorb tie to close any port >5 mm.
- Use Endo GIA or LigaSure for division of the inferior mesenteric vessels.
- Proximal division of the left colon is done before the perineal dissection is completed. This is because the pneumoperitoneum will disappear once the perineal dissection reaches the abdominal cavity.
- During rectal dissection, the uterus can be suspended from the abdominal wall using a Keith needle.
- During anterior perineal dissection, the specimen may be extracted from the pelvis to facilitate division of any remaining anterior attachments of the rectum.
- Use a wound protector for cancer cases (protractor, small or medium).

11.4.4 Laparoscopic Hartmann Procedure

Infrequently a laparoscopic Hartmann procedure may be required for patients with rectal cancer.

The indications for this procedure are generally related to very advanced age or infirmity in whom one does not want to put the patient at risk of a coloanal anastomosis or when anal sphincter tone is inadequate for anastomosis. This has the potential benefit of avoiding a perineal wound for these infirm patients.

11.4.4.1 Step 1. Position and Equipment

As per description of laparoscopic low anterior resection.

11.4.4.2 Step 2. Port Placement

As per description of laparoscopic low anterior resection.

11.4.4.3 Step 3. Exposure of the Operating Field

As per description of laparoscopic low anterior resection.

11.4.4.4 Step 4. Identification of Inferior Mesenteric Vessels and Left Ureter

As per description of laparoscopic low anterior resection.

11.4.4.5 Step 5. Division of the Inferior Mesenteric Artery

As per description of laparoscopic low anterior resection.

11.4.4.6 Step 6. Division of the Inferior Mesenteric Vein

As per description of laparoscopic low anterior resection.

11.4.4.7 Step 7. Mobilization of the Left Colon

As per description of laparoscopic low anterior resection.

It is not necessary to mobilize the left colon completely. The left colon is only mobilized enough to give adequate length to the colonic stoma.

11.4.4.8 Step 8. Mobilization of the Rectum

As per description of laparoscopic low anterior resection.

11.4.4.9 Step 9. Division of the Rectum

As per description of laparoscopic low anterior resection.

11.4.4.10 Step 10. Exteriorization of the Specimen

The specimen can be extracted from a left lower quadrant stoma site, or it can be extracted through a separate Pfannenstiel incision, especially if the bowel and mesentery are bulky. The left colon is divided and the specimen removed and checked for margin.

11.4.4.11 Step 11. Creation of Left Iliac Fossa Colostomy

As per description of laparoscopic abdominoperineal resection.

11.4.4.12 Step 12. Wound Closure

All trocar incisions larger than 5 mm are sutured. The subcutaneous spaces are irrigated, and wounds are sutured with subcuticular 4-0 absorbable sutures.

11.4.5 Laparoscopic Loop Sigmoid Colostomy

When patients presented with obstructing unresectable rectal cancer, palliative options might help the patient. The options include endoscopically placed rectal stents, fulguration of the rectal tumor, and laparoscopic loop colostomy.

11.4.5.1 Step 1. Position and Equipment

As per description of laparoscopic sigmoid colectomy.

11.4.5.2 Step 2. Port Placement (Fig. 11.18)

A 10 mm subumbilical incision is made. The fascia is opened and abdomen entered using

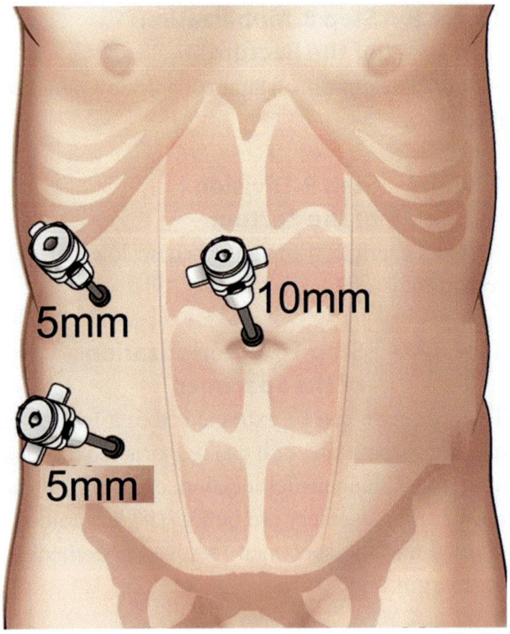

Fig. 11.18 Port placement (loop sigmoid colostomy)

Hasson technique. A purse-string stitch on the fascia and a Rommel tourniquet is used to prevent air leak. A 10 mm port is inserted. Abdomen is insufflated with CO2 to pressure of 12 mmHg. Under direct vision, in the right lower quadrant, a 5 mm port is inserted. Its location is approximately 3 cm medial and superior to the anterior superior iliac spine. Another 5 mm port is placed in the right upper quadrant. If an additional port is required, it can be placed at the planed ostomy site. Make sure at least a hand's breadth distance is present between all ports.

11.4.5.3 Step 3. Exposure of the Operating Field

As per description of laparoscopic sigmoid colectomy.

11.4.5.4 Step 4. Mobilization of the Sigmoid Colon

The surgeon grasps the sigmoid colon and raises it toward the abdominal wall. If the sigmoid colon cannot reach the abdominal wall without tension, then division of lateral attachments of sigmoid colon is necessary.

11.4.5.5 Step 5. Creation of Left Iliac Fossa Colostomy

A skin disk is excised at the left iliac fossa colostomy site. The anterior rectus fascia is opened longitudinally with cautery. The rectus muscle is then split with a long Kelly. The peritoneum is grasped and opened. The sigmoid colon is delivered through the ostomy site and grasped by a Babcock forceps. A stoma rod is passed between the bowel and the mesentery to support the colon.

11.4.5.6 Step 6. Wound Closure

All trocar incisions larger than 5 mm are sutured. The subcutaneous spaces are irrigated, and wounds are sutured with subcuticular 4-0 absorbable sutures.

11.4.5.7 Step 7. Stoma Maturation

The loop colostomy is matured with absorbable sutures in the standard fashion.

11.5 Postoperative Care for Colorectal Surgery Using Fast-Track Care Pathways

For patients undergoing major abdominal surgeries, the traditional postoperative care pathway involves the routine use of nasogastric tubes, prolonged abstinence of oral intake until the patient demonstrates gastrointestinal (GI) function with flatus, copious analgesia, and prolonged bladder catheterization. As a result of this type of postoperative management, patients routinely stay in the hospital for 1–2 weeks following colorectal surgery. There are many unwanted consequences with prolonged hospital stays. On an individual level, patients tend to have increased nosocomial infections and complication with prolonged stay. At the institutional or national level, it means more stress on medical resources which have been limited already. The HCFA data (Medicare) from 1999 to 2000 in the USA demonstrated that approximately 160,000 patients underwent major intestinal and colorectal resection, with a mean postoperative stay of 11.3 days and with a total of 1.8 million bed days. The estimated total postoperative cost was $1.75 billion per annum.

There is increasing effort over the past decade to develop approaches to reduce hospital stay and improve efficiency of provision of care. Postoperative stay is related to pain, ileus, fatigue, stress-induced organ dysfunction, and mechanical factors (such as drains). Multiple studies have been conducted to explore the effect of these factors.

Cheatham ML et al. studied the effect of routine nasogastric tubes after elective laparotomy. A meta-analysis was performed utilizing data from 26 trials and 3,694 patients. Their study revealed that for those patients who didn't manage with nasogastric tubes, there was greater incidence of abdominal distension and vomiting requiring 5 % reinsertion rate of the nasogastric tubes. There were no other complications. Fever, atelectasis, and pneumonia were meaningfully less common and days to first oral intake were meaningfully fewer in patients who didn't manage with nasogastric tubes. They concluded that routine nasogastric decompression is not supported [29].

Postoperative pain management is essential for patients' recovery. The aim for postoperative pain control is to reduce or eliminate pain with minimum side effects as efficiently as possible. Since pain in the postoperative period represents the effect of several different nociceptive mechanisms, several different treatment modalities can be used in combination to optimize analgesia and minimize side effects. This includes opioid analgesia (IV form such as PCA or oral form), NSAIDs, and/or epidurals. Knowing that individual requirements for opioids vary considerably, patient-controlled analgesia (PCA) has become a popular choice for postoperative pain control. These systems, which allow patients administer their own intravenous analgesia and titrate the dose to their own end-point of pain, therefore allow lower doses to be administered.

There are some controversies in terms of the efficacy of epidural anesthesia. It has been suggested by some doctors that the use of local anesthetic through the epidural may improve gastrointestinal function and reduce ileus [30]. Carli et al. showed that thoracic epidural analgesia provides superior quality of analgesia and shortens the duration of postoperative ileus (POI), and this has been confirmed in Cochrane database meta-analysis. However, these and other studies do not demonstrate any shortening of hospital length of stay (LOS) with epidural [31, 32].

NSAIDs have not only analgesic but also anti-inflammatory actions. Their action mechanism is mainly predominantly by inhibition of prostaglandins, the chief mediators of inflammation. It has been demonstrated in several randomized studies that the combination of NSAIDs with opioids improves analgesia and reduces analgesia requirements.

POI is defined as a transient impairment of bowel motility occurring after surgery. It is considered a usual response to surgery. The average ileus duration after major abdominal surgery varies depending on the organ. In general, the small intestine recovers first (12–24 h), then the stomach (24–48 h), and finally the colon (48–120 h). The postoperative ileus duration is connected with the anatomic location of surgery, degree of surgical manipulation, and the magnitude of inflammatory response. The pathogenesis of ileus is not completely understood, but it is generally accepted that there are three major factors causing it: inhibitory sympathetic reflexes initiated from the injury site, local intestinal inflammatory responses, and the use of opioids.

Traditionally, the therapy has primarily involved nasogastric intubation and IV fluids. Some surgeon even uses laxatives or prokinetic agents for the management of postoperative ileus, although studies do not show any consistent clinical benefit to reduce POI with these efforts. Recently, however, as more active researches carried out in this field, some pharmacologic options are emerging for preventing postoperative ileus.

The most promising group of pharmacologic agents to date are peripheral opioid receptor antagonists. These agents selectively inhibit the GI tract mu-opioid receptors without reversing centrally mediated opioid-induced analgesia. Two peripherally acting mu-opioid receptor antagonists have been studied extensively. Alvimopan has been shown to reduce postoperative nausea and vomiting, POI, and the hospital LOS. In the USA, it was recently approved for the POI treatment after abdominal surgery with bowel resection. Methylnaltrexone has also been evaluated for the POI treatment. Phase II data demonstrated that methylnaltrexone was effective for reducing POI and LOS, improving GI recovery. But further studies are necessary to determine the potential role of methylnaltrexone in the prevention of POI [33–39].

Based on the data mentioned above, the concept of "fast-track" or "enhanced recovery" postoperative care was developed to accelerate recovery, reduce hospital stay, and improve morbidity. In essence, multimodal rehabilitation emphasizes on preoperative information, reducing the surgical stress responses and optimizing pain relief, and early mobilization and oral nutrition reduces hospital stay, morbidity, convalescence, and cost.

Basse et al. performed a prospective, nonrandomized study in 30 consecutive patients who undergo fast-track rehabilitation manage and 30 consecutive patients who undergo conventional care manage after colonic surgery. The median hospital stay was reduced from 8 days in the conventional care group to 2 days in the fast-track group. They also demonstrated that fast-track rehabilitation results in earlier normal activities resumption with reduced fatigue without increased needing for nursing care [40].

We performed a prospective, randomized, controlled trial between a pathway of controlled rehabilitation with early ambulation and diet (CREAD) and traditional postoperative care after laparotomy and intestinal resection. Sixty-four patients underwent intestinal or rectal resections were randomly assigned to pathway of CREAD and traditional postoperative care. We reported a significant reduction in the length of stay from 7.1 days in traditional group to 5.4 days in fast-track group. There was undifferentiated in terms of readmission or complication rates, pain score, or quality of life after surgery [41]. In other studies, we reported these pathways reducing mean hospital stay to 4.3 days after open colorectal surgery, including reoperative and pelvic surgery [42].

The application of laparoscopic surgery to colorectal resection can easily be integrated into fast-track protocols. Delaney et al. compared the short-term outcomes in age-matched patients who underwent laparoscopic versus open colectomy managed with CREAD protocol. It was demonstrated that CREAD protocol can be safely done in all age groups. There were some additional benefits to older patients because of reductions in length of hospital stay, morbidity and mortality rates, and direct cost of care. In a separate study, the same authors also demonstrated that CREAD protocol can be applied to complex reoperative pelvic surgeries with a reduction in the length of hospital stay without any increased complications [43]. Most recently, we have shown that these pathways can be used in combination with laparoscopy to give mean hospital stays of under 4 days for laparoscopic colorectal surgery and median stays of 3 days for rectal surgery, with up to 10 % of patients going home 24 h after surgery [44, 45].

In conclusion, current results from the studies of fast-track colonic surgery demonstrate that this technique can improve postoperative organ functions; allow for early rehabilitation with decreased hospital stay, convalescence, and costs; and be applied safely to patients undergoing either open or laparoscopic colorectal surgery.

- *CREAD Protocol for Open Colectomies:*
  - Preoperative information and education.
  - No nasogastric intubation or epidurals.
  - PCA analgesia, supplementary IV Toradol.
  - Encouraged to ambulate five times a day post-op day 1.
  - Liquids ad lib after surgery. Carbohydrate drink daily.
  - Diet from morning post-op day 2.
  - Oral analgesia post-op day 2 if tolerating diet.
  - Foley out post-op day 2.
- *CREAD Protocol for Laparoscopic Colectomies*:
  - Preoperative information and education.
  - No nasogastric intubation or epidurals.
  - PCA analgesia, supplementary IV Toradol.
  - Encouraged to ambulate five times a day post-op day 1.
  - Liquids ad lib after surgery. Carbohydrate drink daily.

  - Diet from morning post-op day 1, chewing gum.
  - Oral analgesia post-op day 1 if tolerating diet.
  - Foley out post-op day 1.
- *Discharge Criteria*:
  - Passing flatus or stool
  - Tolerating fluids and solid diet
  - Comfortable on oral analgesia
  - Happy to be discharged, with adequate home support

References

1. Devesa, et al. Colorectal cancer incidence trends by subsite in urban Shanghai, 1972–1994. Cancer Epidemiol Biomarkers Prev. 1998;7(8):661–6.
2. Dubois, et al. Laparoscopic cholecystectomy: historic perspective and personal experience. Surg Laparosc Endosc. 1991;1(1):52–7.
3. Vecchio R, et al. History of laparoscopic surgery. Panminerva Med. 2000;42(1):87–90.
4. Rane, et al. Port site metastases. Curr Opin Urol. 2008;18(2):185–9.
5. Curet, et al. Port site metastases. Am J Surg. 2004;187(6):705–12.
6. Fleshman, et al. Early results of laparoscopic surgery for colorectal cancer. Retrospective analysis of 372 patients treated by clinical outcomes of surgical therapy (COST) study group. Dis Colon Rectum. 1996;39:S53–8.
7. Hartley, et al. Patterns of recurrence and survival after laparoscopic and conventional resections for colorectal carcinoma. Ann Surg. 2000;232(2):181–6.
8. Lacy, et al. Laparoscopy-assisted colectomy versus open colectomy for treatment of non-metastatic colon cancer: a randomized trial. Lancet. 2002;359(9325):2224–9.
9. COST. A comparison of laparoscopically assisted and open colectomy for colon cancer. N Engl J Med. 2004;350(20):2050–9.
10. Jayne, et al. Randomized trial of laparoscopic assisted resection of colorectal carcinoma: 3-year results of the UK MRC CLASICC trial group. J Clin Oncol. 2007;25(21):3061–8.
11. Hazebroek, et al. COLOR: a randomized clinical trial comparing laparoscopic and open resection for colon cancer. Surg Endosc. 2002;16(6):949–53.
12. Abraham NS, et al. Meta-analysis of short-term outcomes after laparoscopic resection for colorectal cancer. Br J Surg. 2004;91(9):1111–24.
13. Schwenk W, et al. Meta-analysis of short-term outcomes after laparoscopic resection for colorectal cancer. Br J Surg. 2004;91(12):1653–4.
14. Delaney CP, et al. Case matched comparison of clinical and financial outcome after laparoscopic or open colectomy. Ann Surg. 2003;238:67–72.
15. Tjandra JJ, et al. Systematic review on the short-term outcome of laparoscopic resection for colon and rectosigmoid cancer. Colorectal Dis. 2006;8(5):375–88.
16. Delaney CP, et al. Clinical outcomes and resource utilization associated with laparoscopic and open colectomy using a large national database. Ann Surg. 2008;247(5):819–24.
17. de Verteuil RM, et al. Economic evaluation of laparoscopic surgery for colorectal cancer. Int J Technol Assess Health Care. 2007;23(4):464–72.
18. Dowson HM, et al. Systematic review of the costs of laparoscopic colorectal surgery. Dis Colon Rectum. 2007;50(6):908–19.
19. Janson M, et al. Randomized clinical trial of the costs of open and laparoscopic surgery for colonic cancer. Br J Surg. 2004;91(4):409–17.
20. Leung KL, et al. Laparoscopic resection of rectosigmoid carcinoma: prospective randomized trial. Lancet. 2004;363(9416):1187–92.
21. Morino M, et al. Laparoscopic total mesorectal excision: a consecutive series of 100 patients. Ann Surg. 2003;237(3):335–42.
22. Dulucq JL, et al. Laparoscopic rectal resection with anal sphincter preservation for rectal cancer: long-term outcome. Surg Endosc. 2005;19(11):1468.
23. Kim SH, et al. Laparoscopic resection for rectal cancer: a prospective analysis of thirty-month follow-up outcomes in 312 patients. Surg Endosc. 2006;20(8):1197–202.
24. Heriot, et al. Laparoscopic versus open surgery for rectal cancer: a meta-analysis. Ann Surg Oncol. 2006;13(3):413–24.
25. Laurent C, et al. Laparoscopic versus open surgery for rectal cancer: long-term oncologic results. Ann Surg. 2009;250(1):54–61.
26. Bianchi PP, et al. Laparoscopic surgery in rectal cancer: a prospective analysis of patient survival and outcomes. Dist Colon Rectum. 2007;50(12):2047–53.
27. Staudacher C, et al. Total mesorectal excision (TME) with laparoscopic approach: 226 consecutive cases. Surg Oncol. 2007;16 Suppl 1:S113–6.
28. Schiedeck TH, et al. Laparoscopic TME: better vision, better results? Recent Results Cancer Res. 2005;165:148–57.
29. Cheatham ML, et al. A meta-analysis of selective versus routine nasogastric decompression after elective laparotomy. Ann Surg. 1995;221(5):469–76.
30. Kehlet H, et al. Postoperative ileus – an update on preventive techniques. Nat Clin Pract Gastroenterol Hepatol. 2008;5(10):552–8.
31. Carli F, et al. The effect of intraoperative thoracic epidural anesthesia and postoperative analgesia on bowel function after colorectal surgery: a prospective, randomized trial. Dis Colon Rectum. 2001;44(8):1083–9.
32. Turunen P, et al. Epidural analgesia diminished pain but did not otherwise improve enhanced recovery

after laparoscopic sigmoidectomy: a prospective randomized study. Surg Endosc. 2009;23(1):31–7.
33. Behm B, et al. Postoperative ileus: etiologies and interventions. Clin Gastroentero Hepatol. 2003;1(2):71–80.
34. Kurz A, et al. Opioid-induced bowel dysfunction: pathophysiology and potential new therapies. Drugs. 2003;63(7):649–71.
35. Sinatra RS, et al. Peripherally acting mu-opioid-receptor antagonists and the connection between postoperative ileus and pain management: the anesthesiologist's view and beyond. J Perianesth Nurs. 2006;21:S16–23.
36. Kraft, et al. Emerging pharmacologic options for treating postoperative ileus. Am J Health Syst Pharm. 2007;64:S13–20.
37. Kraft, et al. Methylnaltrexone, a new peripherally acting mu-opioid receptor antagonist being evaluated for the treatment of postoperative ileus. Exp Opin Investig Drugs. 2008;17(9):1365–77.
38. Neyens R, et al. Novel opioid antagonists for opioid-induced bowel dysfunction and postoperative ileus. J Pain Palliat Care Pharmacother. 2007;21(2):27–33.
39. Delaney CP, et al. Alvimopan, for postoperative ileus following bowel resection: a pooled analysis of phase III studies. Ann Surg. 2007;245(3):364–5.
40. Jakobsen D, et al. Convalescence after colonic resection with fast-track versus conventional care. Scand J Surg. 2004;93(1):24–8.
41. Delaney CP, et al. Prospective, randomized controlled trial between a pathway of controlled rehabilitation with early ambulation and diet and traditional postoperative care after laparotomy and intestinal resection. Dis Colon Rectum. 2003;46(7):851–9.
42. Delaney CP, et al. 'Fast track' postoperative management protocol for patients with high co-morbidity undergoing complex abdominal and pelvic colorectal surgery. Br J Surg. 2001;88(11):1533–8.
43. Delaney CP, et al. Advantages of laparoscopic colectomy in older patients. Arch Surg. 2003;138(3):252–6.
44. Lindsetmo RO, et al. Laparoscopic rectal resections and fast-track surgery: what can be expected? Am J Surg. 2009;197(3):408–12.
45. Delaney CP, et al. Outcome of discharge within 24 to 72 hours after laparoscopic colorectal surgery. Dis Colon rectum. 2008 Feb;51(2):181-5. Wang, H., Quah, S. Y., Dong, J. M., et al. PRL-3 down-regulates PTEN expression and signals through PI3K to promote epithelial-mesenchymal transition. Cancer Res, 2007. 67: 2922–6.

12 New Neoadjuvant Chemotherapy for Resectable Liver Metastases of Colorectal Cancer

Antoine Brouquet, Stéphane Benoist, and Bernard Nordlinger

12.1 Introduction

Colorectal cancer (CRC) is one of the primary causes of cancer death worldwide, ranking second in Europe and third in the USA and Asia [1, 2]. Nearly 50 % of colorectal cancer patients can develop liver metastases at some point during the course of their disease [1, 3, 4]. Surgical resection remains the only method that can ensure long-term survival in 25–40 % of the patients with colorectal liver metastases so far [5, 6]. Unfortunately, only 15–20 % of patients can undergo surgical resection at the time of diagnosis [4]. In patients with initially unresectable metastases, chemotherapy is the only therapeutic option, but 5-year survivors who are treated by chemotherapy alone are anecdotic. After surgical resection of liver metastatic lesions, recurrences are still observed in a majority of patients [7]. In the case of improving the oncological results in operated patients, the mutlimodality approach should be the standard of care. Neoadjuvant chemotherapy has been evaluated in initially resectable liver metastasis patients. This chapter will summarize the current statistics on the rationale, advantages, and potential disadvantages of neoadjuvant chemotherapy in resectable CRC liver metastasis patients.

12.2 The Rationale for Neoadjuvant Chemotherapy in Patients with Resectable Liver Metastases

After "curative" surgical resection of CRC liver metastasis patients, 5-year survival rates range from 30 % to 50 %. However, recurrences are observed in the majority of patients who undergo liver resection after resection of liver metastases despite progress in developed surgical technique and improved surgical skills [5, 6, 8].

In the case of improving the oncological results, adjuvant treatment which uses fluorouracil (5FU), folinic acid, or floxuridine in systemic chemotherapy or hepatic arterial infusion has been evaluated after resection of CRC liver metastases in several randomized studies [9–13],

A. Brouquet, MD • S. Benoist, MD, PhD
Assistance Publique Hôpitaux de Paris, Université de Versailles, Versailles, France

Hôpital Ambroise Paré, Boulogne, France

B. Nordlinger, MD (✉)
Assistance Publique Hôpitaux de Paris, Université de Versailles, Versailles, France

Hôpital Ambroise Paré, Boulogne, France

Service de Chirurgie Digestive,
Hôpital Ambroise Paré, 9 avenue Charles-de-Gaulle, 92104 Boulogne Cedex, France
e-mail: bernard.nordlinger@apr.ap-hop-paris.fr; bernard.nordlinger@apr.aphp.fr

X. Qin et al. (eds.), *Multidisciplinary Management of Liver Metastases in Colorectal Cancer*, DOI 10.1007/978-94-017-7755-1_12

but definite survival benefit has not yet been confirmed so far. Recently, a meta-analysis showed that, after complete resection of CRC liver metastases, a 5FU-based adjuvant CT vs. no postoperative chemotherapy tended to improve disease-free and overall survival, but the observed increases in survival did not reach statistical significance (27.9 vs. 18.8 months, respectively [$p=0.059$], for disease-free survival and 62.2 vs. 47.3 months, respectively [$p=0.95$], for overall survival) [14]. Ychou et al. has presented a randomized phase III study comparing systemic chemotherapy with 5FU vs. irinotecan-based regimen as adjuvant treatment after complete resection of colorectal liver metastases at the ASCO Annual Meeting 2008 [15]. This study did not show any significant advantage in disease-free survival for the addition of irinotecan to 5FU [15].

Overall, the sole application of adjuvant chemotherapy after liver metastasis resection may not be sufficient to improve long-term prognosis. New approaches are needed. Some of the advantages of preoperative administration of chemotherapy are as follows (Table 12.1):

- To test the chemoresponsiveness of metastases while they are still measurable in the liver, which can help decide which treatment should be given after resection [4].
- To eliminate micrometastatic disease and eradicate dormant cancer cells of liver metastasis.
- To increase the complete resection rate and spare more non-tumorous liver parenchyma if tumor is shrinked during neoadjuvant chemotherapy [16].
- To provide a useful tool to predict long-term survival. Indeed, several studies have demonstrated that response to neoadjuvant chemotherapy was a significant prognostic factor and could provide a better selection of candidates for surgical resection. Allen et al. [17] have compared the outcomes of patients referred for resection of synchronous colorectal liver metastases with previous neoadjuvant chemotherapy vs. without previous neoadjuvant chemotherapy. The 5-year survival was undifferentiated in two groups. Patients with stable disease or disease responding to chemotherapy had a better survival than patients who did not receive chemotherapy (85 % vs. 35 %, $p=0.03$). In another study, tumor progression during neoadjuvant chemotherapy was also related to reduced 5-year survival rate when compared to patients with tumor response or stable disease (8 % vs. 37 % and 30 %, respectively, $p<0.001$) [18]. In this study, tumor progression while on chemotherapy was an independent predictive factor associated with decreased survival and considered by the authors as a contraindication to liver resection. Recently, three studies have evaluated the impact of pathologic response to chemotherapy on outcome after resection [19–21]. Rubbia Brandt et al. have elaborated the tumor regression grading (TRG) system to evaluate tumor response to neoadjuvant chemotherapy. In this study, major histological tumor regression was associated with improved survival [19]. Two other studies have focused on the impact of complete pathologic response on long-term outcome [20, 21]. Results of these two studies are consistent: Complete pathologic response is associated with increased long-term survival rates and pathologic response to chemotherapy is an important prognostic factor.

Table 12.1 Potential benefits and risks of preoperative chemotherapy

Benefits	Risks
Improved progression-free survival	Delayed surgery
Evaluation of chemoresponsiveness	More reversible surgical complications
Selection for surgery	Chemotherapy-associated liver injuries
Fewer "open and close"	Complete response making metastases difficult to find
Low operative mortality	Cost

12.3 Potential Risks of Preoperative Chemotherapy

Neoadjuvant chemotherapy has potential defects (Table 12.1).

Application of preoperative chemotherapy may induce pathologic application in the non-tumorous liver parenchyma [20–30]. There were reports that preoperative chemotherapy has two main types of chemotherapy-associated liver injuries: vascular changes including sinusoidal dilatation and nonalcoholic fatty liver disease related to chemotherapy including chemotherapy-associated steatosis and steatohepatitis (CASH). Application of 5-fluorouracil may increase the risk of steatosis [28]. Application of oxaliplatin-based combination regimens may be associated with an increased risk of vascular lesions in the liver [22, 25, 26, 30]. Irinotecan-containing regimens can increase the risks of steatosis and steatohepatitis [23, 25].

The critical question is whether chemotherapy-associated liver injuries have any clinical significance and in particular if they are associated with an increased risk of liver surgery for metastases. The relation between the type of lesions induced by chemotherapy and their potential clinical consequences has been reported. Kooby et al. showed that steatosis increase the risk of complications, in particular infectious complications, but had no effective impact on mortality [29]. Vauthey et al. showed that steatohepatitis was observed in 20 % of patients with irinotecan-based chemotherapy and may be associated with death due to postoperative liver failure in 7 % of patients with steatohepatitis [25]. Impact of vascular lesions on postoperative course after liver resection is controversial. Nakano et al. have reported that occurrence of sinusoidal injuries could increase the risk of major hepatectomy for colorectal liver metastases [30], whereas in the other report [25], vascular lesions were only associated with an increased risk of operative bleeding but not perioperative morbidity or mortality [25].

The European Organisation for Research and Treatment of Cancer (EORTC) Intergroup phase III study 40983 have compared the outcomes of perioperative chemotherapy with 5FU, leucovorin, and oxaliplatin (six cycles before surgery and six cycles after) to surgery alone in 364 patients [31]. The results of safety showed that in the two treatment arms, the mortality rate was both less than 1 % and was not statistically significant [31]. Morbidity rate was slightly higher in the chemotherapy arm than in the surgery-alone arm (25 % vs. 16 %; $p=0.04$) (Table 12.2), but still in the range of other reports' observation [5, 6, 32]. Intra-abdominal abscesses and transient biliary fistula were more frequent in the chemotherapy arm. Thus, preoperative administration of six cycles of FOLFOX (a kind of Chemotherapy regimen, including Oxaliplatin, Fluorouracil and Leucovorin ivgtt) is safe and feasible. Even though no report clearly demonstrated the correlation between increased morbidity rates and duration of neoadjuvant chemotherapy, there are several arguments to support the

Table 12.2 Postoperative complications in EORTC intergroup trial 40983

	Period CT group	Surgery group
Reversible postoperative complications[a]	40 (25 %)	27 (16 %)
Cardiopulmonary failure	3 (2 %)	2 (1 %)
Bleeding	3 (2 %)	3 (2 %)
Biliary fistula	13 (8 %)	7 (4 %)
Hepatic failure	11 (7 %)	8 (5 %)
Wound infection	5 (3 %)	4 (2 %)
Intra-abdominal infection	11 (7 %)	4 (2 %)
Need for reoperation	5 (3 %)	3 (2 %)
Urinary infection	4 (3 %)	
Pleural effusion	2 (1 %)	1 (1 %)
Pulmonary embolism/deep venous	2 (1 %)	1 (1 %)
Pneumopathy	2 (1 %)	
Neutropenia	1 (1 %)	
Ascites	2 (1 %)	1 (1 %)
Ileus		1 (1 %)
Cardiac arrhythmia		1 (1 %)
Renal failure	4 (3 %)	1 (1 %)
Other		4 (2 %)

Modified from *Lancet* 2008;371:1007–16

[a] $p=0.04$

hypothesis of a cumulative toxicity of chemotherapy on non-tumorous liver parenchyma [24, 26, 30]. Preoperative chemotherapy is safe if it is properly chosen and monitored and if patients are not over chemotherapy-treated before surgery.

The potential risks of liver surgery after administration of combinations of cytotoxic drugs and targeted agents are poorly understood. Anti-EGF agents, particularly cetuximab, which could interfere with surgery have little known side effect. In some researches, it is demonstrated that bevacizumab, an anti-VEGF, can be supervised securely before liver resection of colorectal liver metastases and that bevacizumab's administration is discontinued 6–8 weeks before surgery. The feasibility and benefits of liver surgery after administration of novel, systemic targeted agents will be further elaborated in ongoing prospective clinical studies (EORTC study 40091 (BOS2 (Efficacy of FOLFOX Alone, FOLFOX Plus Bevacizumab and FOLFOX Plus Panitumumab in Patients With Resectable Liver Metastases) study)):

- When there is a response to chemotherapy, certain liver metastases may be no longer visible on imaging and be considered as complete responses. It is significant to wonder whether these metastases are thoroughly eliminated or they are not visible on imaging but still exist. In order to deal with these puzzlers, 66 liver metastases that disappeared on CT scan were reviewed [35]. As a result, in more than 80% of the cases, at the initial site of liver metastases where still existed viable cancer cells, which were disappeared on imaging. It does not mean that complete radiologic responses stand for the cure of the disease [35]. So, to the patients with resectable liver metastases, they should not stop referral to surgeons until their liver metastases have completely disappeared. It is necessary to resect the initial site if the liver metastases were gone, and the surgeon is required to identify this site in the liver, a comparatively difficult and impossible task.
- There will be another theoretical risk if the metastases progressed so seriously that it would become unresectable during preoperative chemotherapy. In the EORTC Intergroup phase III study 40983, in 12 of 182 (7%) patients who accepted systemic chemotherapy, progressive diseases were observed [31]. In about 12 of these patients, four could even have resection of metastases. For the rest, half of the patients cannot have the resection due to the appearance of new extrahepatic lesions which can reappear in any site after immediate surgery. In only one third of cases, the cause of unresectability was the progression of known liver metastases. According to the research on chemotherapy, progression of liver metastases is a factor of poor prognosis after hepatic resection. Most of these patients develop early cancer recurrence. Thus, some authors consider that tumor progression while on chemotherapy is a contraindication for surgery [18].

12.4 Benefits of Preoperative Chemotherapy in Patients with Resectable Liver Metastases

Phase II studies using oxaliplatin, or oxaliplatin- and irinotecan-based regimen, have demonstrated the potential benefit of preoperative chemotherapy.

The EORTC Intergroup phase III study 40983 is a prospective randomized study which randomized 364 patients with one to four potentially resectable liver metastases and compared perioperative chemotherapy (six cycles before surgery and six cycles after) with 5FU, leucovorin, and oxaliplatin to surgery alone [31]. The progression-free survival was the primary endpoint of this study. One hundred and seventy-one patients in each treatment arm were eligible for entry in the protocol. Twenty-two patients, 11 in each arm were mainly too much advanced in disease to enroll. Concerning the tolerance of preoperative chemotherapy, of the 171 patients who were randomized in the perioperative chemotherapy + surgery group, 143 patients (84%) received the full preoperative treatment, i.e., six cycles before liver resection. Partial or complete response

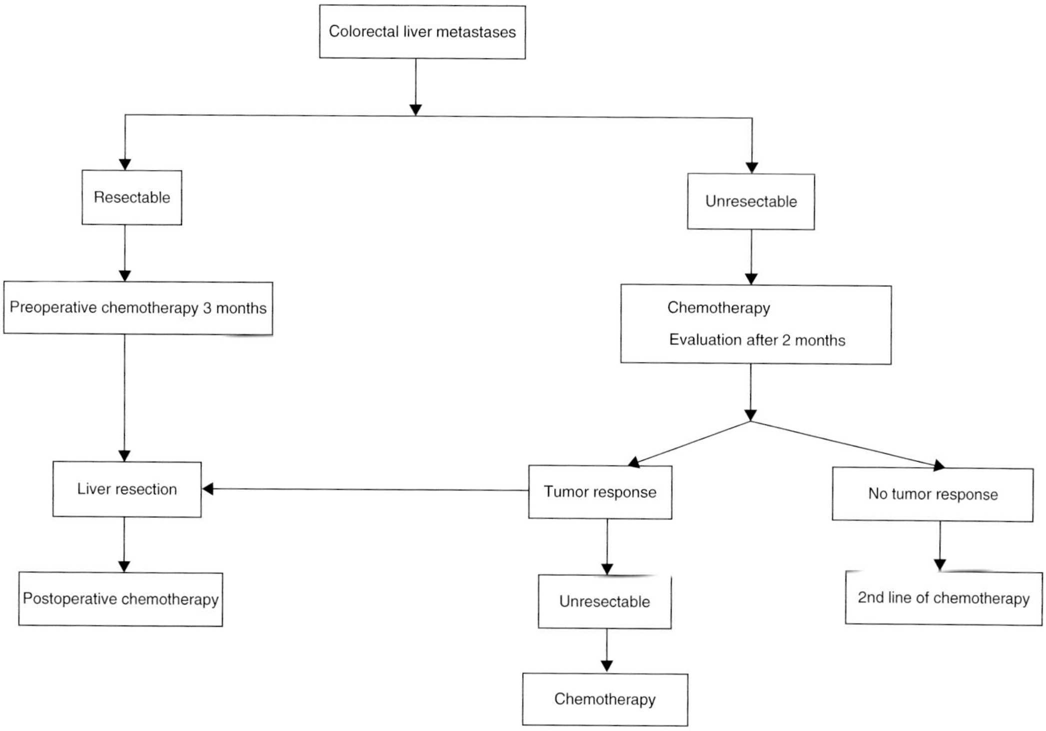

Fig. 12.1 Therapy plan for colorectal liver metastases

according to (Response Evaluation Criteria in Solid Tumors) RECIST criteria was observed in 43 % of patients [27]. Tumor size was decreased by a mean of 25 % after chemotherapy. Eighty-three percent of patients could undergo curative liver resection in each treatment arm. With a median follow-up of 3.9 years, the absolute increased progression-free survival rate at 3 years was 8.1 % in the perioperative chemotherapy + surgery group vs. surgery alone group (36.1 % vs. 28.1 %, respectively; $p=0.041$) in eligible patients. In the 303 patients who actually underwent surgical resection, progression-free survival rate at 3 years was increased by 9.2 % in the perioperative chemotherapy + surgery group vs. surgery alone group (42.4 % vs. 33.2 %, respectively; $p=0.025$). In conclusion this study demonstrated that perioperative FOLFOX4 (a kind of Chemotherapy regimen, L-OHP 85mg/m2 ivgtt for 2h d1, CF 200mg/m2, ivgtt for 2h d1, 5-FU 400mg/m2 iv, 5-FU 600mg/m2 ivgtt for 22h d1/d2) chemotherapy decreased cancer relapse rate by a quarter and was compatible with major surgery.

This study validated the essence of combined chemotherapy and surgery to treat colorectal liver metastases. Most patients who have resectable colorectal liver metastases should consider perioperative chemotherapy as the standard of care (Fig. 12.1).

Conclusion

Combined strategy including chemotherapy and liver resection has become the standard of care for patients with resectable liver metastases. The EORTC study has shown that perioperative chemotherapy could reduce the risk of cancer relapse after surgery. It is easily manageable if patients are well monitored, receive surgery at the right moment, and are not overtreated with chemotherapy.

In the future, it is likely that the addition of targeted therapies to cytotoxic drugs will increase the efficacy of preoperative treatment. The interest of such strategies has to be evaluated in phase III controlled studies such as the BOS2 study organized by the Gastrointestinal Group of EORTC.

In the fast-moving field of combined treatment of colorectal cancer liver metastases, patients should all receive care after multidisciplinary discussion and repeated evaluations.

References

1. Jemal A, Siegel R, Ward E, Hao Y, Xu J, Thun MJ. Cancer statistics, 2009. CA Cancer J Clin. 2009;59:225 [Epub ahead of print].
2. Sung JJ, Lau JY, Goh KL, Leung WK, Asia Pacific Working Group on Colorectal Cancer. Increasing incidence of colorectal cancer in Asia: implications for screening. Lancet Oncol. 2005;6(11):871–6.
3. Stangl R, Altendorf-Hofmann A, Charnley RM, Scheele J. Factors influencing the natural history of colorectal liver metastases. Lancet. 1994;343:1405–10.
4. Leonard GD, Brenner B, Kemeny NE. Neoadjuvant chemotherapy before liver resection for patients with unresectable liver metastases from colorectal carcinoma. J Clin Oncol. 2005;23:2038–48.
5. Nordlinger B, Jaeck D, Guiguet M, Vaillant JC, Balladur P, Schaal JC. Surgical resection of hepatic metastases. Multicentric retrospective study by the French Association of Surgery. In: Nordlinger B, Jaeck D, editors. Treatment of hepatic metastases of colorectal cancer. Paris: Springer; 1992. p. 129–46.
6. Fong Y, Fortner J, Sun RL, Brennan MF, Blumgart LH. Clinical score for predicting recurrence after hepatic resection for metastatic colorectal cancer: analysis of 1001 consecutive cases. Ann Surg. 1999;230:309–18.
7. Scheele J. Hepatectomy for liver metastases. Br J Surg. 1993;80:274–6.
8. Khatri VP, Petrelli NJ, Belghiti J. Extending the frontiers of surgical therapy for hepatic colorectal metastases: is there a limit? J Clin Oncol. 2005;23:8490–9.
9. Lorenz M, Muller HH, Schramm H, et al. Randomized trial of surgery versus surgery followed by adjuvant hepatic arterial infusion with 5-fluorouracil and folinic acid for liver metastases of colorectal cancer. German Cooperative on Liver Metastases. Ann Surg. 1998;228:756–62.
10. Kemeny N, Huang Y, Cohen AM, et al. Hepatic arterial infusion of chemotherapy after resection of hepatic metastases from colorectal cancer. N Engl J Med. 1999;341:2039–48.
11. Kemeny MM, Adak S, Gray B, et al. Combined-modality treatment for resectable metastatic colorectal carcinoma to the liver: surgical resection of hepatic metastases in combination with continuous infusion of chemotherapy-an intergroup study. J Clin Oncol. 2002;20:1499–505.
12. Portier G, Elias D, Bouche O, et al. Multicenter randomized trial of adjuvant fluorouracil and folinic acid compared with surgery alone after resection of colorectal liver metastases: FFCD ACHBTH AURC 9002 trial. J Clin Oncol. 2006;24:4976–82.
13. Langer B, Bleiberg H, Labianca R. Fluorouracil (FU) plus l-leucovorin (l-LV) versus observation after potentially curative resection of liver or lung metastases from colorectal cancer (CRC): results of the ENG (EORTC/NCIC CTG/GIVIO) randomized trial. J Clin Oncol. 2002;20:149a. abstr 592.
14. Mitry E, Fields A, Bleiberg H, et al. Adjuvant chemotherapy after potentially curative resection of metastases from colorectal cancer. A meta-analysis of two randomized trials. J Clin Oncol. 2006;24(18S):3524.
15. Ychou M, Hohenberger W, Thezenas S, et al. Randomized phase III trial comparing infused 5-fluorouracil/folinic acid (LV5FU) versus LV5FU+irinotecan (LV5FU+IRI) as adjuvant treatment after complete resection of liver metastases from colorectal cancer (CPT-GMA-301). J Clin Oncol. 2008;26:LBA4013.
16. Tanaka K, Adam R, Shimada H, Azoulay D, Levi F, Bismuth H. Role of neoadjuvant chemotherapy in the treatment of multiple colorectal metastases to the liver. Br J Surg. 2003;90:963–9.
17. Allen PJ, Kemeny N, Jarnagin W, DeMatteo R, Blumgart L, Fong Y. Importance of response to neoadjuvant chemotherapy in patients undergoing resection of synchronous colorectal liver metastases. J Gastrointest Surg. 2003;7:109–15.
18. Adam R, Pascal G, Castaing D, Azoulay D, Delvart V, Paule B, Levi F, Bismuth H. Tumor progression while on chemotherapy: a contraindication to liver resection for multiple colorectal metastases? Ann Surg. 2004;240:1052–61.
19. Rubbia-Brandt L, Giostra E, Brezault C, et al. Importance of histological tumor response assessment in predicting the outcome in patients with colorectal liver metastases treated with neo-adjuvant chemotherapy followed by liver surgery. Ann Oncol. 2007;18:299–304.
20. Adam R, Wicherts DA, de Haas RJ, et al. Complete pathologic response after preoperative chemotherapy for colorectal liver metastases: myth or reality? J Clin Oncol. 2008;26:1635–41.
21. Blazer 3rd DG, Kishi Y, Maru DM, Kopetz S, Chun YS, Overman MJ, Fogelman D, Eng C, Chang DZ, Wang H, Zorzi D, Ribero D, Ellis LM, Glover KY, Wolff RA, Curley SA, Abdalla EK, Vauthey JN. Pathologic response to preoperative chemotherapy: a new outcome end point after resection of hepatic colorectal metastases. J Clin Oncol. 2008;26(33):5344–51.
22. Rubbia-Brandt L, Audard V, Sartoretti P, et al. Severe hepatic sinusoidal obstruction associated with oxaliplatin-based chemotherapy in patients with metastatic colorectal cancer. Ann Oncol. 2004;15:460–6.

23. Fernandez FG, Ritter J, Goodwin JW, Linehan DC, Hawkins WG, Strasberg SM. Effect of steatohepatitis associated with irinotecan or oxaliplatin pretreatment on resectability of hepatic colorectal metastases. J Am Coll Surg. 2005;200:845–53.
24. Karoui M, Penna C, Amin-Hashem M, et al. Influence of preoperative chemotherapy on the risk of major hepatectomy for colorectal liver metastases. Ann Surg. 2006;243:1–7.
25. Vauthey JN, Pawlik TM, Ribero D, et al. Chemotherapy regimen predicts steatohepatitis and an increase in 90-day mortality after surgery for hepatic colorectal metastases. J Clin Oncol. 2006;24:2065–72.
26. Brouquet A, Benoist S, Julie C, et al. Risk factors for chemotherapy-associated liver injuries: a multivariate analysis of a group of 146 patients with colorectal metastases. Surgery. 2009;145:362–71.
27. Nordlinger B, Benoist S. Benefits and risks of neoadjuvant therapy for liver metastases. J Clin Oncol. 2006;24:4954–5.
28. Peppercorn PD, Reznek RH, Wilson P, Slevin ML, Gupta RK. Demonstration of hepatic steatosis by computerized tomography in patients receiving 5-fluorouracil-based therapy for advanced colorectal cancer. Br J Cancer. 1998;77:2008–11.
29. Kooby DA, Fong Y, Suriawinata A, et al. Impact of steatosis on perioperative outcome following hepatic resection. J Gastrointest Surg. 2003;7:1034–44.
30. Nakano H, Oussoultzoglou E, Rosso E, et al. Sinusoidal injury increases morbidity after major hepatectomy in patients with colorectal liver metastases receiving preoperative chemotherapy. Ann Surg. 2008;24:118–24.
31. Nordlinger B, Sorbye H, Glimelius B, EORTC Gastro-Intestinal Tract Cancer Group; Cancer Research UK; Arbeitsgruppe Lebermetastasen und-tumoren in der Chirurgischen Arbeitsgemeinschaft Onkologie (ALM-CAO); Australasian Gastro-Intestinal Trials Group (AGITG); Fédération Francophone de Cancérologie Digestive (FFCD), et al. Perioperative chemotherapy with FOLFOX4 and surgery versus surgery alone for resectable liver metastases from colorectal cancer (EORTC Intergroup trial 40983): a randomised controlled trial. Lancet. 2008;371:1007–16.
32. Belghiti J, Hiramatsu K, Benoist S, Massault P, Sauvanet A, Farges O. Seven hundred forty-seven hepatectomies in the 1990s: an update to evaluate the actual risk of liver resection. J Am Coll Surg. 2000;191:38–46.
33. Gruenberger B, Tamandl D, Schueller J, et al. Bevacizumab, capecitabine, and oxaliplatin as neoadjuvant therapy for patients with potentially curable metastatic colorectal cancer. J Clin Oncol. 2008;26:1830–5.
34. Ribero D, Wang H, Donadon M, et al. Bevacizumab improves pathologic response and protects against hepatic injury in patients treated with oxaliplatin-based chemotherapy for colorectal liver metastases. Cancer. 2007;110:2761–7.
35. Benoist S, Brouquet A, Penna C, et al. Complete response of colorectal liver metastases after chemotherapy: does it mean cure? J Clin Oncol. 2006;24:3939–45.

Surgical Techniques for Metastatic Hepatic Carcinoma

13

Jia Fan

13.1 Introduction

Hepatic metastasis of colorectal cancer is a critical factor affecting prognosis of colorectal cancer. For about 25 % of patients, hepatic metastasis had occurred when colorectal cancer was confirmed; for 40–50 % of patients, it would occur within 3 years after surgery for colorectal cancer [1]. Surgical therapy is the only means by which radical treatment can be achieved. With the improvement of surgical techniques today, the 5-year survival rate has increased to 45–60 %, from 30 to 35 % in the 1990s [2].

13.1.1 Indications and Contraindications for Surgery

It is generally accepted that surgical indications for hepatic metastasis of colorectal cancer include the following: (1) primary foci can be resected radically (R0); (2) hepatic metastatic foci can be resected and sufficient hepatic function can be preserved; if the hepatic metastatic foci and primary foci of colorectal cancer are to be resected separately at different stages, the volume of the residual liver should be ≥30 %; if the hepatic metastatic foci and primary foci of colorectal cancer are to be resected simultaneously, the volume of the residual liver should be ≥50 %; (3) the foci of extrahepatic metastasis can be resected or ablated; and (4) the patients have good cardiopulmonary function and can tolerate surgical treatment.

Surgical contraindications: uncontrollable extrahepatic lesion, e.g., unresectable primary foci, local recurrence of primary foci, peritoneum involvement, extensive lymphatic metastasis (lymphatic metastasis in the retroperitoneal region, mediastinum, or porta hepatis), or extensive pulmonary, bony, or central nervous system metastasis [3]. For patients with extrahepatic metastasis, hepatectomy can still be considered under the following conditions: pulmonary metastasis that can be resected or locally ablated; solitary extrahepatic lesions that can be resected or locally ablated, e.g., foci occurred in spleen or adrenal, or locally recurred foci; foci of hepatic metastasis can be resected although they directly invade ambient tissues, e.g., diaphragm or adrenal.

At present, the size, amount, and site of hepatic foci are no longer the factor restricting surgery. In a retrospective analysis on 131 patients with hepatic metastasis of colorectal cancer whose foci were resected, Imamura et al. [4] found that 5-year survival rates were 51 %, 46 %, and 25 %, respectively, for patients with 1–3, 4–9, and ≥10

J. Fan
Zhongshan Hospital, Fudan University, Shanghai, China
e-mail: fan.jia@zs-hospital.sh.cn

X. Qin et al. (eds.), *Multidisciplinary Management of Liver Metastases in Colorectal Cancer*, DOI 10.1007/978-94-017-7755-1_13

foci. According to a multi-factor analysis, there was a significant difference in the survival time for the patients with ≥10 metastatic foci and those with one to three foci, but there was not any significant statistical difference in survival time for the patients with four to nine foci and those with one to three foci. Therefore, for patients with <10 metastatic foci, surgical resection is still suggested if the functional compensation can be achieved by residual livers.

13.1.2 Selection of Operation Opportunity

For patients of colorectal cancer confirmed with hepatic metastasis, there was a dispute on selection of simultaneous resection or sequential surgery. In the 1990s, apprehensions about simultaneous resection included the following: (1) the incision for resection of colorectal cancer was different from that for hepatectomy; (2) resection of colorectal cancer might contaminate abdominal cavity, resulting in cross-sectional infection of the liver or subphrenic infection; and (3) simultaneous resection of colorectal cancer with hepatectomy might lead to a large operation wound and a higher morbidity and mortality rate. Therefore, generally, primary colorectal foci were resected first, and hepatectomy would be carried out after postoperative chemotherapy for 3–4 months.

In recent years, with the progress of postoperative treatment and operation technique, this conventional opinion has been changed. According to a retrospective study of Capussott et al. [5], the rates of morbidity, mortality, and anastomotic leakage were similar between the group of simultaneous resection and the group of sequential surgery; the operation time and the utilization ratio of red cell suspension and plasma for the group of simultaneous resection were more than that for the group of sequential surgery, but the hospitalization time for the group of sequential resection was longer than that for the group of simultaneous resection; a follow-up visit indicated that there was no difference in a 10-year survival rate. A similar result was obtained by Martin et al. [6] after a retrospective analysis on 230 patients treated with surgical resection against hepatic metastasis of colorectal cancer. The mortality rates of simultaneous resection and sequential resection were 2.2 % and 2.8 % respectively ($P > 0.05$). Peeters et al. [7] found that after resection of primary foci for patients with hepatic metastasis of colorectal cancer, the ratio of apoptosis to proliferation of cancer cells in hepatic metastatic foci was unbalanced, and the growth rate of tumor was speeded; therefore, they supported simultaneous resection. It is suggested in the Practice Parameters for Colon Cancer prepared by Standards Practice Task Force of the American Society of Colon and Rectal Surgeons [8] that: "If the hepatic metastatic foci can be resected completely and the incisal margin ≥1 cm; the incision is applicable to hepatectomy; the amount of the resected liver <50 %; the physical condition of patients allow the operation; the operator is skillful, they can be resected simultaneously." At present, it is accepted that simultaneous resection of hepatic metastatic foci and primary foci are safe.

13.1.3 Preoperative Evaluation

Preoperative evaluation involves the possibility of resection of hepatic and extrahepatic metastatic foci, the liver function, and the general body state. The evaluation of resectability of hepatic metastatic foci and extrahepatic metastatic foci depends mainly on imaging examination. Type B ultrasonic is preferred for hepatic metastatic foci. Contrast-enhanced CT is helpful for confirmation of lesion; detection of the size, amount, site of metastatic foci and the relation between metastatic foci and the bile duct and blood vessels in the liver; and measurement of volume of tumor, the part of the liver to be resected, and the residual liver. MRI has the advantage in detection of foci <1 cm; the enhanced MRI has a sensitivity of 80–90 % and a high specificity for detection of hepatic metastatic foci. PET/CT examination has an obvious advantage in sensitivity and specificity, which is helpful for detection of extrahepatic metastasis; moreover, it is the most correct method for staging of colorectal cancer in the progressive stage. Kong et al. [9] compared the detection results of PET/CT, contrast-enhanced CT, and enhanced MRI in foci of hepatic metastasis of colorectal cancer; in terms of each focus, the enhanced MRI could find out smaller metastatic foci, while PET/CT could find out more metastatic foci. With regard to the patients, the sensitivity and specificity of PET/CT and enhanced MRI both reached 98 and 100 %. In terms of detection of extrahepatic foci, PET/CT had an incomparable advantage over CT, which had changed the operation scheme for 17 % of patients. As neoadjuvant chemotherapy could lower the intake of 18F-fluorodeoxyglucose (18F-FDG) by hepatic metastatic foci, resulting in a lower sensitivity of PET/CT, it was suggested that PET/CT should be carried out before neoadjuvant chemotherapy [10, 11].

Few patients of hepatic metastasis of colorectal cancer are combined with hepatocirrhosis; although most of patients have good liver function, attention must be paid to the toxicity of chemotherapeutic drug to the liver. Vauthey et al. [12] reported that liver injury occurred to 22.7 % of patients receiving chemotherapy, for which the rate of liver failure and 90-day mortality increased; moreover, irinotecan was related to steatohepatitis. Rubbia-Brandt et al. [13] reported that oxaliplatin might lead to injury of sinus hepaticus. Therefore, before operation, evaluation should be carried out carefully on hepatic reserve function. Evaluation of hepatic reserve function includes (1) routine test of liver function, including serum bilirubin level, albumin level, leukocyte ratio, aminotransferase level, prealbumin level, and coagulation function test; it is generally accepted that, in terms of Child-Pugh score, patients of Class A have good tolerance to operation, while those of Class B are restricted to some extent, who could tolerate hepatolobectomy only after sufficient preoperative preparation; patients of Class C have bad tolerance to various operations, who should be restricted strictly. (2) Quantified hepatic reserve function test: at present, it is generally accepted that indocyanine green (ICG) excretive test is a sensitive index for estimation of hepatic reserve function; the ICG retention value at 15 min (ICGR-15) <20 % is the safety margin for hepatolobectomy; for those with ICGR15 of 20–29 %, the hepatic segmental resection can be carried out; for those with ICGR15 of 30–39 %, local resection can be carried out.

13.1.4 Selection of Operation Mode

Selection of operation mode for hepatic metastasis of colorectal cancer depends on the size, amount, and site of metastatic foci, the relation of metastatic foci with blood vessels and the bile duct, and the liver function and the residual liver volume of patients. Besides preoperative evaluation, exploration during operation and application of iconography also play important roles in selection of operation mode. By means of ultrasonic exploration in operation, information can be obtained on distribution of metastatic foci in the liver and possibility of resection. Zacherl et al. [14] reported that the sensitivity of ultrasonic exploration during operation to metastatic hepatic carcinoma was up to 95.2 %, higher than 84.9 % of that of MRI, which changed the operation scheme of 22.8 % of patients. It was suggested that the probe should move along the surface of the liver slowly for carefully scanning section by section, which could avoid omission. During the scanning of the porta hepatis, attention should be paid as to whether or not abnormal resonance occurs in the main portal vein, its left and right branches, or the hepatic duct. During the scanning of the secondary porta hepatis, attention should be paid as to whether or not abnormal resonance occurs inside and along the hepatic vein and its branches. Finally, the size and border of tumor, the possible subfoci, and the anatomical relation of tumors with portal vein, hepatic duct and hepatic vein should be observed to determine the best margin of excision for tumors, which should not only comply with the principle of radical correction of tumors, but also be helpful for reservation of livers as much as possible. The portal vein, hepatic duct, and hepatic vein must be reserved; a scanning technique should be applied to determine the distance between their border and the tumor, the projection on hepatic surface, and their depth to hepatic surface, in order to avoid accidental injury during resection of liver parenchyma. In addition, during hepatectomy, especially hemihepatectomy, if there is any question on anatomical character of the bile duct, intraoperative cholangiography can be applied to determine the position of the bile duct and avoid injury.

13.1.4.1 Incisal Margin

An incisal margin >1 cm is suggested in the Guidelines for Resection of Colorectal Cancer Liver Metastases of the UK [3]. Pawlik et al. [15] indicated that the recurrence rate was 51 % and the 5-year survival rate was 17.1 % for patients with positive incisal margin; for patients with negative incisal margin, there was no significant difference in the recurrence rates of tumors for those whose incisal margins were 1–4, 5–9, and ≥10 mm, respectively; i.e., the recurrence rates of tumors were 39 %, 41 %, and 39 %, and the 5-year rates were 62.3 %, 71.1 %, and 63.0 %, respectively; among the patients recurred, only 3.6 % recurred at the incisal margin. Hamady et al. [16] also found that among the patients with negative incisal margin, 1, 3, and 10-mm incisal margins had no significant influence on postoperative recurrence and long-term survival. Therefore, if a negative result is obtained in a pathological test of incisal margin, it can be concluded that the operation is successful. However, as the negative pathological result can hardly be represented by that observed by eyes, the "1 cm" rule is still a basic principle for surgical treatment of hepatic metastasis of colorectal cancer. For metastatic foci at complicated anatomical sites close to great vessels, e.g., those at the caudate lobe, porta hepatis, or secondary porta hepatis, the "1 cm" rule is hardly to be obeyed; even so, a negative pathological result should be ensured.

13.1.4.2 Anatomical Resection and Non-anatomical Resection

For anatomical resection, the hepatic segment is the basic unit of hepatectomy, including lobe or segment hepatectomy; for non-anatomical resection, the anatomical limit of the hepatic segment does not act as an incision line, e.g., a wedge resection. The advantage of anatomical resection is that functional unit of the liver is resected completely, and the positive rate of the incisal margin is lower than that of non-anatomical resection. Dematteo et al. [17] suggested that anatomical resection would lead to a higher survival rate than non-anatomical resection. However, Rorzi et al. and Sarpel et al. [18, 19] indicated that there was no significant difference in recurrence rates and survival time of patients who received either anatomical resection or non-anatomical resection. Moreover, as more liver parenchyme were reserved in non-anatomical resection, a better tolerance to postoperative chemotherapy could be achieved, and resection after recurrence is possible. According to our experience, anatomical resection is applicable to big foci, multiple foci, deep foci, or foci at the left lateral site. To peripheral small foci, either anatomical resection or non-anatomical resection is applicable.

13.1.4.3 Resection of Multiple Metastatic Foci at Left and Right Lobes of the Liver

Strategies of surgical treatment for this kind of patients include the following:

1. Direct resection: if the volume of residual liver is over 30 %, either hepatic segmentectomy or non-anatomical can be applied to resect all foci completely.
2. Portal vein embolization combined with resection: if the expected volume of residual liver is less than 30 %, the portal vein where main tumors are located should be embolized first, and then resection should be carried out after proliferation of contralateral liver.
3. Resection combined with ablation: after resection of main tumors, if the number of residual foci is not over three and the size of one single focus is less than 3 cm, residual tumors can be treated by radiofrequency ablation; if the size of one single focus is over 3 cm, crymotherapy can be used.
4. (4) Two-step resection: a part of tumors are resected first, and the second operation should be carried out to resect the residual foci after compensatory hypertrophy of liver.
5. Chemotherapy combined with resection.

13.1.5 Re-resection for Recurrence of Hepatic Metastasis of Colorectal Cancer After Resection

The postoperative recurrence rate of hepatic metastasis of colorectal cancer is about 56.7 %, among which 36.4 % are intrahepatic recurrence [2]. Petrowsky et al. [20] reported a bicentric prospective study on 126 patients who received re-resection treatment due to recurrence after resection of hepatic metastatic foci of colorectal cancer; the 1-year, 3-year, and 5-year survival rates were 86 %, 51 %, and 34 %, respectively, similar to that of patients without recurrence after first resection of hepatic metastatic foci, while incidence of complications and mortality after operation were comparable to that after the first operation. Adam et al. [21] reported a follow-up study on 60 patients who received three times of the resection of hepatic metastatic foci; results indicated that the incidence of complication after operation was 25 %, and the 5-year survival rate was 32 %, significantly higher than those who did not receive surgery treatment after recurrence of hepatic metastatic foci after the second resection. However, because of adhesion, change of morphology and ratio of hepatic lobe due to hypertrophy of the residual liver, and change of the anatomical position of blood vessels and bile duct, the difficulty of re-resection after recurrence is significantly higher. Therefore, indications should be treated strictly; in principle, indications for re-resection are identical to that of the first resection. For patients recurred after operation, especially those who experience careful evaluation and have low tumor load, re-resection is applicable.

13.2 Hepatolobectomy

13.2.1 Right Hemihepatectomy

Open the hilar plate to reveal the branches of the left and right hepatic ducts. Incise peritoneum at the right side of the hepatoduodenal ligament to reveal the common bile duct and posterior portal vein. Resect bile cyst. Dissociate the right branch of the hepatic artery, which is usually located over the level of the cystic duct and behind the common hepatic duct, and then ligate it. The right branch of the posterior portal vein appears. Incise peritoneum behind the portal vein; dissociate the right branch of the portal vein slightly under direct viewing with the help of a curved clamp. Note: Do not injure the first branch of the right posterior branch, which goes downward and supplies the right half of the caudate lobe. It should be ligated and disconnected separately if the separation of the right branch of the portal vein is affected. Clamp with blunt-pointed straight blood vessel forceps, and disconnect the right branch of the portal vein. As the right branch of the portal vein is relatively short, simple ligation is not recommended in order to avoid a resultant narrow confluence. Close the residual end with a successive suture by 5-0 Prolene or Endo-GIA™ stapler. If the anterior and posterior branches of the portal vein occur separately, they should be treated separately. After disconnection of the right branch of the portal vein, the border of the left and right part of the liver appeared.

Be careful during anatomizing the right hepatic duct, especially when the tumor is close to portal fissure. Opening omphaloschisis can reveal an anatomic character of the hepatic hilar region better. Sometimes the bile duct of the right front lobe or right back lobe merges into the confluence of the left and right hepatic ducts separately, or merges into the left hepatic duct, which should be identified carefully and disconnected separately. If the right hepatic duct cannot be identified, disconnection is not recommended, and the completeness should be maintained. As there are lots of varieties in the right hepatic duct, extrahepatic separation may lead to severe injury; our experience is that intrahepatic disconnection should be carried out when liver parenchyma is disconnected.

Intrahepatic vessel ligature technique is an alternative of extrahepatic anatomization of the porta hepatis, which is applicable especially when the tumor is far from the porta hepatis. As hepatic triads are coated with tough Glisson's sheath, anatomize along the sheath to resect the portal triads, and ligate it. Thus, the separation time of the porta hepatis can be minimized, and the possibility that contralateral blood vessels and the bile duct are injured is decreased.

The right hepatic vein can be dissociated outside the liver, or treated inside the liver during separation of liver parenchyma. It is safer to treat the hepatic vein in liver parenchyma, while control of the right hepatic vein outside the liver may decrease the bleeding during disconnection of the liver and the massive hemorrhage during breakage of the vein. It is recommended to control the right hepatic vein outside the liver for giant tumors near the inferior vena cava. During anatomizing the right hepatic vein, the central venous pressure should be controlled to less than 5 mmHg, and Trendelenburg position of patients should be kept to avoid air embolus. Disconnect the hepatorenal ligament, right triangular ligament and right coronary ligament, and turn the right liver to the left; dissociate naked area, and push the adrenal gland away. If the adrenal gland contacts the liver closely, it is recommended to undermine upward along the loose gap between the right margin of the inferior vena cava and adrenal gland; thus, a tunnel is formed. Cut off with clamp, and ligate both ends and the suprarenal vein. Then the inferior vena cava appears. To dissociate the right hepatic vein, the venous ligament covering the inferior vena cava must be disconnected. If the venous ligament is thin, it can be cut directly. However, in most cases, it is thick, inside which there are blood vessels from the right posterior hepatic lobe to the inferior vena cava; therefore, it can be cut with clamp, and both ends should be sutured with 4-0 Prolene; alternatively, it can also be cut with Endo GIA to avoid massive hemorrhage. The anatomical gap between the right hepatic vein and the inferior vena cava will appear after cutting the venous ligament. Undermine along this gap, and go out of the gap between the liver and the right hepatic vein. If the gap is small and the separation is difficult to carry out, short hepatic veins should be cut and sutured upward stepwise, so that the front wall of the inferior vena cava will be dissociated completely, and the right hepatic vein will appear clearly. Disconnect the right hepatic vein with clamp, suture both ends with 4-0 Prolene, or disconnect with Endo GIA. During resection of the right lobe, it is unnecessary to control the middle hepatic vein outside of the liver.

During dissociation of the liver parenchyma, the Pringle method should be used to block the hepatic portal. It should be carried out upward along the boundary of the left and right lobes (interlobar plane). Crash liver parenchyma with a blunt-pointed vascular clamp, or reveal intrahepatic vessels by CUSA; ligate and disconnect one by one. With intensive separation of liver parenchyma, the middle hepatic vein appears. Dissociate along the right edge of the middle hepatic vein, and disconnect the branches of the middle hepatic vein from Segments V and VIII. Continue the separation and the right portal triads will appear in which the right hepatic duct is involved; if the right hepatic duct has not been treated outside, disconnect and suture it. Dissociate upward, the front wall of the inferior vena cava and the right hepatic vein will appear; if the right hepatic vein has not been cut outside, cut it off and suture. Insert the left hand behind the right hepatic lobe, and put the finger under the inferior vena cava; thus, the inferior vena cava will not be injured, and the stress at the incision of liver parenchyma will increase, which is a help for dissociation.

For effusion of blood at the cross section of the liver, suture or argon knife treatment is suitable. Cover it with white gauze after complete hemostasis, or inject methylene blue through bile vesica to detect whether or not a biliary leakage occurs. If it occurs, suture properly. Intraoperative cholangiography through the cystic duct is helpful for identification of the abnormal biliary tract, biliary tract injury, and biliary leakage, which can decrease the incidence of complications. The cross section can be treated by spraying fibrin glue or covering with great omentum; do not force to suture. After resection of the right hepatic lobe, there will be a large space under the right diaphragm; therefore, the falciform ligament and round ligament should be sutured here to stabilize the residual left hepatic lobe, and prevent it from turning right to twist the bile duct and portal vein. Moreover, drainage should be carried out under the right diaphragm.

As for giant tumors at the right hepatic lobe, it is difficult to disconnect liver parenchyma after dissociation of the right hepatic lobe; moreover, excessive overturning and pressure of tumors will promote spreading of cancer cells. To this kind of cases, anterior approach can be applied; i.e., the liver should be disconnected before dissociation. Firstly, the hepatic portal should be anatomized and feeding on blood should be blocked, as mentioned above. Then dissociate liver parenchyma downward from the front, until the right hepatic vein appears; cut it. Go further gradually to the front wall of the inferior vena cava, and then dissociate the right side of the inferior vena cava; disconnect and suture short hepatic veins that may exist. Dissociate the perihepatic ligament, and remove the right hepatic lobe.

13.2.2 Right Trisegmentectomy

It is also named as extended right hemihepatectomy, and the range to be resected includes Segments IV, V, VI, VII, and VIII. It is applicable to patients with giant or multiple tumors at the right lobe and Segment IV, whose reserve function of liver is good and the left exterior lobe has proliferated. The initial step is identical to that of right hemihepatectomy. Lower the hilar plate; anatomize the omphaloschisis leftward further after controlling the blood stream feeding to the right hepatic lobe. Disconnect liver parenchyma bridge that may exist between Segments III and IV, and incise peritoneum at the base of Segment IV with a sharp dissection; extend to the omphaloschisis. Thus the hilar plate can be lowered, and the left hepatic duct can be dissociated from the base of Segment IV. Anatomize the base of the omphaloschisis; do not injure the left hepatic artery and left branch of the portal vein. Anatomize the right side of the omphaloschisis upward continuously, and two branches of the portal vein supplying Segments IVa and IVb will appear. If the tumor is close to the omphaloschisis, it is advised to dissociate or suture these two blood vessels at the right side of the omphaloschisis. If the tumor is away from the omphaloschisis, it can be treated during dissociation of liver parenchyma.

Dissociation of the liver parenchyma starts from the left bottom of Segment IVb, and continue downward to the base of the omphaloschisis along the right side of the falciform ligament. Once the blood vessels supplying Segments IVa and IVb are disconnected, Segment IV will be devascularized. Continue the separation along the right side of the falciform ligament toward the inferior vena cava. With the progress of anatomization, intrahepatic veins will appear. Track along the intrahepatic vein to the confluence of the inferior vena cava, ligate and disconnect to achieve the maximum cleaning range against tumors. If the right hepatic vein has not been cut outside, it can be disconnected inside then.

If the tumor is big and occupies Segment IV, it may push the left hepatic duct at the base of Segment IV. If so, the left hepatic duct is difficult to dissociate from the base of the hepatic portal and omphaloschisis; usually, a part of the left hepatic duct should be resected to ensure there is no tumor at the incisal margin. After removal of the sample, according to the range and length of defect, end-to-end anastomosis should be carried out to both ends of the left hepatic duct and common hepatic duct, or the left hepatic duct jejunum Roux-en-Y anastomosis can also be carried out, to rebuild the bile duct.

13.2.3 Left Hemihepatectomy

Raise the round ligament, and lift the quadrate lobe; scissor the peritoneum at the hepatic portal from the bottom of the quadrate lobe to the base of the omphaloschisis. Push the hilar plate downward. Incise the peritoneum at the left side of the omphaloschisis base, and the left hepatic artery will appear. Dissociate, double ligate, and disconnect. Pay attention to the hepatogastric ligament; if the accessory hepatic artery from the left gastric artery occurs, ligation is necessary. Continue the anatomization at the base of the omphaloschisis to reveal the left branch of the portal vein and the branch of the caudate lobe. If the caudate lobe is to be resected simultaneously, the fracture of the portal vein should be located at the close end of the caudate lobe branch. If the caudate lobe is not to be resected, the far end of the caudate lobe branch coming from the portal vein should be dissociated to reserve the caudate lobe branch. During the dissociation, if hemorrhage occurs due to injury of the portal vein, it can be blocked by the Pringle method, and sutured with 5-0 Prolene. The left hepatic duct is usually located above the left branch of the portal vein; dissociate and set suture line around it; dissociate at the entry of the omphaloschisis. Then the ischemia line is clear from the gallbladder fossa to the left lateral wall of the inferior vena cava; mark the incisal line with an electric knife.

Disconnect the left triangular ligament, and dissociate the left exterior hepatic lobe (Segments II and III). Note: The spleen should be protected. The front wall of the superior and inferior vena cava and the common trunk or branches of left and middle hepatic veins should be revealed by anatomization. Turn the left exterior lobe to the right, and disconnect the hepatogastric ligament to reveal the venous ligament. Incise the venous ligament near the left hepatic vein to reveal the triangular anatomic gap at the confluence of the left hepatic vein into the inferior vena cava; (the left hepatic vein is at the front, the inferior vena cava is at the back, and the top of Segment II is at the bottom). Dissociate carefully along the triangular gap to form a tunnel inside the space of the left and middle hepatic vein and the front wall of the inferior vena cava. Perforate the clamp through the space between the left and middle hepatic veins; thus, the common trunk of the left and middle hepatic veins can be dissociated. If the left and middle hepatic veins are separated, they can also be dissociated separately first, and then disconnected with clamp; the residual end should be closed with 4-0 Prolene; alternatively, Endo GIA disconnection may also be applied.

Block the hepatic portal, and dissociate the liver parenchyma along the interlobar plane, incise inclined toward the venous ligament at the left side of the inferior vena cava, and finally dissociate the left hepatic lobe above the caudate lobe.

13.2.4 Extended Left Hemihepatectomy

It means resection of Segments II, III, IV, V, and VIII, which is applicable when the giant tumor at the left lobe goes beyond the interlobar plane and invades Segments V and VIII, or multiple tumors are located at the left lobe and Segments V and VIII. The difficulty of this operation includes the judgment of the incisal plane at right liver parenchyma, and the control of hemorrhage and the biliary tract complications. Preoperative anatomical evaluation is very important; if necessary, A computed tomography angiography (CTA) or magnetic resonance angiography (MRA) should be used to know the involvement of blood vessels.

The initial anatomization is identical to that of left hemihepatectomy. Dissociate the liver completely. The ligation site of the left hepatic artery, left hepatic duct, and portal vein depends on the fact that whether or not the caudate lobe is to be resected. If the caudate lobe is to be resected, disconnection should be carried out near the left and right branches; otherwise, it should be carried out at the base of the omphaloschisis to reserve blood supply of the caudate lobe. The anatomization of the left and middle hepatic veins and the inferior vena cava is the same as that of left hemihepatectomy. If the caudate lobe is to be resected simultaneously, dissociate it from the inferior vena cava at the left side.

It is one of the difficulties of this operation to identify the incisal plane of liver parenchyma. This incisal plane starts from the project of the right hepatic vein on the hepatic surface, and spreads flatly to the gallbladder fossa. If the tumor is not adjacent to the right vessel pedicle, blunt anatomization can be carried out along the Glisson's sheath of the right anterior lobe to dissociate the vessel pedicle of the right anterior lobe. After clamping, the border of the right interlobar fissure will appear. Dissociate the liver parenchyma upward and flatly inward along the incisal plane. Hemorrhage, if occurs, mainly comes from branches of the right hepatic veins, which can be decreased by lowering central venous pressure. If the tumor is so big that the vessel pedicle is pushed and the dissociation cannot be carried out along the anatomical interface, it should be carried out along the interface of the liver parenchyma that shrunk due to pressure of tumor. If the middle and left hepatic veins have not been disconnected before, disconnection should be carried out if they are met during dissociation of the liver parenchyma. Remove the sample, and treat the coarse fracture of the liver carefully. Discontinuous blocking of the hepatic portal may be carried out to find out whether hemorrhage occurs out of branches of the hepatic artery and portal vein; if so, suture and stanch it. As this operation may lead to a high possibility of the biliary fistula, after complete hemostasis, rinse the fracture, and cover the fracture with white gauze for several minutes before finding out biliary fistula; ligate or suture the opening of the bile duct. Stanch the fracture of the liver by spraying fibrin glue or by argon knife; cover it with omentum.

13.2.5 Hepatic Left Lateral Lobectomy

Anatomize the hepatic triads supplying Segments II and III at the left side of the omphaloschisis; disconnect them respectively; this method is applicable to patients whose tumor is adjacent to the omphaloschisis. For those whose tumor is located at periphery, the liver parenchyma can be dissociated backward along the left side of the round ligament and falciform ligament, and vessels met during this process should be treated one by one. With the disconnection of the hepatic tissues, the left hepatic vein will appear at the rear, which should be treated intrahepatic. If the tumor is adjacent to the left and middle hepatic veins, extrahepatic treatment of the left hepatic vein is recommended.

13.2.6 Caudate Lobectomy

Caudate lobectomy includes three main steps: (1) Control of feeding of blood flow: Anatomize the base of the omphaloschisis to reveal the blood vessels of the caudate lobe starting from the left posterior of the hepatic artery and portal venous, and then ligate and disconnect them. (2) Anatomization of the short hepatic veins: Dissociate the left exterior lobe, fold, and spread rightward. Disconnect the fibrous tissue extending from the left edge of the caudate lobe toward the rear of the inferior vena cava, and dissociate the left edge of the caudate lobe. Anatomize the short hepatic vein, ligate or disconnect after clamping, and dissociate the gap between the caudate lobe and the inferior vena cava from left to right, until the caudate lobe is dissociated completely. However, it is recommended to anatomize short hepatic veins from the right side under the following conditions: (a) When the caudate lobe is occupied by large block of tumors, which is hard to lift, and it is difficult to reveal short hepatic veins; (b) when the tumor is located at the caudate process, on the right side of inferior vena cava; (c) when right hemihepatectomy or extended right hemihepatectomy is to be combined. Turn the right lobe to the left, ligate and disconnect short hepatic veins upward gradually from the rear of the caudate process to the hepatic vein; extend leftward, until the caudate lobe is dissociated from the inferior vena cava completely. Some surgeons split the liver along the interlobar plane, dissociate the liver along the right edge of Segment IV, and resect the caudate lobe through the liver. Selection of entry route for operation depends on the site and size of tumor, the means of combined resection, and adhesion of operation fields in the past. (3) Disconnection of liver parenchyma.

Another difficulty of single resection of the caudate lobe is that when the tumor is big or located at a higher position, adjacent to or invading the hepatic vein, inferior vena cava, and the confluence of them, it should be noted that the back wall of left or middle hepatic veins should not be broken; otherwise great hemorrhage may occur. It is recommended to dissociate the hepatic vein along the anatomical space of the left and middle hepatic veins and the inferior vena cava at the caudate lobe; during dissociation of liver parenchyma, the Atrauma Bulldog Clamp should be used to block the left and middle vein temporarily. Alternatively, dissociate the inferior vena cava above and below the liver, and prepare a blocking area; if necessary, block the blood flow of the whole liver; thus, the resection is safer. Right hemihepatectomy or extended right hemihepatectomy can also be combined.

If the tumor invades the wall of the inferior vena cava, resect the involved wall of the inferior vena cava along with tumors; small defects can be repaired directly, while the bigger ones can be rebuilt with the help of autogenous or artificial blood vessels. As for those patients with chronic blocking of the inferior vena cava, well-developed collateral circulation has usually been established; rebuilding is not necessary after resection.

13.3 Hepatic Segmentectomy

The following three methods are involved in hepatic segmentectomy: (1) Orientate the vessel pedicle and fissures of the liver according to the mark on the surface of the liver and intraoperative Type B ultrasonic, and determine the border of the hepatic segments. Then dissociate liver parenchyma, vessel pedicle, and bile duct of the corresponding hepatic segments, and disconnect them. Although this method is simple, it has defects: (a) the borders of some the hepatic segments are difficult to determine, especially that of Segments VII and VIII and when the liver is twisted; (b) during separation of liver parenchyma, the vessel pedicle of the hepatic segment is not controlled, resulting in hemorrhage, and thus the hepatic portal should be blocked. (2) Control the vessel pedicle of hepatic segment to be resected first. This method is applicable especially to right lobe segmentectomy, e.g., resection of Segments VII and VIII, and that of Segments V and VIII. Open the peritoneum outside of the right branch of the portal vein, and reveal the right branch and the right anterior branch and right exterior branch of the portal vein. Lowering the hilar plate can increase the length of these branches outside of the liver. Block the branches of the portal vein and arteries of the segments to be resected, and the color of the hepatic segments will change; dissociate liver parenchyma along the border of the ischemia line, and finally ligate the broken pedicles of the arteries and portal vein. This method has two advantages: (a) The border of the hepatic segment is defined clearly; (b) separation of liver parenchyma at the border will lead to little hemorrhage. (3) Resection under the guide of ultrasonic. Orientate the portal vein supplying tumors with the help of ultrasonic; puncture the portal vein, and inject methylene blue or congo red to dye the liver parenchyma corresponding to this portal vein. Insert a balloon catheter, and inflate the balloon to block the portal vein selectively; anatomize the hepatic artery at the hepatic portal and block it; thus, the boundary of the hepatic segment to be resected will be clearer. Dissociate liver parenchyma intensively from the top, block it for 10–15 min, and then loosen it for 3–5 min; finally, disconnect the vessel pedicle and bile duct. This method is similar to the anatomic resection, but a high level of ultrasonic skill is needed.

13.3.1 Hepatic Segmentectomy for Segments II and III

Simple hepatic segmentectomy for Segments II and III is just applicable to the cases in which hepatic tissues are expected to be reserved as much as possible. If the corresponding portal pedicle is not blocked, the boundary of the segments is difficult to determine. It is recommended to lift the round ligament and left hepatic lobe, anatomize the omphaloschisis, and dissociate the branches of the portal vein supplying Segments II and III, respectively. Ligate the vessel pedicle of corresponding segments to reveal the boundary. Dissociate liver parenchyma along the ischemia line. Anatomize and block the left hepatic vein; thus hemorrhage can be decreased further during incision of the liver. If simple resection of Segments II and III are carried out, the left hepatic vein should be kept.

13.3.2 Hepatic Segmentectomy for Segment IV

Firstly, disconnect the round ligament, falciform ligament, and the possible liver parenchyma bridge that may exist between Segments III and IV, and incise the peritoneum at the base of Segment IV with sharp dissection; lower the hilar plate to reveal the left branch of left portal veins. Open the peritoneum covering the left branch of the portal vein, and dissociate upward along the omphaloschisis; then the two branches of portal veins supplying Segments IVa and IVb will reveal. The IVb branch can be dissociated and disconnected before incision of the liver. IVa branch is located deeply; moreover, it is short and wide; sometimes it is difficult to dissociate; therefore, it can be treated during disconnection of the liver parenchyma.

Dissociation of the liver parenchyma starts from the left side, along the right side of the falciform ligament or the omphaloschisis, where the hepatic tissues are thin; disconnect all blood vessels supplying Segment IV. Dissociate along the interlobar plane from the middle point of the cholecystic bed; in this incisal plane, the left branches of the middle hepatic vein will be met; ligate and disconnect them; it should be noted that the middle hepatic vein should be protected. The bottom of Segment IV should be treated at last; disconnect the liver parenchyma flatly near the inferior vena cava, and converge the left and right incisal planes.

13.3.3 Hepatic Segmentectomy for Segments V and VIII

Control of hemorrhage is the key factor that ensures the smooth progress of mesohepatectomy. Lower the hilar plate first, and then extend to the right portal triads. Open the peritoneum near the portal pedicle, dissociate branches of the portal vein and hepatic artery at the right anterior lobe, and clamp them. Dissociate the right hepatic lobe, reveal the right hepatic vein, and clamp the entry of the right hepatic vein to the inferior vena cava temporarily to decrease hemorrhage. For those patients whose tumors are adjacent to or involve the hepatic vein or the inferior vena cava, the possibility of hemorrhage or air embolus is high; therefore, the inferior vena cava above and below the liver should be dissociated before incision of the liver; wind the inferior vena cava; when necessary, block the blood flow of the whole liver.

Dissociation of liver parenchyma starts from the left side and continue along the interlobar plane (right side of the middle hepatic vein); in this incisal plane, branches of the middle hepatic vein will appear; if so, ligate and disconnect them; continue until the front wall of the inferior vena cava is reached. Disconnect along the right interlobar fissure (left side of the right hepatic vein). After complete resection of Segment VIII, the lateral walls of the right and middle hepatic veins will appear; after resection of Segment V, the ligated branches of the right and middle hepatic veins and the vessel pedicle of Segment V will appear.

13.3.4 Hepatic Segmentectomy for Segment VIII

Segment VIII is located at the top of the liver, of which the left boundary is the interlobar plane (in which the middle hepatic vein is located), and the right boundary is the right interlobar fissure (in which the right hepatic vein is located); moreover, the inferior vena cava is behind it, and its lower boundary is the plane of the right branch of the portal vein. Therefore, it is difficult to carry out individual hepatic segmentectomy for Segment VIII, except for isolated small metastatic focus.

Disconnect the liver parenchyma along the boundary, and lift hepatic tissues gradually. The incisal plane should be vertical to the surface of the liver and should not contact the surface of tumor. During separation of boundaries at two sides, do not hurt the middle and right hepatic veins. It is difficult to reveal hepatic veins before removal of hepatic tissues; thus, it is not easy to repair. During disconnection of the lower liver parenchyma, vessel pedicle of Segment VIII will appear. Marriotti et al. suggested to split the liver along the left side of the middle hepatic vein so that Segment VIII is easier to dissociate.

13.3.5 Hepatic Segmentectomy for Segments IV+V+VIII

Hepatic segmentectomy for Segments IV+V+VIII is also named as mesohepatectomy, which is the combination of hepatic segmentectomy for

Segment IV and the right anterior lobe. At first, lower the hilar plate, and spread to the left and right side. Anatomize the umbilical gap, and disconnect the branch of the portal vein supplying Segment IV. Dissociate the middle hepatic vein, and ligate it near the inferior vena cava. If the tumor is not adjacent to the main trunk of the right portal vein, under the precondition that the removal of tumor is not affected, the right anterior branch can be dissociated and ligated first, and then the incisal line can be marked correctly according to the ischemia line. If the right anterior branch is difficult to dissociate or adjacent to tumors, the Pringle method can be adopted; i.e., disassociate the liver parenchyma first, and then treat the right anterior branch in the liver.

The dissociation of liver parenchyma starts from the right side of falciform ligament, and then continues along the right interlobar fissure; ligate and disconnect the branches of right hepatic veins of Segments V and VIII, and the incisal plane at the left side will be met. After resection, the inferior vena cava will appear; ligate and disconnect the middle hepatic vein, but reserve the left and right hepatic veins. Treat the two disconnected planes carefully and do not force to fold and suture them.

13.3.6 Hepatic Segmentectomy for Segments VI and VII

Segments VI and VII, located at the right posterior of the right hepatic vein, form the right posterior lobe of the liver. Anatomize the right posterior branch of the portal vein. The incisal line near the cholecystic bed is helpful for the identification of the right posterior branch; 70 % of the right posterior branches are located in it. Dissociate the right posterior branch of the portal vein, and block it temporarily, which will lead to color change of corresponding hepatic tissues; mark the incisal line along the ischemia line. If the Segments VI and VII are to be resected simultaneously, the right posterior branch of the portal vein should be disconnected then. If the Segment VI or VII are to be resected individually, the right posterior branch of the portal vein should be maintained. Dissociate the right lobe of the liver, and disconnect a part of the short hepatic vein to dissociate the right hepatic vein.

The disconnection of liver parenchyma should be carried out along the right side of the right hepatic vein. The root of the right hepatic vein can be blocked to decrease hemorrhage. Identify and protect the main trunk of the right hepatic vein. Ligate and disconnect the branch of the right posterior lobe. After individual resection of Segments VI and VII, the fracture planes can usually be folded and sutured.

13.4 Irregular Hepatectomy

13.4.1 Sufficient Dissociation of Liver

Disconnect the perihepatic ligament, and dissociate the liver sufficiently; thus, the tumor will appear completely, the hemorrhage can be controlled easily, and the fracture plane is easy to close.

13.4.2 Design of Incisal Line of Liver

The design of the incisal line of liver should consider both the radical treatment of tumor and the safety of resection. The distance between the incisal margin and tumor should be more than 1 cm. The critical blood vessels and bile duct in the liver should be avoided. Moreover, the volume of the residual liver should be over 30 %, and the inlet and outlet of blood vessels of the residual liver should not be affected.

Wedging resection can be designed for tumors at edge of the liver, e.g., those located in Segments II, III, IVb, V, VI, and VII; incise the capsula fibrosa with an electric knife at a distance of 2–3 cm from the edge of the tumor to label the incisal line. For tumors at the center of the liver, e.g., those located in Segments IVa or VIII or intrasegment, fusiform, or lip form incision can be designed. As the incisal line is inclined from the surface of the liver to the base of the tumor during disconnection of liver parenchyma, the incisal range at the surface of the liver should be large enough for tumors at deep sites, to ensure the distance between the incisal margin and tumor at the base should be over 1 cm.

13.4.3 Suture and Traction at Both Sides of Incisal Line

Suture and traction at both sides of the incisal line of the liver can decrease the hemorrhage during disconnection of liver parenchyma at the surface. Moreover, traction will help the appearance during separation of liver parenchyma, and avoid pushing tumors, which is also the exhibition of non-tumor technique.

13.4.4 Control of Blood Flow In and Out of the Liver

As irregular resection is not carried out along the fissures of the liver, the hepatic portal is often to be blocked to decrease hemorrhage. Usually, the time of individual blocking should not over 15–20 min at an interval of 3–5 min.

13.4.5 Disconnection of Liver Parenchyma

The direction of liver parenchyma disconnection is inclined from the sides of tumor to the base of tumor; ligate and disconnect the vessels, and large vessels should be sutured. The direction of the incisal plane should be controlled to avoid incision of tumor, and critical vessels should also be protected. If necessary, Type B ultrasonic can be used for orientation.

13.4.6 Treatment of Fracture Plane

The bleeding points at the fracture plane should be sutured for hemostasis. Rinse to clean the plane, and then check whether or not a biliary leakage occurs. If there is enough volume of the residual liver and suture does not affect the blood stream supplying to and backflow from the residual liver, the fracture plane can be folded to suture. Alternatively, after thorough hemostasis, spraying fibrin glue or covering the fracture plane with hemostatic gauze is also applicable.

13.5 Portal Vein Embolization

13.5.1 Indications

Patients with normal hepatic reserve function (the ICG retention value at 15 min, ICGR-15 <10 %), of whom >60 % of the liver with function (i.e., hepatic tissues without tumors) is resected.

Patients with slight decrease of hepatic reserve function (ICG-R15 10–20 %), of whom 40–60 % of the liver with function is resected; or those combined with obstructive jaundice.

13.5.2 Contraindication

Patients with moderate to severe decrease of hepatic reserve function (ICG-R15 >20 %). These kinds of patients are often combined with moderate to severe hepatocirrhosis, whose proliferation of the liver is prohibited or elongated.

13.5.3 Portal Vein Embolization Technique

There are several routes for the portal vein embolization technique: (1) percutaneous portal vein embolization (PTPE): Puncture the intrahepatic portal vein under the guide of ultrasonic, and insert catheters by means of the Seldinger technique; (2) for portal vein embolization through ileocolic vein, make a small incision at the abdomen, and insert catheters through the branch of ileocolic vein; (3) portal vein embolization through the right gastroepiploic vein; and (4) portal vein embolization through the middle colic vein.

The mixture of gelatin sponge, thrombin, and cardiografin can act as the embolic agent. Application of iodipin can reveal the shape of the portal vein in the postoperative plain film for a long time. It is reported that fibrin glue, butyl-2-cyanoacrylate, and 99 % ethanol or steel ring can also be used.

Direct portovenography through the inserted catheter can reveal the anatomic character and variation of the intrahepatic portal vein. Under the guide of an X-ray, inject embolic agents slowly to embolize the branch of the portal vein of the hepatic lobes to be resected, until the portal vein of the hepatic lobe to be resected is blocked. Embolic agents should be injected separately to the portal veins of the right anterior lobe and right posterior lobe; the main trunk at the right side of portal vein should not be embolized, to prevent the backflow of embolic agent to the left branch of the portal vein. Please pay more attention to the case that the secondary branch starts near or from main trunk of the portal vein; under this condition, a balloon catheter should be used to prevent the backflow of embolic agent into the contralateral portal vein. After portal vein embolization, portovenography or ultrasonography should be used to ensure the portal vein at the reserved side is unblocked. The portal vein pressure before and after embolization should be measured.

After operation, hepatic function and blood flow in the portal vein of the unembolized lobe should be monitored periodically. CT scanning should be carried out 2–3 weeks after operation to examine the volume of embolized hepatic lobes to that of unembolized ones. Hepatectomy is usually carried out 2–4 weeks after embolization.

References

1. O'Reilly DA, Poston GJ. Colorectal liver metastases: current and future perspectives. Future Oncol. 2006;2(4):525–31.
2. De Jong MC, Pulitano C, Ribero D, et al. Rates and patterns of recurrence following curative intent surgery for colorectal liver metastasis: an international multi-institutional analysis of 1669 patients. Ann Surg. 2009;250(3):440–8.
3. Garden OJ, Rees M, Poston GJ, et al. Guidelines for resection of colorectal cancer liver metastases. Gut. 2006;55 Suppl 3:iii1–8.
4. Imamura H, Seyama Y, Kokudo N, et al. Single and multiple resections of multiple hepatic metastases of colorectal origin. Surgery. 2004;135(5):508–17.
5. Capussotti L, Vigano' L, Ferrero A, et al. Timing of resection of liver metastases synchronous to colorectal tumor: proposal of prognosis-based decisional model. Ann Surg Oncol. 2007;14(3):1143–50.
6. Martin 2nd RC, Augenstein V, Reuter NP, et al. Simultaneous versus staged resection for synchronous colorectal cancer liver metastases. J Am Coll Surg. 2009;208(5):842–50.
7. Peeters CF, de Waal RM, Wobbes T, et al. Outgrowth of human liver metastases after resection of the primary colorectal tumor: a shift in the balance between apoptosis and proliferation. Int J Cancer. 2006;119(6):1249–53.
8. Otchy D, Hyman NH, Simmang C, et al. Practice parameters for colon cancer. Dis Colon Rectum. 2004;47(8):1269–84.
9. Kong G, Jackson C, Koh DM, et al. The use of 18F-FDG PET/CT in colorectal liver metastases – comparison with CT and liver MRI. Eur J Nucl Med Mol Imaging. 2008;35(7):1323–9.
10. Lubezky N, Metser U, Geva R, et al. The role and limitations of 18-fluoro-2-deoxy-D-glucose positron emission tomography (FDG-PET) scan and computerized tomography (CT) in restaging patients with hepatic colorectal metastases following neoadjuvant chemotherapy: comparison with operative and pathological findings. J Gastrointest Surg. 2007;11(4):472–8.
11. Adie S, Yip C, Chu F, et al. Resection of liver metastases from colorectal cancer: does preoperative chemotherapy affect the accuracy of PET in preoperative planning? ANZ J Surg. 2009;79(5):358–61.
12. Vauthey JN, Pawlik TM, Ribero D, et al. Chemotherapy regimen predicts steatohepatitis and an increase in 90-day mortality after surgery for hepatic colorectal metastases. J Clin Oncol. 2006;24(13):2065–72.
13. Rubbia-Brandt L, Mentha G, Terris B. Sinusoidal obstruction syndrome is a major feature of hepatic lesions associated with oxaliplatin neoadjuvant chemotherapy for liver colorectal metastases. J Am Coll Surg. 2006;202(1):199–200.
14. Zacherl J, Scheuba C, Imhof M, et al. Current value of intraoperative sonography during surgery for hepatic neoplasms. World J Surg. 2002;26(5):550–4.
15. Pawlik TM, Vauthey JN. Surgical margins during hepatic surgery for colorectal liver metastases: complete resection not millimeters defines outcome. Ann Surg Oncol. 2008;15(3):677–9.
16. Hamady ZZ, Cameron IC, Wyatt J, et al. Resection margin in patients undergoing hepatectomy for colorectal liver metastasis: a critical appraisal of the 1cm rule. Eur J Surg Oncol. 2006;32(5):557–63.
17. DeMatteo RP, Palese C, Jarnagin WR, et al. Anatomic segmental hepatic resection is superior to wedge resection as an oncologic operation for colorectal liver metastases. J Gastrointest Surg. 2000;4(2):178–84.

18. Zorzi D, Mullen JT, Abdalla EK, et al. Comparison between hepatic wedge resection and anatomic resection for colorectal liver metastases. J Gastrointest Surg. 2006;10(1):86–94.
19. Sarpel U, Bonavia AS, Grucela A, et al. Does anatomic versus nonanatomic resection affect recurrence and survival in patients undergoing surgery for colorectal liver metastasis? Ann Surg Oncol. 2009;16(2):379–84.
20. Petrowsky H, Gonen M, Jarnagin W, et al. Second liver resections are safe and effective treatment for recurrent hepatic metastases from colorectal cancer: a bi-institutional analysis. Ann Surg. 2002;235(6):863–71.
21. Adam R, Pascal G, Azoulay D, et al. Liver resection for colorectal metastases: the third hepatectomy. Ann Surg. 2003;238(6):871–83.

Laparoscopic Management of Colorectal Liver Metastases

14

Thomas Satyadas, Zahra Shafaee, and Brice Gayet

14.1 Introduction

Colorectal cancer is the third most common cancer worldwide, with a lifetime risk of approximately 5 %. The most common site for haematogenous metastasis is the liver. Approximately 10–20 % of patients with colorectal adenocarcinoma will have synchronous hepatic metastasis at the time of diagnosis, and 20–25 % of the patients will develop metachronous metastasis later in life. Without treatment, the prognosis of colorectal cancer with liver metastasis is poor, and the 5-year survival rate is less than 5 %. At present, liver resection offers the best chance of survival for patients with colorectal cancer liver metastasis. Currently the 5-year survival rate following curative resection of colorectal liver metastasis approaches 45–60 %. Many reasons have contributed to the better results of colorectal liver metastasis. Improved patient selection in a multidisciplinary team setting, increased understanding of liver surgery and anaesthesia, technological improvements, advances made in diagnostic and interventional radiology and advances made in the field of chemotherapy are to name a few contributory factors.

Since the initial laparoscopic liver resection in the early 1990s, there has been a slow progress in the number of liver resections performed laparoscopically. Increasing expertise and experience in liver and laparoscopic surgery and advances in technology, there has been an exponential rise in the number of liver resections performed laparoscopically. Recent world review suggests that there are almost 3,000 laparoscopic liver resections reported in the world literature.

The use of laparoscopy in colorectal liver metastasis also includes staging of the disease to look for peritoneal disease and with the use of laparoscopic ultrasound to identify and confirm the location and number of lesions as suggested by the preoperative imaging. This would be a valid tool as it would prevent patients from having an unnecessary laparotomy if the metastatic lesions are deemed unresectable. There is also a role for laparoscopy in radiofrequency ablation in the treatment of colorectal liver metastasis. Laparoscopic ablation is found to have less local recurrence than percutaneous with the obvious advantages over open ablation. Laparoscopic radiofrequency ablation of the liver metastasis can be done as an adjunct to resection of other lesions in order to preserve functional residual liver volume. Current evidence does not support the use of radiofrequency ablation as the primary

T. Satyadas • Z. Shafaee • B. Gayet (✉)
Department of Digestive Disease, Institut Mutualiste Montsouris, Université Paris-Descartes, Paris, France
e-mail: brice.gayet@imm.fr

X. Qin et al. (eds.), *Multidisciplinary Management of Liver Metastases in Colorectal Cancer*,
DOI 10.1007/978-94-017-7755-1_14

treatment for fit patients who have lesions which are amenable to resection.

This chapter would discuss mainly about laparoscopic liver resection for colorectal liver metastasis.

14.2 Preoperative Imaging

This is the same as in open hepatic resection for colorectal liver metastasis and involves ultrasound with or without contrast, triple-phase contrast CT scan, MRI scan and PET scan.

14.2.1 Ultrasound Scan (USS)

Ultrasonography is cheap and provides detailed information about the number, size and relation of metastatic lesions with the hepatic vasculature. The sensitivity can be increased by the use of contrast-enhanced ultrasound. However, ultrasound is operator dependent.

14.2.2 CT Scan

Computed tomography is routinely performed as part of staging for patients with colorectal liver metastasis. CT scans of the chest, abdomen and pelvis with intravenous contrast are obtained. A triphasic CT scan of the liver will further characterize the hepatic metastasis. Arterial phase images are useful in cases of neuroendocrine metastasis, primary hepatomas, hepatic adenomas and haemangiomas. This phase also outlines the arterial anatomy of the liver. Portal venous phase is the most useful for the evaluation of colorectal liver metastasis. Metastasis from colorectal cancer usually respects the liver capsule and intersegmental planes and pushes structures away rather than invades directly into them. However, one should be aware that there are reports of colorectal liver metastasis with intrabiliary growth. Invasion of the vena cava and diaphragm is rare, and even if imaging studies suggest invasion of these structures, surgical exploration is indicated.

14.2.3 Magnetic Resonance Imaging (MRI)

MRI is most useful to evaluate the relationship of the tumours to the hepatic vasculature and biliary system. MRI is particularly used to characterize benign lesions like hepatic adenoma, haemangioma and focal nodular hyperplasia. In cases of fatty infiltration due to obesity or prior chemotherapy and in cases of cirrhosis, MRI might be able to delineate lesions better than a contrast CT scan.

14.2.4 Positron Emission Tomography (PET) Scan

PET scan is being used to localize the distribution of the metastatic lesions. The most common tracer used is 18F-fluorodeoxyglucose (FDG). This glucose analogue cannot continue down the glycolytic pathway and accumulates within glucose-avid cancer cells. However, PET scans are not very sensitive for lesions less than 1 cm in size.

14.3 Principles of Resection

The principles of laparoscopic hepatic resection for colorectal liver metastasis remain the same as open resection. Patient fitness for the procedure, preservation of liver remnant with at least 30 % of functioning hepatic reserve following resection and to have R0 resection with a 1 cm margin.

Patient selection for laparoscopic hepatic resection also depends on the expertise and experience of the surgeon and team performing the procedure and looking after the patient. In the initial development of a laparoscopic liver resection programme, it is better to tackle small solitary lesions in the anterolateral segments (II, III, IVb, V and VI). As experience and expertise builds up, the indications can be expanded to perform more complex resections. It is important that the surgeon has advanced skills in liver and laparoscopic surgery prior to contemplating the initiation of the programme. It is also paramount that the surgeon has a very good experience of using laparoscopic intraoperative ultrasound in order to achieve an optimal result for the patient. At present, there are no laparoscopic specific contraindications in our unit; however, this is due to the extensive experience and expertise of the senior author.

Laparoscopic anatomical resection, although technically more challenging, has the advantages of lower rates of positive resection margin and less blood loss and less transfusion requirements. However, when there are multiple lesions in different segments of the liver, multiple liver conserving nonanatomical resections with a 1 cm margin can be a good alternative to preserve a larger functioning liver remnant.

14.4 Laparoscopic Management of Colorectal Liver Metastasis

The exponential rise in laparoscopic liver resections since 2005 was reported in a world review of laparoscopic liver resections in 2009. There were almost 3,000 laparoscopic liver resections in the world literature, and of them almost 45 % were for benign lesions. Of the malignant lesions which were resected laparoscopically, 35 % were for colorectal liver metastasis. Since the initial laparoscopic liver resection was reported in 1992, there has been slow progress in the number of liver resections performed laparoscopically.

Initial valid concerns were about the safety and efficacy of laparoscopic liver resection, coupled with the oncological safety of the procedure when performed for malignant lesions. A meta-analysis of eight nonrandomized studies comparing open and laparoscopic liver resection confirmed the safety and feasibility aspects of the laparoscopic liver resections. There was also significant reduction in morbidity for laparoscopic liver resections compared to open, if you look at the five studies published since 2003 which were included in the meta-analysis. Evidence suggests that laparoscopic liver resections can be safely performed by appropriately trained surgeons in a cost-effective fashion, with a reduction in the length of stay. There is also the advantage of less blood loss intraoperatively, with some studies showing a less transfusion requirement. The oncological safety has been assessed by different studies including a comparative study between open cases from Paul Brousse hospital and laparoscopic cases from Institut Mutualiste Montsouris, the authors' institution. At present there are no concerns regarding the oncological safety of laparoscopic liver resections for both primary and metastatic lesions of the liver.

There still persist some valid concerns about situations where there is uncontrolled haemorrhage and gas embolism. With all the skill mix one can attain with experience and advanced training in liver and laparoscopic surgery, profuse haemorrhage is still a distinct possibility. Surgeons should be prepared for this and should be mindful about the fact that conversion to open surgery or hand-assisted surgery is not to be deemed as a failure and be ready to convert at the appropriate time. Gas embolism leading to a clinical instability has been reported with the use of argon, and it should be emphasized that argon is 17 times less soluble than CO_2 in blood. With the current evidence, it would be better to the use of laparoscopic argon in liver surgery.

Our senior author has the experience of performing more than 200 laparoscopic liver resections for colorectal liver metastasis. This includes 59 major resections and 31 repeat hepatectomies at the Institut Mutualiste Montsouris

14.5 Operative Technique

A team approach is crucial in the provision of high-quality services to the patient. All the members of the team including nursing staff should be aware of their specific roles and should be briefed preoperatively. Nursing staff and residents should be given appropriate and regular training to be able to provide the best services to the patient.

14.5.1 Operating Room Setup

Patient is placed supine in the modified lithotomy position with legs abducted and the arms tucked on the side. Video monitor and the robotic arm for the camera are placed as shown in picture 1. The surgeon stands between the legs of the patient, the assistant on the left side and the scrub nurse on the right side of the patient. There should be flexibility in the system so that the surgeon swaps with the positions of the scrub nurse and the assistant as and when required. Patient positioning is slightly changed from the standard supine position when resection is performed for lesions in the posterosuperior segments of the liver especially resections of segments VII, VII and IVa. For this type of resections, a lateral approach is utilized, and to facilitate this, the patient's right side is elevated and the right arm is rotated to the left and padded and secured.

Nasogastric tube is not routinely inserted and neither is a urinary catheter unless it is a major hepatectomy.

14.5.2 Access

The patient is dressed and draped as for any liver resection. Pneumoperitoneum is achieved with a Veress needle. Trocar positioning would depend on the type of resection performed. A 10 mm zero degree telescope is used. The intra-abdominal pressure is raised to 20 mmHg prior to insertion of the first trocar to further elevate the anterior abdominal wall to prevent injury during the blind insertion of trocar. This is facilitated by using the aspiration technique of the anterior abdominal wall with a syringe and green needle to make sure that there is no inadvertent entry into abdominal structures. The camera is placed close to the vascular axis of dissection which is usually the hepatic pedicle. A useful guide is halfway between the right subcostal margin and the umbilicus at the midclavicular line. For left hepatic lobectomy, the camera port will be inserted at the same level in the midline. Two working trocars are inserted four fingerbreadths apart from the camera port. The working ports are always inserted at slightly different levels to provide the optimal ergonomics. An assist 5 mm port is placed further laterally to help with traction and exposure. A liver retractor might be required, and another 5 mm port will be utilized for this purpose. The retractor can be mounted on a multi-joint holder placed on the right side as cephalad as possible.

14.5.3 Technical Aspects

General exploration of the abdominal cavity is undertaken, and any suspicious peritoneal lesion would be biopsied for frozen section. Thorough and systematic laparoscopic ultrasound is performed to confirm the lesions with specific emphasis on the intrahepatic venous anatomy to plan resection and aid transection. In the cases of major hepatic resection, a tape is placed around the hepatic pedicle to perform Pringle manoeuvre as and when required. In the early phase of learning curve, the placement of a hand port in the upper abdomen, early in the case, would be beneficial in dealing with profuse haemorrhage if that happens, and the same incision can be used to remove the resected specimen. Preparation of the hand port early in the case has the advantage of having a hand ready for manual pressure if there is severe bleeding. Once the team has gone past the learning, one could dispense with this practice.

The senior author uses harmonic scalpel, bipolar diathermy forceps and monopolar scissors for dissection and parenchymal transection. The major pedicles and hepatic veins are dealt with vascular staplers.

In cases of wedge resections, it is important to start the resection at least more than 2 cm away from lesion as on intraoperative ultrasound (IOUS). There is invariably a coning effect due to the two-dimensional nature of laparoscopic surgery and the rigidity of non-flexibility in majority of laparoscopic instruments in use at present. In order to prevent the coning effect leading to a compromise in margin clearance, it is extremely important to start the resection quite wide (>2 cm) from the lesion edge on IOUS.

For major hepatic resections, dissection is carried out as in open hepatic resections. Lowering of the hilar plate is done, and this invariably causes some bleeding. It is important to deal with even the slightest of bleeding straightaway so that it does not interfere with optimal optics straightaway or later in the operation. Time spent to aspirate even the slightest of bleeding allows to dealing with the bleeding area immediately and precisely. We do not use saline for wash as we feel that it is not necessary and only suction is used.

In cases where one has to do a cholecystectomy as part of the procedure, the cystic duct is disconnected from the hepatic duct, but the gallbladder is left on the liver as this allows to using it as a handle to move things around during dissection and transection.

For a right hepatectomy, the right portal vein is dissected out and either clipped and sutured with Prolene or tied and sutured with Prolene. The bile duct is cut after clipping it with hemolock. Similar manoeuvres are done for resection of the liver on the left as well. The hepatic veins are dissected as in open surgery, and, for example, in a case of right hepatectomy, the right hepatic vein is transected only after the parenchyma has been dealt with completely. Hepatic venous transection is done with vascular staples.

During the transection of any type of hepatectomy, it is important to keep checking with IOUS, the margin clearance and the proximity of the inflow structures and the drainage vein. This will allow for better planning of the transection and as one can look out for the structures and deal with it appropriately, thereby reducing blood loss.

Almost always specimens are removed by a suprapubic incision, always in a bag. Residual bleeding is dealt with bipolar diathermy and suture ligation with Prolene. Drains are not used routinely, and if necessary in the postoperative phase, percutaneous drains are inserted under image guidance. Closure of all port sites larger than 5 mm is done with PDS.

In our centre, the indications, contraindications and technique for resections are the same as open surgery. The senior author has had extensive experience doing major hepatectomies, posterior segmental resections and repeat hepatectomies laparoscopically. However, we would recommend that in the initial stages of developing a laparoscopic liver resection programme for colorectal metastatic disease, to limit oneself to small solitary lesions in the anterolateral segments and to build enough experience and expertise.

15 Surgery for Nonresectable Metastatic Colorectal Cancer

René Adam, Emir Hoti, and Francois Faitot

15.1 Introduction

Forty to 50 % of patients who have been diagnosed with colorectal cancer will go on to develop liver metastases [1]. No less than 20–30 % of patients will present synchronous liver metastases at the time of the first operation, and another 15–20 % will develop liver metastases on the subsequent follow-up [1].

The surgical resection of hepatic metastases is the only treatment which provides a long-term survival. Currently, the 5-year survival rates after potentially curative surgery range from 37 to 58 %, and 10-year survival rates can range from 20 to 25 % [2]. On the contrary, the untreated patients had very poor prognosis with the majority patients succumbing to their disease within 12 months of diagnosis. 5-year survival in untreated patients is greatly rare, with only 0.9 % reported rates [3].

The surgical resection is the only treatment which can provide the prospect of long-term survival; it should always be considered as the first line in the treatment arsenal. The resection involves removal of the lesion(s), leaving at least 30 % tumor-free and well-vascularized parenchyma. Based on the most reported results of recent series of patients who undergo surgical resection of liver metastases, the mortality between 0 % and 3.7 % and the postoperative morbidity ranges from 15 to 46 % [4].

Despite the surgical technique advances, only 15–25 % of newly patients who have been diagnosed with colorectal liver metastases can benefit from surgical resection, the rest unresectable patient either as a result of multiple hepatic lesions or extrahepatic tumor invasion, hence are not suitable. To solve this problem, surgeons and oncologists have developed a variety of strategies involving both chemotherapy and surgery with the objective to increase the resectability rate and therefore improve their outcome.

In this regard, in surgeons' point of view, there has been a paradigm shift in the definition of resectability for patients with multiple liver metastases in the past 10 years. The presence of multiple metastases is no longer considered a contraindication to resection. Our results have demonstrated that although the 5-year survival in patients who have resection of four or more metastases is 30 % compared to the survival of 45 % in patients with no more than three lesions, resection remains the only option to increase their long-term survival [5].

R. Adam, MD, PhD (✉) • E. Hoti • F. Faitot
AP-HP Hôpital Paul Brousse, Centre Hépato-Biliaire, 12 Avenue Paul Vaillant Couturier, Villejuif 94804, France

Liver Transplant Unit, Saint Vincent's University Hospital, Dublin 4, Ireland

Inserm, Unité 785, Villejuif 94804, France

Université Paris-Sud, UMR-S 785, Villejuif 94804, France
e-mail: rene.adam@pbr.aphp.fr

X. Qin et al. (eds.), *Multidisciplinary Management of Liver Metastases in Colorectal Cancer*,
DOI 10.1007/978-94-017-7755-1_15

The most important factors known to influence the outcome after the surgical treatment are the extent of hepatic involvement at the time of diagnosis, spread of tumor in the extrahepatic sites, and abnormal hepatic function. Thus, in such patients, the tumor burden is the major determining factor in the choice of the treatment type. In circumstances where adverse factors are present resulting in an unresectable disease, the best treatment strategy would be a combined oncosurgical approach, which includes chemotherapy, portal vein embolization, and ultimately multistage hepatic resections. The objective of this combination is to increase the rate of resection of patients with CRM who are initially considered as having unresectable disease. In this regard, improved response rates to chemotherapy among CRM patients have certainly had a great impact. Our experience has demonstrated that a 5-year survival can be achieved in 33 % of patients who respond sufficiently to chemotherapy [6]. In addition, the effects of the chemotherapy can be further augmented by the addition of portal vein embolization or local ablative treatments [7, 8]. Furthermore, the extension of the indications for resection of liver lesions, without lowering the survival results, has been influenced also by the development of a newer multi-step strategy, whose multiple steps have a common purpose – the cure of patients with multinodular metastatic disease.

15.2 Patient Evaluation

15.2.1 Patient Selection for Surgery

To decide which patient will tolerate liver resection, several factors including patient comorbidities have to be considered. Age is not an independent factor for increased operative risk [9]. This is very important considering that an increasing proportion of patients being evaluated for surgery for malignant disease are elderly. On the other hand, scores like the American Society of Anesthesiologists (ASA) [10] or the preoperative Acute Physiology and Chronic Health Evaluation score are closely related to the incidence of postoperative complications. It has been shown that patients with an ASA score >1 have more than triple mortality and double morbidity compared with those patients with an ASA of 1 [10]. Therefore, the main goal of the preoperative evaluation is to confirm patients with high operative risk, so those with a prohibitive risk can be precluded from surgery, whereas those with manageable comorbidities can have these conditions addressed preoperatively in an attempt to decrease their operative risk.

15.2.2 Preoperative Imaging

The complex decision to determine resectability requires a detailed imaging to determine the tumor location, exclude unresectable extrahepatic metastases, and assess the adequacy of the liver volume after surgery. Despite the number of imaging modalities (three-dimensional CT scanning, CT angiography, magnetic resonance angiography MRI, and CT volumetry), difficulties still exist, especially when trying to differentiate between metastases and benign liver lesions or to detect small metastatic lesions. The current approach to address these pitfalls is to use a multimodal strategy [11]. For example, although helical CT scanning provides information for the entire chest and abdomen during a single breath hold, up to 25 % of the lesion can still be missed [12]. MRI on the other hand, is currently the most effective imaging modality in detecting and characterizing liver lesions and is often ordered prior to liver resection to characterize indeterminate lesions seen on a CT scan as it has a higher sensitivity to detect and characterize small lesions [13]. Using a liver-specific contrast agent, MRI has equivalent sensitivity to CT angiography [14]. Positron emission tomography (PET) is another useful modality for detecting liver metastases, especially when combined with CT scanning. However, it is no more sensitive than MRI in detection, and it lacks the special resolution and the ability to characterize lesions.

15.2.3 Assessment of Hepatic Functional Reserve

The functional hepatic reserve can be assessed by Child-Pugh score and hepatic biological blood tests; however, to date, the only test which has proven to have a good predictive value is the indocyanine green (ICG) clearance test [15]. In candidates for liver resection with retention of less than 20 % of ICG at 15 min, up to 60 % of the volume of the parenchyma can be resected. Special attention should be addressed to the specific pathologic changes of the liver parenchyma (vascular changes and/or chemotherapy-associated steatohepatitis) progressively being observed following administration of preoperative chemotherapy.

15.2.4 Selection of the Type of Resection

The principles of colorectal metastases' hepatic resection (including the oncological goal which is to resect all metastatic lesions with tumor-free margins) are no different than any other hepatic surgery. The aim of surgery should be to remove all metastases with negative histologic margins; thus, the surgical procedure selection of a particular patient should be individualized based on the size, number, and location of the metastatic lesions, their relation to main vascular pedicles, and the volume of future liver parenchyma. Resection should spare as much as possible the nontumoral parenchyma, bearing in mind that new recurrences could eventually develop for which surgery could possibly be indicated again. Lastly, no difference has been demonstrated between anatomical and non-anatomical resection.

15.3 Management of Nonresectable Colorectal Liver Metastases

15.3.1 Downstaging Chemotherapy

15.3.1.1 Systemic Neoadjuvant Chemotherapy

The improved efficacy of chemotherapy agents has allowed a subset of initially unresectable patients to undergo liver surgery after "tumor downstaging" (Fig. 15.1). By performing liver resection, a remarkable proportion of patients who otherwise would have a poor prognosis can achieve survival.

The efficacy of FOLFOX and FOLFIRI has been confirmed in large single-center series. These regimens are considered effective in facilitating hepatic resection in selected, initially nonresectable patients. Increasingly, however, the trend is to use a combination of three chemotherapy agents (all cytotoxic agents or two cytotoxic agents and one biologic agent). For example, in the phase III CRYSTAL trial, which included 1,217 patients, combined use of cetuximab with FOLFIRI (5-fluorouracil, irinotecan, leucovorin) increased response rates (59 % vs. 43 %, $P=0.004$) and PFS (HR 0.68, CI 0.50–0.94, $P=0.02$) in patients with K-ras wild-type (wt) tumors and increased R0 resection rates of patients with initially unresectable metastatic CRC (4.8 % with FOLFIRI + cetuximab vs. 1.7 % with FOLFIRI alone [includes both K-ras wt and mutant tumor status]) [16]. The OPUS trial has obtained similar results (FOLFOX ± cetuximab vs. standard chemotherapy alone). The response rate in patients with K-ras wild-type tumors was 61 % with the addition of cetuximab vs. 37 % with standard chemotherapy [17]. Another randomized phase II multicenter study (the CELIM study) of cetuximab plus FOLFOX6 or cetuximab plus FOLFIRI in the neoadjuvant setting of nonresectable metastatic CRC confined to liver found response rates of 68 % in the FOLFOX6 arms and 57 % in the FOLFIRI arms. In a combined

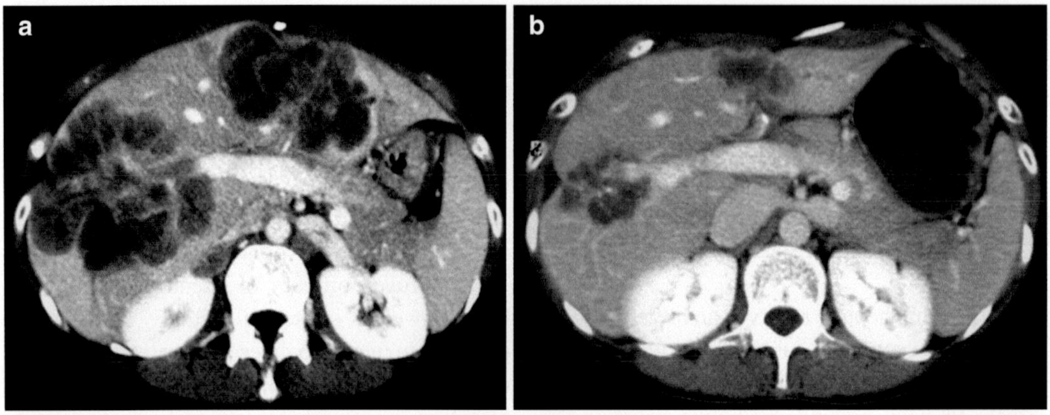

Fig. 15.1 Results of chemotherapy: CT scan demonstrating. (**a**) Tumor burden prechemotherapy treatment; (**b**) tumor burden postchemotherapy treatment

analysis of both arms, response rate was 70 % in patients with wild-type K-ras tumors. R0 resections were performed in 34 % of patients [18].

In addition, surgeons have begun to examine combinations of three times cytotoxic chemotherapy plus antibody treatment with bevacizumab or cetuximab. Randomized trials have shown that combination of a biologic agent with an oxaliplatin- or irinotecan- based regimen can increase efficacy and also the rate of secondary resection of metastatic lesions [19]. The combination of cetuximab with a chronomodulated FOLFOXIRI regimen resulted in an 85 % response rate and a 75 % resection rate. However, dose reduction was necessary because of unacceptable rates of diarrhea, and a less conservative definition of nonresectability was used [20]. Further studies are needed to show an advantage over FOLFOXIRI or chemotherapy plus cetuximab.

As for initially nonresectable CRLM to conventional systemic therapy, a number of studies have shown very significantly results. A retrospective study evaluated 151 initially nonresectable CRLM patients to first-line conventional chemotherapy, who then underwent combining therapy with cetuximab [21]. After a median of six cycles of combining therapy with cetuximab, 25 (16 %) of those patients underwent surgery. After a median of 16 months follow-up, 23 of the 25 patients (92 %) were alive and 10 (40 %) were disease-free. Median OS durations from initiation of cetuximab therapy were 20 months and PFS durations were 13 months. Similarly, in a single-arm study, initially unresectable CRLM patients to tritherapy with fluorouracil/leucovorin, irinotecan, and oxaliplatin, 82 % of patients could have R0 resection. Complete clinical remission rate postoperative was 79 %, and 2-year survival rate was 83 % following triple cytotoxic chemotherapy [22].

15.3.1.2 Intra-arterial Chemotherapy

The interest in using intra-arterial chemotherapy in neoadjuvant setting has also progressively increased as it has been demonstrated to have a high response rate in both the first- and second-line settings. In a Clavien et al. study, 6 (26 %) of 23 previously treated patients were induced resectability using HAI-FUDR with or without leucovorin. The actuarial 3-year survival rates were 84 % for neoadjuvant therapy responders compared to 40 % for nonresponders [23]. In a Memorial Sloan-Kettering hospital study [24], 44 patients with extensive liver metastases using HAI-FUDR and dexamethasone plus oxaliplatin-based systemic chemotherapy as part of two phase I trials in 44 extensive liver metastases patients. The study population in this trial had a high number of patients with more than four metastases, metastases greater than 5 cm, more than 25 % liver involvement with tumor, a CEA level greater than 10 ng/dl, and previous chemotherapy exposure. Despite these negative parameters, the objective response rate was 82 %; therefore, 9 (20 %) of the 44 patients underwent complete gross resection of tumor and a median survival for all patients of 26 months. The current, original data from several clinical trials using the oxaliplatin or irinotecan via HAI have been promising.

15.3.2 Adjunctive Techniques Employed to Reduce the Liver Volume to Be Resected Tumor Ablation Techniques

The use of ablative techniques enables the possibility to avoid resection of healthy parenchyma around tumors, thus permitting treatment of a greater number of lesions. Efficacy of these local ablative techniques is considered superior to that of chemotherapy alone.

Radiofrequency ablation (RFA) – This technique uses heat (200 to 2 MHz) to destroy solid organ tumors. It is considered as a curative treatment for hepatocellular carcinoma smaller than 3 cm. It has also been proven to be an effective technique to treat colorectal liver metastases (Fig. 15.2). Risk factors for failure of RFA are tumor volume (>3 cm), centrally located metastases and proximity to large vessels [25, 26], age above 55 years, and percutaneous approach. Morbidity is low (range 0–33 %) but, when occurring, can be very deleterious. RFA procedure when performed in combination with surgery increases the resectability and curability for patients in whom hepatic resection alone is not curative. It has reported that adding RFA to liver resection could be well tolerated with a perioperative morbidity and mortality comparable to those seen after resection alone [27]. For metastases considered as unresectable, RFA combined with hepatic resection can achieve a median survival as high 37 months [28].

Cryotherapy – This method causes destruction of tumoral cells by direct cellular freezing and indirectly through vascular thrombosis and tissue anoxia (Fig. 15.3). It has proven to be effective in liver metastases of colorectal cancer in terms of survival, and results of such treatment combined with hepatic resection for patients not eligible for hepatic resection alone have shown a 5-year survival rate of 24 %, better than those obtained by

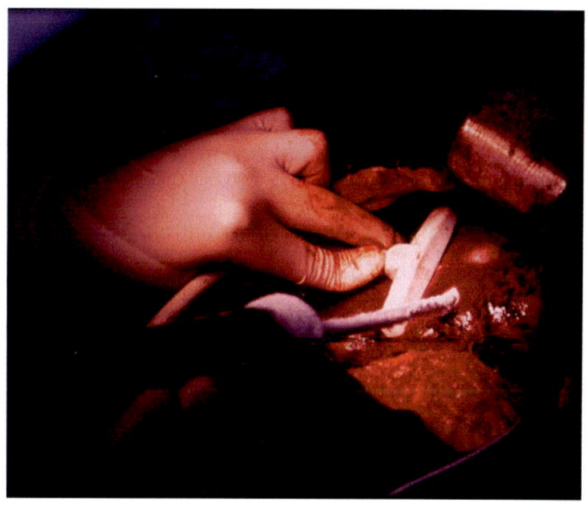

Fig. 15.3 Intraoperative cryotherapy ablation as adjunctive procedure to liver resection

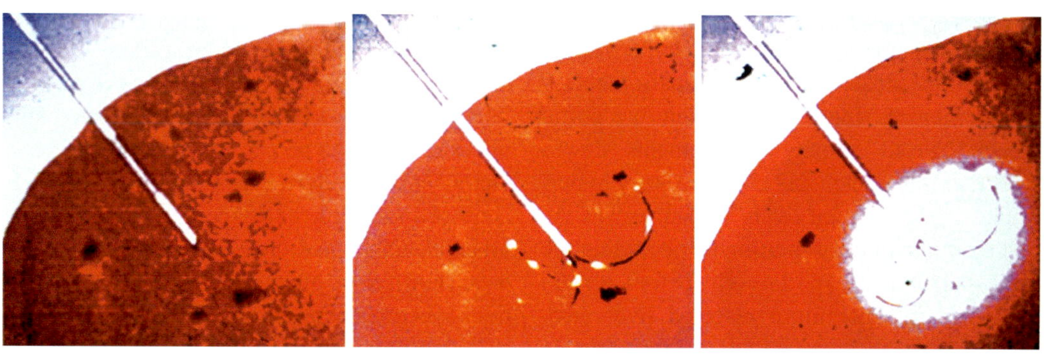

Fig. 15.2 Schematic demonstration of the tumor radiofrequency ablation (*RFA*) used as adjunctive procedure to liver surgery

palliative chemotherapy [8, 29]. Local recurrence at the site of cryotherapy occurs in 5–44 % of patients, and it has been found that the rate increases when treating multiple lesions (>8), large lesions (>3 cm), or tumors located to major blood vessels (blood warmth may impair the freezing process). Recurrence rate is however higher than after liver resection and RFA. Edge cryotherapy is utilized in some centers to achieve a 1 cm margin after hepatectomy. However, with the emergence of radiofrequency ablation, the use of cryotherapy in liver metastases has become limited.

15.3.3 Techniques Employed to Improve Remnant Liver Volume

15.3.3.1 Preoperative Portal Vein Embolization

The first cause of mortality after liver resection remains liver failure. This complication appears when the liver remnant volume is too small to cope with the postoperative metabolic demands. Criteria defining this state are encephalopathy, hyperbilirubinemia, and coagulopathy, which are frequently associated with renal insufficiency. It is accepted that the risk of liver failure is considerable when remnant liver is less than 30 % (normal parenchyma) and less than 40 % (pathological parenchyma). In this context, embolizing one side of the portal venous system that induces the contralateral liver lobe hypertrophy (the future remnant liver) can reduce the incidence of postoperative liver failure.

This phenomenon (unilateral hypertrophy) was initially observed in intrahepatic cholangiocarcinomas, where compression of a portal branch caused atrophy of segments downstream to this branch and compensatory hypertrophy of the remnant liver. Makuuchi was the first to utilize this observation by occluding the right branch of the portal vein before a right hepatectomy. The future resected liver atrophied while the future remnant liver grew in size. Many products have been used to occlude the portal vein including gelatin sponge, coils, cyanoacrylate, and alcohol. None has shown an advantage in inducing atrophy or hypertrophy of the liver. Recently, transient portal vein embolization with reabsorbable occlusive products has been successfully developed and employed [30].

There are several ways of occluding the portal vein. Portal vein embolization can be done percutaneously under radioscopic control (Fig. 15.4) by punctioning the contralateral branch of the portal vein to be embolized (e.g., left branch of PV). The product is injected or deployed in the contralateral side (e.g., right branch of PV) in the same direction of the bloodstream. The ipsilateral approach is another alternative method performed by punctioning the right portal vein and injecting the product in counter stream direction.

Surgical approaches have also been described. An ileocolic vein approach is sometimes performed through a mini-laparotomy. The catheter is pushed to the desired portal branch through the superior mesenteric vein accessed by an ileocolic vein.

Finally, portal vein occlusion can be performed as a part of a two-step resection (see Two-Stage Hepatectomy). There are reports of laparoscopic portal vein ligation in the same operative time as primary resection [31]. The results are comparable to those of radiological or laparotomy PVE/PVL. Mortality of PVE or PVL is exceptional. Morbidity is mainly due to the so-called post-embolization syndrome which is characterized by nausea and vomiting.

Standard chemotherapy does not seem to impact compensatory hyperplasia after PVE [32]. Similarly bevacizumab does not impact regeneration after PVE procedure [33]. Regeneration failure after PVE can be considered as a predictive factor for liver failure after hepatectomy as PVE is a stress test for liver regeneration. Indocyanine green clearance and three-dimensional CT scan have shown to be effective monitoring investigations for compensatory liver hypertrophy. Timing of hepatectomy after portal vein embolization is highly variable. Most frequently, the interval

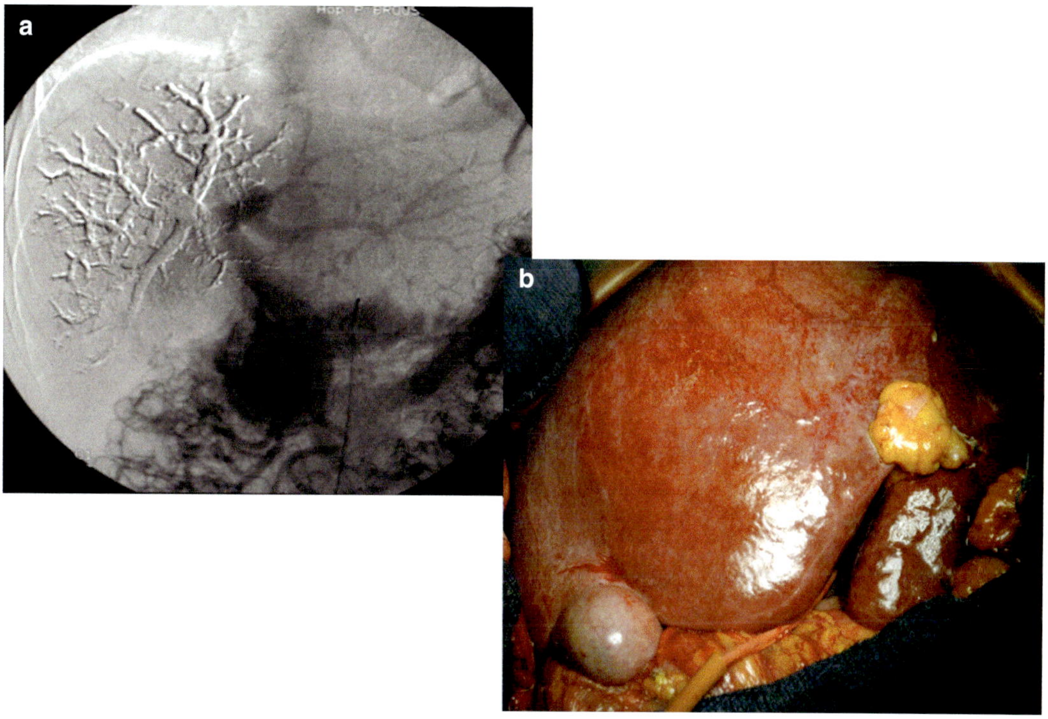

Fig. 15.4 (**a**) Radiological demonstration of percutaneous portal vein embolization; (**b**) intraoperative demonstration of the right lobe atrophy with a contralateral lobe hypertrophy

between the two procedures is 3–6 weeks. During this interval, chemotherapy must be resumed except for bevacizumab. Indeed there are studies underlining the risk of tumor growth in the future remnant liver though literature is controversial. Elias was the first to report a growth of metastases in the non-embolized lobe after PVE in the waiting time before surgery. Others have reported growth of metastases in the embolized lobe. However, these studies only compare pre- and post-PVE volumes and therefore do not show an increase in growth speed after PVE. To prevent the growth of metastases in the future remnant liver, association of PVE to chemoembolization, as practiced for hepatocellular carcinoma by Japanese teams, may be a treatment option. Indeed, the arterial buffer response activated after PVE could be responsible for the growth of the metastases in both lobes via an increased oxygen and nutrient support. Nevertheless, morbidity of this procedure especially biliary necrosis could be considerable, and a very careful evaluation of this strategy is always necessary. The most important figure is how this potential growth could impact on curability of the patients. In a recent meta-analysis, it is shown that, after PVE, 17 % of the embolized patients do not undergo liver resection, two thirds of which due to disease progression [34].

15.3.3.2 Two-Stage Hepatectomy

Principles

This strategy is reserved for extremely difficult cases of multinodular, bilobar disease, not manageable with standard liver resections, often requiring more than 70 % of the functional parenchyma to be sacrificed. The main principle of this strategy is sequential resection by two-staged hepatectomies. The objective of first hepatectomy is to render the eventual remnant liver parenchyma tumor-free, as a result of which, the second liver resection becomes feasible and potentially curative. The success of this procedure depends upon liver regeneration between the two interventions, which in turn allows the second resection to be performed with acceptable risks. Generally, patients can be classified into three possible groups: patients with multinodular, unilobar metastatic disease who require resection of up to 70 % of the functional parenchyma; patients with multinodular, bilobar metastatic disease, whose resection leaves no more than three nodules in the remnant liver; and lastly patients with multiple bilobar lesions, in which a planed resection would live more than three nodules or any nodule larger than 3 cm in the remnant liver. For the first group, preoperative portal vein embolization followed by liver resection provides the best surgical treatment, whereas liver resection combined with intraoperative local ablation therapy is the choice for the second group of patients. On the other hand, patients belonging to the later group would be best treated with two-stage hepatectomy; hence, it is this group of patients which would benefit the most from the recently developed strategy.

Preoperative and Intraoperative Assessment

Patients' evaluation should include liver US, contrasted CT, or MR imaging of the abdomen and pelvis (preferred investigative modalities). It is essential for planning the resection extensiveness by determining the intrahepatic extent of the disease and its relation with important vascular and biliary structures. Local recurrence at the primary site should be excluded by performing a colonoscopy.

The functional capacity of the liver should be measured by the indocyanine green (ICG) test, to determine the necessary remaining liver volume after hepatic resection. Usually, to perform a safe hepatic resection, in the patients with absence of prolonged chemotherapy and normal ICG clearance, the remnant liver should have >30 % of functional parenchyma. For another, the functional parenchyma volume should be >40 % in patients with prolonged chemotherapy or abnormal ICG clearance.

During the intervention, the abdominal cavity is carefully explored, and if any extrahepatic tumor deposit or suspicious lymph node(s) is suspected, a frozen-section histological examination should be performed. The second step involves a manual palpation and intraoperative US examination of the liver to determine the degree of the metastatic disease affecting it. Intraoperative US is a mandatory part of the operation as it can give additional information in up to 89 % and may contribute to change therapeutic plans in up to 42 % of the cases [35]. Its guidance is invaluable, particularly when precise mapping of the anatomical relationship between metastases and main hepatic vessels is required. Its sensitivity approaches 90 %, and if there are no contraindications to surgery, the hepatic resection should begin.

Technical Aspects

Types of Resection

Depending on the pattern of the metastatic disease, different approaches can be used to decide which lobe is operated on first and often this decision is made intraoperatively. From a general point of view, the type of resection performed during the first stage can be one of the two described below.

Left metastatic resection (anatomical or nonanatomical) and right PVE – This approach consists of metastatic clearance on the left liver combined with right portal vein embolization. In addition, in patients with a primary colorectal tumor in place, a colectomy is performed during the same intervention (first stage). The initial steps of this procedure are identical to those of standard hepatectomies. However, considering that the ultimate intention is to proceed with a second liver resection, minimum dissection at the site to be resected during the second stage should be performed in order to minimize the fibrotic adhesions. Therefore, the division of triangular ligament and excessive dissection of hilar structures of the contralateral lobe is avoided. Following the mobilization of the concerned site of the liver and the control of the portal structures, the resection of the metastases commences, aiming not only to achieve the oncological target (complete clearance of tumor lesions from the left lobe with microscopically free margins) but also at the maximal conservation of the tumor-free liver parenchyma. The resection of the liver is done in the usual fashion by using either ultrasonic dissector or Kelly clamp with intermittent inflow occlusion combined with the use of low central venous pressure anesthesia. Major supplying vessels are ligated along the parenchyma transection, taking care in minimizing in maximum the blood loss which has been proven to be an independent risk factor in the postoperative outcome [4]. Following the resection, the procedure continues with the exposure of the right branch of the portal vein. The exposure is obtained by a lateral approaching of the free edge of the hepatoduodenal ligament. Knowing that position of the portal vein is posterior helps to direct the dissection toward it, minimizing excessive tissue disruption. Obtaining the control of the right branch of PV just distal to the bifurcation is followed by its ligation/division and by absolute alcohol injection (10–15 cc) into the distal end. This step has a double purpose: first, it triggers the growth of the remnant parenchyma of the left lobe, and second it prevents a cavernous transformation of the right portal system [36]. Important point of this maneuver is to ligate the vein before the injection in order to prevent proximal spilling of the alcohol which can result in thrombosis of the common portal trunk. Our practice is to check the result of embolization intraoperatively by US/Doppler examination. Demonstration of the absence of flow in the portal system as well as visualization of a newly formed thrombus would confirm the result of the procedure. The procedure is terminated after the completion of the embolization. A drain is left in the resected site of the liver, and the abdomen is closed with nonabsorbable sutures (interrupted). Subsequently, after an interval of 3–4 weeks (interval to allow liver regeneration), chemotherapy is commenced, following which the second resection (stage) is performed, aiming at a complete metastatic clearance by resecting the right lobe or individual segments harboring the remaining metastatic lesions. Our approach in deciding the appropriate time for the second liver resection is based on the amount of liver regeneration and the control of remnant tumor by chemotherapy. Although this technique is advantageous as it limits the dissection only at the hepatic pedicle, its applicability can at times be limited by the tumor volume, often making the use of local ablation therapies (RFA, cryotherapy) necessary.

Right hepatectomy – In circumstances whereby the right lobe harbors several large or multiple small tumor lesions with a less extensive involvement of the left lobe, a right hepatectomy can be done as the first stage. Indeed, this intervention involves the same steps as for a standard right segmental or lobe resection (surgical incision, IOUS, mobilization of the right lobe and control of the portal inflow followed by the resection of the concerned area). Performing the right hepatectomy first allows removal of the main tumoral mass. The subsequent second stage (resection of the remaining metastases of the left lobe) is delayed until the left liver has undergone sufficient regeneration; however, two important issues are associated with this approach, firstly due to a more extensive nature this intervention leads to formation of dense adhesions which in turn make the second stage technically more difficult. Secondly, it exposes the remaining metastases in the left liver to high growth stimulation, potentially surpassing the growth of the nontumoral hepatic parenchyma, potentially making impossible to proceed with the second stage.

Intraoperative Portal Vein Embolization

As mentioned in the earlier paragraph, our preferred approach is to perform PVE during the first-stage resection, be it right hepatectomy or metastasectomy (procedure described in the paragraph of the Surgical Technique). This maneuver is reserved mainly for cases which are anticipated to have a small liver volume after the second (stage) liver resection. It is important to remember that larger liver volumes are required for patients who have received high doses of chemotherapy [37] (40 % of the total volume as opposed to 30 % for non chemo patients), hence making the PVE for the extended resections often a necessity. A point to stress out is that to achieve the desired end result (growth of the opposite lobe), the operating surgeon has to make sure that both the branches of the right portal vein (anterior and posterior sector) should be embolized. This is done by a careful intraoperative US mapping of the portal branches before and after alcohol injection, with the objective to demonstrate lack of portal flow and thrombus formation. The use of PVE in the published two-stage resection series ranges between 46 and 100% [38, 39]. In our series, we used PVE in 74% of the patients; Shimada et al. [40] in his series used PVE in 83% of patients as opposed to the 100% use in the series of Jaeck et al. [39]. Although some of the authors perform the PVE postoperatively [39], our preference is to perform the embolization of the PV during the first-stage intervention. The embolization itself does not add significant morbidity and can possibly increase the 5-year survival.

Interval Adjuvant Chemotherapy

Chemotherapy is an important part of this treatment strategy. Our approach involves administration of chemotherapy before and between the two stages. The role of the "downstaging" preoperative chemotherapy as a determinant in the postoperative outcome and its efficacy has been demonstrated by previous studies [6]. The chemotherapy given between the two stages usually started 3–4 weeks after the first intervention, in order to avoid suppression of the liver regeneration which normally takes place after the resection. The type of chemotherapy protocol is the same as the one administered in the preoperative period, unless the tumor size or the levels of tumor markers have increased, in which case a new regime is commenced. Although the influence of chemotherapy (between two stages) on the survival benefits as well as morbidity and mortality remains to be better evaluated, we utilize it based on the rationale that it inhibits the tumor growth. In our latest series update among 31 patients who received chemotherapy between the two resections, only one had evidence of disease progression before the second-stage operation [41]. Similarly, Jaeck et al. in their series observed the same (halt of the disease progress) in patients who received chemotherapy after the first resection [39].

Surgical Results

Using a very selective approach, our experience has demonstrated a completion rate for the second-stage hepatectomy of 69%. In other studies, the completion rate ranges from 70 to 100% [39, 42, 43]. In the reported series, the mortality and morbidity after the second resection range from 0% [39, 40, 43] to 15% [38] and 18% [43] to 56% [39], respectively. The 3-year survival rate was 54% in the series reported by Jaeck et al. which is higher than the survival rate reported by Togo et al. (3-year survival of 45%), with the former author attributing the good results to a very careful patient selection and also to administration of chemotherapy between the two operative stages.

In our initial report [38], the 3-year survival was 35%, and the mortality and morbidity rates were 15% and 45%, respectively. However, in a recent updated series reported by our group [41], the mortality after the second hepatectomy had improved considerably (6.5% versus 15%), whereas the morbidity rates remained at the same range (48% versus 45%). The actuarial 3- and 5-year overall survivals were 47% and 28%.

15.3.4 Extreme Liver Surgery

When metastases are located in direct vicinity or invade inferior vena cava or the confluence of the hepatic veins, liver resection is highly dangerous. The risk of massive hemorrhage and gas embolism is high, precluding resection in many cases. However, technical improvements, now, have enabled liver surgeons to operate on such patients.

Preoperative evaluation is crucial to identify patients who would require vascular reconstruction (reimplantation or graft replacement). Ultimately the final decision whether to operate or not on these patients would entirely depend on the risk to benefit ratio. Therefore, these interventions would be performed only when the surgeon anticipates that performing such radical procedures outweighs the risk involved. Total vascular exclusion (TVE) of the liver is achieved by associating inflow and outflow occlusion. Portal triad

Fig. 15.5 Schematic demonstration of liver resection combined with total vascular exclusion, veno-venous bypass and hypothermic perfusion

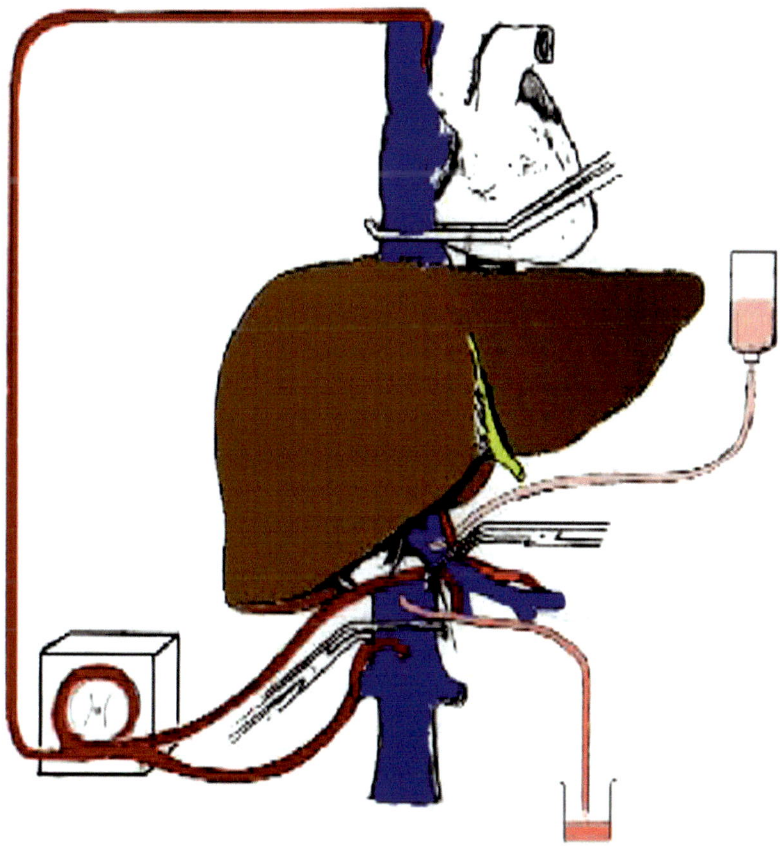

clamping is the first step of this procedure followed by interruption of the outflow achieved either by clamping the concerned hepatic vein(s) or by clamping the vena cava above and below the liver. The first method is the preferred one as it does not interrupt the venous return to the heart. On the other hand, when this strategy is not applicable (i.e., tumor too close to the hepatic or portal veins), the exclusion of the liver by clamping the supra- and infra-hepatic vena cava is done, in which case a veno-venous bypass is required in order to prevent cardiac and renal complications (Fig. 15.5).

Maximal hepatic ischemia time is estimated to 60 min. Over this limit, in situ hypothermia must be used to avoid ischemic suffering of the remnant liver parenchyma. Topical cooling or hypothermic perfusion can be performed depending on the situation. In situ perfusion is performed via a catheter placed downstream of the portal clamp with a conservation solution chilled at 4 °C. In this regard, it was the work conducted by our team [44], which identified three predictive factors for a TVE >60 min (tumors >10 cm, portal vein embolization, anticipated vascular reconstruction) whose presence could be used as criteria to plan the hypothermic perfusion as early as the preoperative stage for patients who require major liver resection with vascular reconstruction for colorectal liver metastases.

Conclusion

Resectability of colorectal liver metastases has improved by the development of a number of novel therapies.

The presence of poor prognostic factors no longer limits the indications for liver resection. It is essential to require close cooperation between oncologists and surgeons for treating unresectable colorectal liver metastases patients.

Combined chemotherapy regimens including 5FU, leucovorin, oxaliplatin, and/or irinotecan can significantly downstage metastatic liver lesions capacitating curative rescue resection leading to improved long-term survival. In addition, cetuximab and bevacizumab may produce a higher resectability rate resulting in a higher number of patients who undergo potential curative surgery.

Different surgical techniques such as portal vein embolization and two-stage hepatectomy at times associated with local ablation (RFA or cryotherapy) are nowadays widely available in order to achieve a respectable situation.

Own to vascular exclusion and reconstruction techniques, tumor involvement of the hepatic, portal, or caval vein(s) no longer prohibits the indication for liver resection.

Overall surgery should be performed in resectable liver metastases as soon as possible.

References

1. Jaeck D, Bachellier P, Guiguet M, et al. Long term survival following resection of colorectal matastases. Br J Surg. 1997;84:977–80.
2. Simmonds PC, Primrose JN, Colquitt JL, et al. Surgical resection of hepatic metastases from colorectal cancer: a systematic review of published studies. Br J Cancer. 2006;94:982–99.
3. Wagner JS, Adson MA, Van Heerden JA, et al. The natural history of hepatic metastases from colorectal cancer. Ann Surg. 1984;199:502–8.
4. Jarnagin WR, Gonen M, Fong Y, et al. Improvement in perioperative outcome after hepatic resection: analysis of 1803 consecutive cases over the past decade. Ann Surg. 2002;236:397–406.
5. Adam R. Current surgical strategies for the treatment of colorectal cancer liver metastases. Eur J Cancer. 2004;7:21–6.
6. Adam R, Delvart V, Pascal G, et al. Rescue surgery for unresectable colorectal metastases downstaged by chemotherapy. Ann Surg. 2004;240:644–58.
7. Azoulay D, Castaing D, Smail A, et al. Resection of nonresectable liver metastases from colorectal cancer after percutaneous portal vein embolization. Ann Surg. 2000;231:480–6.
8. Adam R, Akpinar E, Johann M, et al. Place of cryosurgery in the treatment of malignant liver tumors. Ann Surg. 1997;225:39–50.
9. Mentha G, Huber O, Robert J, et al. Elective hepatic resection in the elderly. Br J Surg. 1992;79:557–9.
10. Belghiti J, Hiramatsu K, Benoist S, et al. Seven hundred forty seven hepatectomies in the 1990s: an update to evaluate the actual risk of liver resection. J Am Coll Surg. 2000;191:38–46.
11. Sica GT, Ji H, Ross PR. CT and MR imaging of hepatic metastases. AJR Am J Roentgenol. 2000;174: 691–8.
12. Scott DJ, Guthrie JA, Arnold P, et al. Dual phase helical CT versus portal venous phase CT for detection of colorectal liver metastases: correlation with intraoperative sonography, surgical and pathological findings. Clin Radiol. 2001;56:235–42.
13. Kamel IR, Bluemke DA. MR imaging of liver tumors. Radiol Clin North Am. 2003;41:51–65.
14. Bipat S, van Leeuwen MS, Comans EF, et al. Colorectal liver metastases: CT, MR and PET for diagnosis: meta-analysis. Radiology. 2005;237:123–31.
15. Ozawa K. Hepatic function and liver resection. J Gastroenterol Hepatol. 1990;5:296–309.
16. Van Cutsem E, Köhne CH, Hitre E, et al. Cetuximab and chemotherapy as initial treatment for metastatic colorectal cancer. N Engl J Med. 2009;360:1408–17.
17. Bokemeyer C, Bondarenko I, Makhson A, et al. Fluorouracil, leucovorin, and oxaliplatin with and without cetuximab in the first-line treatment of metastatic colorectal cancer. J Clin Oncol. 2009;27:663–71.
18. Folprecht G, Gruenberger T, Hartmann JT, et al. Cetuximab plus FOLFOX6 or cetuximab plus FOLFIRI as neoadjuvant treatment of nonresectable colorectal liver metastases: a randomized multicenter study (CELIM study). 2009 ASCO Gastrointestinal Cancers Symposium, San Francisco, 15–17 Jan 2009, (abstr 296).
19. Falcone A, Masi G, Loupakis F, et al. FOLFOXIRI (irinotecan, oxaliplatin, and infusional 5FU/LV) in combination with bevacizumab (BV) in the first line treatment of metastatic colorectal cancer (mCRC): a phase II study by GONO group. 2008 ASCO annual meeting proceedings. J Clin Oncol. 2008;26:15S. (abstr 4031).
20. Garufi C, Torsello A, Tomolo S, et al. POCHER (preoperative chemotherapy for hepatic resection) study with cetuximab plus chronomodulated CPT-11/5-fluorouracil (5-FU)/leucovorin (FA)/oxaliplatin(L-OHP) in colorectal liver metastases. 2008 ASCO gastrointestinal cancers symposium, Orlando, 25–27 Jan 2008. (abstr 367).
21. Adam R, Aloia T, Lévi F, et al. Hepatic resection after rescue cetuximab treatment for colorectal liver metastases previously refractory to conventional systemic therapy. J Clin Oncol. 2007;25:4593–602.
22. Ychou M, Viret F, Kramar A, et al. Tritherapy with fluorouracil/leucovorin, irinotecan and oxaliplatin: a phase II study in colorectal cancer patients with non resectable liver metastases. Cancer Chemother Pharmacol. 2008; 62:195–201.
23. Clavien PA, Selzner N, Morse M, et al. Downstaging of hepatocellular carcinoma and liver metastases from colorectal cancer by selective intra-arterial chemotherapy. Surgery. 2002;131:433–42.

24. Leonard JD, et al. Liver resection after hepatic arterial infusion plus systemic oxaliplatin combinations in pre treated patients with extensive unresectable colorectal liver metastases. J Clin Oncol. 2004;22: 3542–5.
25. Berber E, Siperstein A. Local recurrence after laparoscopic radiofrequency ablation of liver tumors: an analysis of 1032 tumors. Ann Surg Oncol. 2008; 15(10):2757–64.
26. van Duijnhoven FH, et al. Factors influencing the local failure rate of radiofrequency ablation of colorectal liver metastases. Ann Surg Oncol. 2006; 13(5):651–8.
27. Abdalla EK, Vauthey JN, Ellis LM, et al. Recurrence and outcomes following hepatic resection, radiofrequency ablation, and combined resection ablation for colorectal liver metastases. Ann Surg. 2004;239:818–25.
28. Curley SA, Izzo F, Delrio P, et al. Radiofrequency ablation of unresectable primary and metastatic hepatic malignancies: results of 123 patients. Ann Surg. 1999;230:1–8.
29. Brooks AJ, Wang F, Alfredson M, et al. Syncronous liver resection and cryotherapy for colorectal metastases: survival analysis. Surgeon. 2005;3:265–8.
30. Lainas P, et al. Liver regeneration and recanalization time course following reversible portal vein embolization. J Hepatol. 2008;49(3):354–62.
31. Are C, et al. Feasibility of laparoscopic portal vein ligation prior to major hepatectomy. HPB (Oxford). 2008;10(4):229–33.
32. Goere D, et al. Chemotherapy does not impair hypertrophy of the left liver after right portal vein obstruction. J Gastrointest Surg. 2006;10(3):365–70.
33. Zorzi D, et al. Chemotherapy with bevacizumab does not affect liver regeneration after portal vein embolization in the treatment of colorectal liver metastases. Ann Surg Oncol. 2008;15(10):2765–72.
34. de Graaf W, et al. Induction of tumor growth after preoperative portal vein embolization: is it a real problem? Ann Surg Oncol. 2009;16(2):423–30.
35. Bloed W, Van Leeuwen MS, Borel Rinks IH. Role of intraoperative ultrasound of the liver with improved preoperative hepatic imaging. Eur J Surg. 2000;166: 691–5.
36. Azoulay D, Castaign D, Krissat J, et al. Percutaneous portal vein embolization increases the feasibility and safety of major liver resection for hepatocellular carcinoma in injured liver. Ann Surg. 2000;232:665–72.
37. Fusai G, Davidson BR. Strategies to increase the resectability of liver metastases from colorectal cancer. Dig Surg. 2003;20:481–96.
38. Adam R, Laurent A, Azoulay D, et al. Two stage hepatectomy: a planned strategy to treat irresectable liver tumors. Ann Surg. 2000;232:777–85.
39. Jaeck D, Oussoultzoglou E, Rosso E, et al. A two stage hepatectomy procedure combined with portal vein embolization to achieve curative resection for initially unresectable multiple and bilobar colorectal liver metastases. Ann Surg. 2004;240:1037–51.
40. Shimada H, Tanaka K, Masui H, et al. Results of surgical treatment for multiple (≥5 nodules) bipolar hepatic metastases from colorectal cancer. Langenbecks Arch Surg. 2004;389:114–21.
41. Adam R, Miller R, Pitombo M, Wichterts WA, et al. Two stage hepatectomy approach for initially unresectable colorectal hepatic metastases. Surg Oncol Clin N Am. 2007;16:525–36.
42. Garcea G, Polemontivi N, O'Leary E, et al. Two stage liver resection and chemotherapy for bilobar colorectal liver metastases. Eur J Surg Oncol. 2004;30:759–64.
43. Togo S, Nagano Y, Masui H, et al. Two stage hepatectomy for multiple bilobular liver metastases from colorectal cancer. Hepatogastroenterology. 2005;52:913–9.
44. Azoulay D, Eshkenazy R, Andreani P, et al. In situ hypothermic perfusion of the liver versus standard total vascular exclusion for complex liver resection. Ann Surg. 2005;241:277–86.

16 Chemotherapy in Patients with Initially Unresectable Liver Metastasis of Colorectal Cancer

Benoist Chibaudel, Christophe Tournigand, Annette Larsen, and Aimery de Gramont

16.1 Introduction

Colorectal cancer is the fourth most frequently diagnosed cancer and the second leading cause of death from cancer in Western countries [1]. Colorectal cancer incidence is also rising in other parts of the world, especially in Asia. Death from colorectal cancer has slightly reduced over the past 30 years, partly own to the advance of treatment modalities.

Approximately 50–60 % of colorectal cancer patients will develop colorectal metastases. Over 70 % of patients with metastatic colorectal cancer (MCRC) show synchronous metastases. Of note, salvage metastatic surgery can be performed in up to 15 % of patients with initially unresectable metastatic colorectal cancer [2, 3].

The basic principle for the optimal management of metastatic colorectal cancer patients is more than based upon the results of the randomized studies. The different features of the disease must be considered and incorporated:

- Patients are heterogeneous regarding prognostic factors, and some are too frail to receive the most active treatments.
- Prolonged survival makes continuous chemotherapy cumbersome, difficult, and expensive.
- Surgery can rescue and cure some patients.
- Oxaliplatin has a limiting cumulative toxicity.
- Several regimens are available for a multi-line strategy.
- Individual results of first- or second-line trials do not fully acknowledge what was done either before or after the study.
- Study endpoints are debatable.
- Molecular targeted drugs failed to replace chemotherapy but are usefully combined with chemotherapy.
- Biomarkers which can be either prognostic or predictive.

Three prognostic risk groups have been identified in patients who undergo 5-fluorouracil (5-FU)-based treatment for MCRC, depending on four baseline parameters: WHO performance status (PS), white blood cell (WBC) count, alkaline phosphatase, and a number of metastatic sites [4]. WHO PS>1 and increased LDH level at baseline appear to be the strongest parameters associated with poor prognosis in recent trials [3, 5–7]. New biomarkers can predict sensitivity or nonsensitivity to therapies such as KRAS or BRAF status [8–12].

In addition our knowledge is built on clinical trials conducted in selected populations who are

B. Chibaudel • C. Tournigand • A. Larsen
A. de Gramont (✉)
Hôpital Saint-Antoine, APHP, Université Paris VI, Paris, France

GERCOR, Groupe Coopérateur Multidisciplinaire en Oncologie, Paris, France

INSERM CDR UMR S938, Paris, France
e-mail: aimery.de-gramont@sat.aphp.fr

X. Qin et al. (eds.), *Multidisciplinary Management of Liver Metastases in Colorectal Cancer*, DOI 10.1007/978-94-017-7755-1_16

younger and suffering less comorbidities than the general population of MCRC.

16.2 First-Line Therapy

16.2.1 Combination or Sequential Therapy

Active chemotherapy drugs in MCRC are fluoropyrimidines, oxaliplatin, and irinotecan. Fluoropyrimidines can be applied either alone or in combination with two other drugs, but should fluoropyrimidine monotherapy, doublets, or triplets, be used as first-line therapy?

Registered studies have demonstrated that combination therapies were better than monotherapy in terms of response rate (RR), progression-free survival (PFS), and in some trials overall survival [5, 7, 13].

Three other studies researched the results of monotherapy versus combination therapy.

The CAIRO 1 study randomized 820 patients [14]. Capecitabine followed by irinotecan, followed by XELOX, was the first arm, and XELIRI followed by XELOX was the second arm. The FOCUS study randomized 2,135 patients in five different arms: modified LV5FU2 followed by irinotecan (arm 1), FOLFIRI (arm 2), mFOLFOX6 (arm 3), FOLFIRI (arm 4), and mFOLFOX6 (arm 5) [15]. Both studies showed that there was no survival advantage for the frontline combination. However, both trials performed unfavorable median survivals compared with pivotal trials with the same regimens, 17.4 and 16.3 months for the combination and sequential therapy in the CAIRO 1 trial, respectively, 15.4 and 16.7 months for the combination therapy, 15.0 and 15.2 months for monotherapy followed by combination therapy, and 13.9 months for sequential monotherapy in the FOCUS trial. Two pitfalls explained the poor survival and were common in the two studies: salvage surgery was not administered and a low proportion of patients (19–55 % according to arms) underwent the three active drugs, fluoropyrimidines, oxaliplatin, and irinotecan. A third France study which randomized 410 patients showed similar results [16].

A lower toxicity is the advantage of monotherapy. However, if combinations are applied later in the process of the disease, worse toxicity could manifest more frequently than that in the first-line therapy. Of note, poor prognosis patients most likely cannot benefit from monotherapy. And on this basis, as soon as the sensitivity is not predicted, we believe that frontline monotherapy should be administered in patients who are unable to receive a combination or refuse intravenous chemotherapy. The patients who have no poor prognostic factor with non-operable sites could also receive fluoropyrimidines alone.

16.2.2 Oxaliplatin-Based or Irinotecan-Based Regimen?

Tournigand et al. randomized metastatic colorectal cancer patients. The first arm was irinotecan or oxaliplatin; the second arm was both given in combination with a simplified LV5FU2 infusion [3]. This trial was the first study for directly comparing the addition of oxaliplatin or irinotecan in combination with infusional 5-FU and leucovorin. In the final results about response rates and PFS, there is no difference between FOLFIRI and FOLFOX6 as first-line therapy. The FOLFIRI regimen as second-line therapy after progression on FOLFOX6 was less active than FOLFOX6 after progression on FOLFIRI. Of note, the second-line therapy was administrated in more than 70 % of the patients, and 13 % of the patients had R0 surgery of metastases on FOLFOX arm and FOLFIRI arm, respectively. The median overall survival of both arms was over 20 months. These results show that sequential regimen treatment optimizes outcome for patients.

The matter of debate focuses on the choice between oxaliplatin-based and irinotecan-based regimen. The choice can also be influenced by fluoropyrimidine regimen, especially in combination with irinotecan: IFL (irinotecan with 5FU bolus). It was shown to be worse and more toxic than FOLFOX [17, 18]. The result from Tournigand study performing FOLFIRI showed it could be more active than irinotecan with the standard LV5FU2 or IFL or XELIRI [7, 13, 19].

However, the Tournigand study also reported FOLFIRI first-line is less grade 3–4 toxicity and more active of FOLFOX second-line (ORR 15 % vs 4 %, PFS second-line 4.9 vs. 2.3 months), while FOLFOX first line are less patients who have serious adverse events and more patients could undergo surgery of metastases (22 % vs. 9 %). Nevertheless, less grade 3–4 toxicity is due to there is no clinically relevant in grade 3 neutropenia which is in most cases and the salvage surgery was not designed or powered to evaluate in this study. Another advantage of FOLFOX is that the same result of patients was achieved in the FOLFOX6 arm which received 44.5 % less combination chemotherapy cycles (1,081 cycles) than in the FOLFIRI arm (1,562 cycles) (unpublished data). The cumulative oxaliplatin-based neurosensory toxicity could explain this result. Most patients stopped oxaliplatin due to neurotoxicity rather than tumor progression. The potential of FOLFOX could be improved if we could manage the neurotoxicity or reintroduce FOLFOX after recovery from neurotoxicity.

Eventually, if this argumentation is true, the most active doublets may be the elements of chemotherapy.

16.2.3 Optimization of Chemotherapy for Metastatic Colorectal Cancer

16.2.3.1 Oxaliplatin Stop-and-Go Strategy

One potential approach to achieve more active and less neurotoxicity of oxaliplatin is to administer the FOLFOX regimen for a defined time span; before severe neurotoxicity emerged stop therapy, and reintroduce the regimen after recovery from neurotoxicity. This approach is encouraged due to the observation that reintroducting oxaliplatin was found to be clinically effective in a series of patients who stopped oxaliplatin due to neurotoxicity and recovered before reintroduction [20].

The OPTIMOX1 trial has evaluated the oxaliplatin stop-and-go strategy [6]. This study randomized the metastatic colorectal cancer patients. The first arm was FOLFOX4 until progression; the second arm was the OPTIMOX1 strategy, which consisted in six cycles of FOLFOX7 chemotherapy [21] followed after evaluating probabilities of salvage surgery by maintenance therapy with the simplified LV5FU2 regimen without oxaliplatin. After 12 cycles of LV5FU2 chemotherapy, FOLFOX7 was reintroduced in patients who have stable disease or response. This enrolled 620 patients, including an exploratory cohort of 95 elderly or poor prognosis patients. Median progression-free survival and survival times of FOLFOX4 arm were 9.0 and 19.3 months, respectively, compared with 8.7 and 21.2 months, respectively, in FOLFOX7/sLV5FU2 arm. This difference, however, was not statistically significant. Lesser grade 3 or 4 toxicity was experienced in the investigational arm. Including oxaliplatin reintroduction, grade 3 sensory neuropathy was observed in 17.9 % and 13.3 % of the FOLFOX4 arm and FOLFOX7/sLV5FU2 arm patients, respectively. In the investigational arm, 40 % of the patients reintroduced oxaliplatin, and 69.4 % of these patients achieved response or stabilization. The OPTIMOX1 study provided that better tolerated and similar efficacy could be achieved in a short induction with oxaliplatin followed by maintenance therapy than continuous administration of the drug until progression or the cumulative neurotoxicity developed.

The OPTIMOX1 study has also demonstrated that oxaliplatin reintroduction was related to improved prognosis in patients with advanced colorectal cancer [22]. The influence of reintroducing oxaliplatin on OS was potentially dissimulated by the fact that majority of the patients did not undergo the planned oxaliplatin reintroduction or received oxaliplatin after second-line therapy in both arms. The oxaliplatin reintroduction had an independent and significant impact on OS (HR = 0.56, P = 0.009) as demonstrated by a Cox model fitted with all effective baseline factors plus time-dependent variables reflecting tumor progression, reintroduction of oxaliplatin, and use of second-line irinotecan. It was also demonstrated that the centage of oxaliplatin reintroduction patients had an effective impact on OS. Centers which more than 40 % of the patients underwent oxaliplatin reintroduction had an oriented HR for OS of 0.59 compared with centers which patients had no oxaliplatin reintroduction.

The Combined Oxaliplatin Neuropathy Prevention Trial (CONCEPT) compared a continuous administration of FOLFOX to a desultory administration of eight cycles of FOLFOX plus bevacizumab, followed by eight cycles of maintenance LV/5FU plus bevacizumab, and FOLFOX reintroduction plus bevacizumab for eight cycles. PFS of continuous administration arm was 7.3 months compared to 12.0 months in the stop-and-go strategy arm ($P=0.044$) [23].

16.2.3.2 Complete Stop of Chemotherapy

The treatment for colorectal cancer has evolved from approximately 1 year with 5-FU alone to 16–20 months for FOLFOX4, to more than 20 months administered all available drugs. The gradual prolongation of median survival in colorectal metastasis patients and the hardness to keep patients a long time on therapy led to evaluate chemotherapy discontinuation in prospective trials are frequently. In order to study several reasons, including lengthy sustained responses or stabilization, toxicity, and the patient's decision to discontinue treatment, advanced colorectal cancer patients were employed in CFIs.

Two studies have been designed for evaluating CFIs after 5-FU therapy alone [24, 25]. 354 patients were randomized in the largest study. The median duration of CFI was 2.8 months; there was not worse survival and less toxicity in patients of stop therapy arm, compared to patients of continuous therapy arm [25]. However, only 37 % of the eligible patients reintroduced their treatment.

Recently, the OPTIMOX2 study compared chemotherapy holiday to maintenance therapy with leucovorin and 5-FU, following six cycles of FOLFOX chemotherapy in the first-line treatment of MCRC [26]. Median PFS and OS of maintenance arm were 8.6 and 23.8 months, respectively, and 6.6 and 19.5 months in CFI arm, respectively. Median duration of patients in maintenance arm and chemotherapy-free interval arm were 4.8 months and 3.9 months, respectively. The MRC COIN study compared a continuous oxaliplatin-based chemotherapy until disease progresses to a complete stop-and-go strategy after 3 months of an oxaliplatin-based treatment [27]. As in the OPTIMOX2 study, median overall survival was lower in the CFI arm than in the control arm (14.4 vs. 15.8 months), but not significantly (HR = 1.084): "a small advantage in survival at the expense of toxicity and time on treatment." However, we believe that we cannot decide chemotherapy holidays before therapy is initiated in advanced colorectal cancer patients. Patients with advanced disease who are on FOLFOX therapy or underwent salvage surgery biased the results. Chemotherapy discontinuation can bring benefit to majority of the patients. Our standards for chemotherapy discontinuation were defined from patients in the OPTIMOX1 and OPTIMOX2 studies: a normal CEA level within 3 months on chemotherapy and 6 months duration of chemotherapy before CFI predicted a prolonged survival [28].

Ongoing studies are further evaluating chemotherapy discontinuation especially the role of targeted therapies alone like the DREAM trial.

16.2.4 Addition of Targeted Therapy

Targeted therapies are discussed in another chapter. Here we will briefly review the recent studies that in our opinion impact or may impact the management of MCRC.

16.2.4.1 VEGF Inhibition

Combination bevacizumab meaningfully improved the PFS of chemotherapy alone. This has been demonstrated with irinotecan-based chemotherapy, 5-FU alone, and oxaliplatin-based chemotherapy. The benefit was greater with irinotecan than with oxaliplatin, and this could be explained either to a better synergy or to a more prolonged administration of bevacizumab in the irinotecan trial [29–31]. Of note, bevacizumab administrated can obtain more benefit in first-line than in second-line therapy, and it is not observed in third-line therapy [32, 33].

16.2.4.2 EGFR Inhibition

Cetuximab has been researched in combination with oxaliplatin-based and irinotecan-based therapy. Results were initially disappointing. However, when it has been revealed that cetuximab only responded to patients with wild-type KRAS tumors, the prolongation of PFS was more convincing. For patients with KRAS wild-type tumors, the combination cetuximab to either FOLFIRI (CRYSTAL) or FOLFOX (OPUS) displayed an improvement in median PFS (9.9 vs. 8.7 months, $p=0.02$ and 7.7 vs. 7.2 months, $p=0.01$) [34, 35]. However, in the COIN trial, the prolongation of PFS was not observed in patients receiving either FOLFOX or XELOX plus cetuximab, but this study was prospectively analyzed according to the KRAS status which was not the case of the previous studies [27].

Of note, the benefit of cetuximab is maintained or even enlarged in second-line or third-line therapy what could observe a survival benefit, which demonstrated that if the objective is survival, to use the drug as salvage therapy might be a better choice [36, 37]. However, in all trials, there is an improved response rate in patients with wild-type KRAS tumors, suggesting a role in patients amenable to surgery which will be discussed thereafter.

The benefit of panitumumab in survival in wild-type KRAS tumors in third-line therapy has also been demonstrated [38]. Two newly performed large trials in first-line and second-line therapy have shown that PFS was prolonged in patients receiving either FOLFOX (first line) or FOLFIRI (second line) plus panitumumab [39, 40].

16.2.4.3 Double VEGF and EGF Inhibition

The double inhibition with monoclonal antibodies plus chemotherapy, bevacizumab plus panitumumab in the PACCE trial, and bevacizumab plus cetuximab in the CAIRO2 study failed to improve the results achieved with chemotherapy plus bevacizumab alone, showing even worst results for the combination [41, 42]. Obviously, the combination of these monoclonal antibodies should not be used.

The ongoing DREAM study is evaluating the combination of bevacizumab plus erlotinib in maintenance therapy.

There is no definitive answer for the most active targeted therapy in first-line therapy. Looking at hazard ratios and benefit in median survival, the combination of bevacizumab plus chemotherapy, especially 5-FU and irinotecan, takes the lead (Fig. 16.1).

16.2.5 Salvage Surgery After Tumor Shrinkage

Salvage surgery can be performed in patients with advanced colorectal cancer when chemotherapy achieves tumor shrinkage [43]. In phase

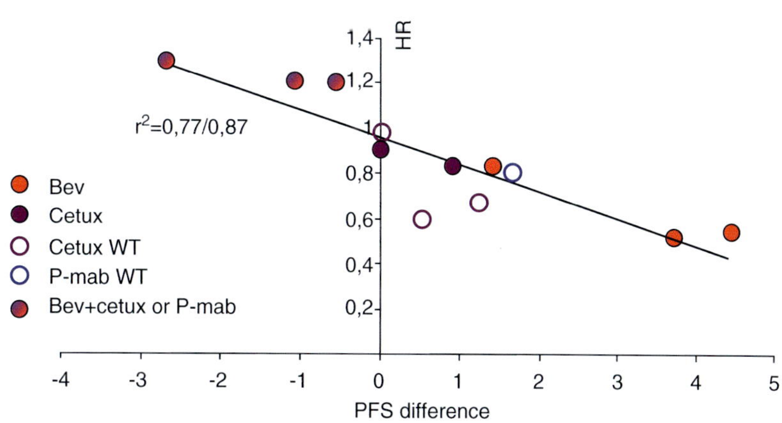

Fig. 16.1 The hazard ratio and the advantage in median PFS observed in the published trials using the monoclonal antibodies, bevacizumab, cetuximab, and panitumumab

III studies, up to 15 % of the patients can benefit from an R0 resection. These patients have a 5-year survival rate of approximately 25 %. These results approach the results achieved in patients with initially resectable metastases [44].

The frequency of salvage surgery depends on the response rate of chemotherapy and on the geographic localization. Obviously, the higher resection rates are observed in trials performed in the Mediterranean countries. Differences in management, multidisciplinary approach, and surgeon experience explain the observed discrepancy. A positive correlation was found between tumor response and resection rate [45]. We confirmed this paper looking only at randomized studies. In the Mediterranean countries, the response rate to achieve a 10 % R0 resection rate is 54 % (Fig. 16.2).

These findings support the use of regimens achieving a high response rate in patients with metastases localized in operable sites.

Response rate over 50 % in first-line therapy has been reported in several randomized studies. FOLFOX4 achieved 50 % (range in trials 34–58 %) [5, 6, 18, 29, 35, 46], FOLFOX6 54 % (range 46–54 %) [3, 15], FOLFIRI 56 % (range 39–56 %) [3, 15, 19, 34, 46], and FOLFOXIRI 60 % (range 53–60 %) [2, 47]. Targeted therapies combined to chemotherapy slightly increase response rates. In patients with wild-type KRAS, response rate was 57.3 % with both FOLFIRI plus cetuximab and FOLFOX plus cetuximab and 55.0 % with FOLFOX plus panitumumab [27, 34, 39].

Of note, the response rate in the bevacizumab trials is not increased as much as in the cetuximab or panitumumab trials, but it is also known that the classical definition of response does not fully reflect the efficacy of antiangiogenic agents.

Finally, should we use the most active regimen frontline to all patients to increase the resection rate? The benefit of a 10 % increase in response rate, which at best is what can be achieved with targeted therapies combined with the most active regimens, should translate in a 2 % increase in R0 resection and ultimately in less than 1 % cure. On the other hand, 100 % of the patients are exposed to a more toxic regimen. Furthermore, such an attitude may compromise the strategy in case of nonresectable metastases as second-line therapies are driven by the choice of the first-line therapy. The correct answer might be to improve patient and tumor selection using optimal biomarkers and imagery to propose the most active regimen only to patients most likely to benefit from this strategy.

To conclude the first-line strategy and regimens, the most relevant ongoing trials are presented in Table 16.1.

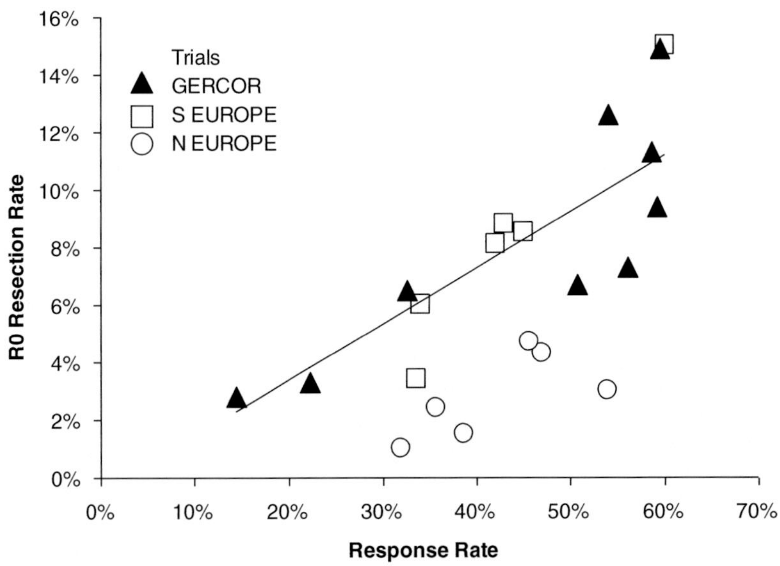

Fig. 16.2 Correlation between response rate and R0 resection rate in patients with metastatic colorectal cancer. *Straight line* represents the regression line in GERCOR and south European countries randomized trials

Table 16.1 Ongoing randomized phase III trials in first-line MCRC

Study	Country sponsor	*N*	Primary endpoint	Design
Continuous chemotherapy/maintenance therapy/chemotherapy discontinuation				
MACRO	Spain	475	PFS	Continuous combination (XELOX-bev)
				6 cycles XELOX-bev then maintenance with bev
OPTIMOX3 – DREAM	France	650	PFS	6-month induction chemotherapy then maintenance with bev
				6-month induction chemotherapy then maintenance with bev+erlotinib
CAIRO3	The Netherland	635	PFS2	Maintenance with chemo-bev
				Chemotherapy discontinuation
SWS-SaKK-41/06	Switzerland	238	TTP	Maintenance bev
				Chemotherapy discontinuation
OASIS	USA	800	PFS	FOLFOX-bev then FOLFIRI-bev
				FOLFOX-bev then LVFU-bev
Which targeted therapy in combination with chemotherapy				
CALGB-C80405	USA	2300	OS	FOLFOX or FOLFIRI + bev
				FOLFOX or FOLFIRI + cetux
				FOLFOX or FOLFIRI + bev + cetux
FIRE-3	Germany	568	ORR	FOLFIRI + cetux
				FOLFIRI + bev
Horizon II	AstraZeneca	1050	PFS	FOLFOX/XELOX+ placebo
				FOLFOX/XELOX+ cediranib
Horizon III	AstraZeneca	1614	PFS	FOLFOX/XELOX+ bevacizumab
				FOLFOX/XELOX+ cediranib
A6181122	Pfizer	720	PFS	FOLFIRI
				FOLFIRI + sunitinib
Which regimen of chemotherapy				
CT/05.16	Greece	330	PFS	FOLFIRI + bev
				XELIRI + bev
2008-03-012	Korea	334	PFS	XELOX
				SOX (S1-oxaliplatin)
GONO-TRIBE	Italy	450	PFS	FOLFIRI + bev
				FOLFOXIRI + bev

16.3 Second- and Third-Line Therapy

Second-line therapy could be administered in most patients when resistance or toxicity closes the first-line therapy. The second-line treatment could be imposed by the choice of the first-line therapy. The knowledge of the most active second-line administrations must not lead to use a suboptimal first-line regimen.

Exposure to all available agents has been reported which could be more significant than the number of lines [48]. Nevertheless, showed by the date between the percentage of patients who received all the available drugs and the median survival, if all eligible patients receive all the available chemotherapy drugs (80 % if we consider that 20 % would have surgery or be unable to receive all drugs), the median survival would be limited to 22 months. However, the median survival would be over 22 months by using targeted agents in the new strategies or using the oxaliplatin in stop-and-go strategy late. This approach argue against the basic one.

Second-line therapies are effective. Classical doublets are active after LV/5FU or capecitabine ineffectively. After failure of FOLFIRI, FOLFOX is still active, but irinotecan or FOLFIRI appears less active after failure of FOLFOX [3]. New irinotecan-based chemotherapy regimens such as FOLFIRI3, ground on an effective interaction between irinotecan given after 5FU infusion [49], should be more active than FOLFIRI in second-line therapy, but these results have not been demonstrated in randomized trials [50, 51].

Targeted therapies have also improved the effect of second-line therapy. Bevacizumab combination with FOLFOX4 after failure of 5FU/irinotecan has increased response rate, PFS, and overall survival [32]. The survival also is prolonged by continuing bevacizumab after progression on first-line therapy, and this result is provided in prospective trials [52]. PTK-ZK combination with FOLFOX after failure of 5FU/irinotecan has shown prolongation of PFS [53]. Cetuximab combination with irinotecan after failure of 5FU/oxaliplatin has demonstrated prolongation of PFS compared with chemotherapy alone even though the outcomes in the subset of patients who were tested for KRAS were not convincing [54, 55]. The median PFS also were prolonged approximately 2 months in FOLFIRI combination with panitumumab [40]. However, the dimensions of the PFS benefit remain modest and uniformly below 3 months, and the OS benefit is shown only in the bevacizumab trial [30]. Crossover in the chemotherapy-alone arms is an acceptable hypothesis to explain the unconformity between PFS and OS.

Majority of patients are even able and glad to accept therapy after two lines of treatment. The BOND trial in which a significant proportion of patients were not only intractable to irinotecan-based chemotherapy but also to oxaliplatin-based chemotherapy has shown cooperation between irinotecan and cetuximab. The effect of irinotecan plus cetuximab overmatches the effect of monoclonal antibody only [37]. Since it was shown that anti-EGFR monoclonal antibodies, cetuximab and panitumumab, were also active alone in third-line versus best supportive care, results magnified in the patients with wild-type KRAS [36, 38]. It is remarkable that bevacizumab is not active in third-line therapy [33].

When to use cetuximab or panitumumab would be a significant practical question for the most part of patients who have nonresectable neoplasms, even in case of tumor shrinkage. As the only active third-line therapies lie on anti-EGFR monoclonal antibodies, there is no third-line therapy for patients with mutated KRAS tumor, and their administration in first- or second-line therapy in patients with wild-type KRAS tumor has the immediate consequence to preclude patients of receiving a third-line therapy. Without the exact data and prospective trial can clarify this unintelligible question. However, there is a nonquestionable survival advantage in third-line therapy. There is also a lack of survival advantage in second-line therapy in the EPIC trial where 50 % of the control patients administered cetuximab in third-line therapy. There is no survival benefit in first-line therapy in the COIN trial and in the preliminary results of the PRIME trial [27, 39]. The CRYSTAL trial has reported the only significant improvement in overall survival (3.5 months) in a first-line trial.

However, the significant results came from a retrospective analysis of a subset of the patients, and the proportion of patients who have accepted the therapy of cetuximab after the first-line in the experimental group has not been covered. According to these data, introduction of the systematic use of anti-EGFR antibody in first-line therapy in patients with unresectable metastases is not enough.

Conclusion

Chemotherapy in metastatic colorectal cancer therapy is not restricted to the most active regimen. It is a portion of a global strategy based on biomarkers, comorbidities, sites of the disease, and previous adjuvant therapy. Furthermore, it should include several lines of therapy and more recently salvage surgery and chemotherapy-free

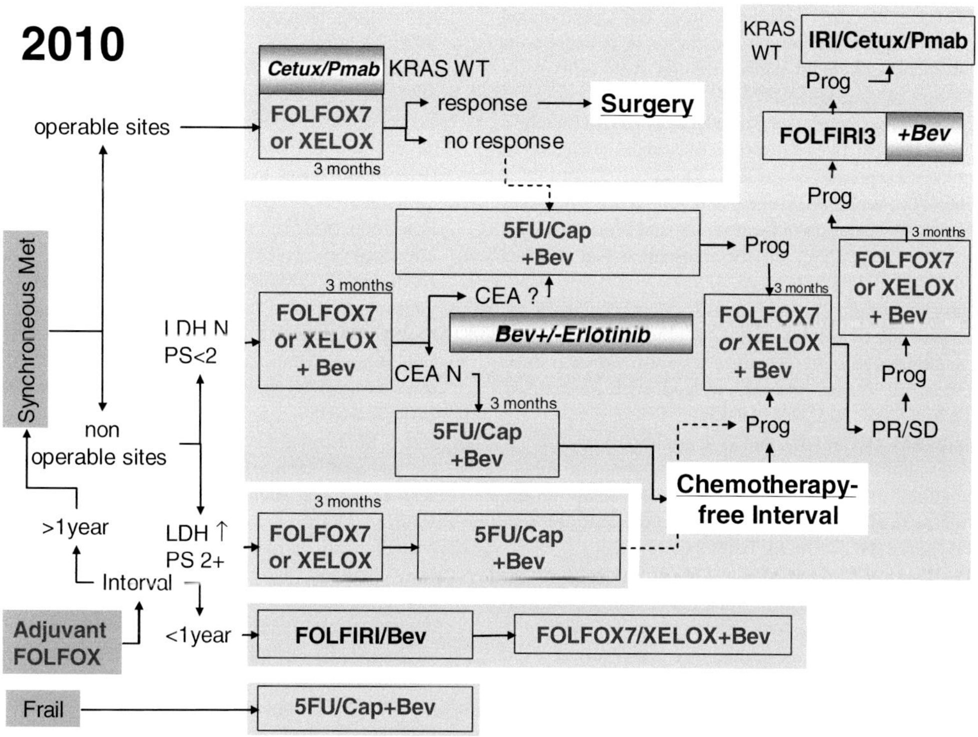

Fig. 16.3 Algorithm to treat patients with advanced unresectable colorectal cancer in Saint-Antoine Hospital (Paris). Start with the *gray boxes* (clinical trials with targeted therapies are in italic). Abbreviations: *5-FU* 5-fluorouracil, *Cap* capecitabine, *CEA* carcinoembryonic antigen, *LDH* lactate dehydrogenase, *PS* performance status, *PR* partial response, *SD* stable disease, *FOLFIRI* folinic acid, fluorouracil, irinotecan, *FOLFOX* oxaliplatin, fluorouracil, and leucovorin, *XELOX* capecitabine plus oxaliplatin, *Bev* bevacizumab, *Cetux* cetuximab, *Pmab* panitumumab, *KRAS WT* KRAS wild type

intervals. The aim is to achieve a 30-month median overall survival. An algorithm, Fig. 16.3, taking into account all these parameters, is proposed.

References

1. Atlanta: American Cancer Society (2009) Open November 2009. American Cancer Society. Cancer Facts & Figures 2009. http://www.cancer.org/downloads/STT/500809web.pdf.
2. Falcone A, Ricci S, Brunetti I, et al. Phase III trial of infusional fluorouracil, leucovorin, oxaliplatin, and irinotecan (FOLFOXIRI) compared with infusional fluorouracil, leucovorin, and irinotecan (FOLFIRI) as first-line treatment for metastatic colorectal cancer: the Gruppo Oncologico Nord Ovest. J Clin Oncol. 2007;25:1670–6.
3. Tournigand C, Andre T, Achille E, et al. FOLFIRI followed by FOLFOX6 or the reverse sequence in advanced colorectal cancer: a randomized GERCOR study. J Clin Oncol. 2004;22:229–37.
4. Kohne C-H, Cunningham D, Di Costanzo F, et al. Clinical determinants of survival in patients with 5-fluorouracil- based treatment for metastatic colorectal cancer: results of a multivariate analysis of 3825 patients. Ann Oncol. 2002;13:308–17.
5. de Gramont A, Figer A, Seymour M, et al. Leucovorin and fluorouracil with or without oxaliplatin as first-line treatment in advanced colorectal cancer. J Clin Oncol. 2000;18:2938–47.
6. Tournigand C, Cervantes A, Figer A, et al. OPTIMOX1: a randomized study of FOLFOX4 or FOLFOX7 with oxaliplatin in a stop-and-go fashion in advanced colorectal cancer-a GERCOR study. J Clin Oncol. 2006;24:394–400.
7. Saltz LB, Cox JV, Blanke C, et al. Irinotecan plus fluorouracil and leucovorin for metastatic colorectal cancer. Irinotecan Study Group. N Engl J Med. 2000;343:905–14.

8. Lièvre A, Bachet JB, Boige V, et al. KRAS mutations as an independent prognostic factor in patients with advanced colorectal cancer treated with cetuximab. J Clin Oncol. 2008;26:374–9.
9. Lièvre A, Bachet JB, Le Corre D, et al. KRAS mutation status is predictive of response to cetuximab therapy in colorectal cancer. Cancer Res. 2006;66:3992–5.
10. Ince WL, Jubb AM, Holden SN, Holmgren EB, Tobin P, et al. Association of k-ras, b-raf, and p53 status with the treatment effect of bevacizumab. J Natl Cancer Inst. 2005;97:981–9.
11. Khambata-Ford S, Garrett CR, Meropol NJ, et al. Expression of epiregulin and amphiregulin and K-ras mutation status predict disease control in metastatic colorectal cancer patients treated with cetuximab. J Clin Oncol. 2007;25:3230–7.
12. Jubb AM, Hurwitz HI, Bai W, et al. Impact of vascular endothelial growth factor-A expression, thrombospondin-2 expression, and microvessel density on the treatment effect of bevacizumab in metastatic colorectal cancer. J Clin Oncol. 2006;24:217–27.
13. Douillard JY, Cunningham D, Roth AD, et al. Irinotecan combined with fluorouracil compared with fluorouracil alone as first-line treatment for metastatic colorectal cancer: a multicentre randomised trial. Lancet. 2000;355:1041–7.
14. Koopman M, Antonini NF, Douma J, et al. Sequential versus combination chemotherapy with capecitabine, irinotecan, and oxaliplatin in advanced colorectal cancer (CAIRO): a phase III randomised controlled trial. Lancet. 2007;370:135–42.
15. Seymour MT, Maughan TS, Ledermann JA, et al. Different strategies of sequential and combination chemotherapy for patients with poor prognosis advanced colorectal cancer (MRC FOCUS): a randomised controlled trial. Lancet. 2007;370:143–52.
16. Bouché O, Castaing M, Etienne PL, et al. Randomized strategical trial of chemotherapy in metastatic colorectal cancer (FFCD 2000–05): preliminary results of toxicity, observance and survival. J Clin Oncol. 2007;18S:4069.
17. Goldberg RM, Sargent DJ, Morton RF, et al. A randomized controlled trial of fluorouracil plus leucovorin, irinotecan, and oxaliplatin combinations in patients with previously untreated metastatic colorectal cancer. J Clin Oncol. 2004;22:23–30.
18. Goldberg RM, Sargent DJ, Morton RF, et al. Randomized controlled trial of reduced-dose bolus fluorouracil plus leucovorin and irinotecan or infused fluorouracil plus leucovorin and oxaliplatin in patients with previously untreated metastatic colorectal cancer: a North American Intergroup Trial. J Clin Oncol. 2006;24:3347–53.
19. Fuchs CS, Marshal J, Mitchell E, et al. A randomized, controlled trial of irinotecan plus infusional, bolus, or oral fluoropyrimidines in first-line treatment of metastatic colorectal cancer: results from the BICC-C study. J Clin Oncol. 2007;25:4779–86.
20. Plantade A, Afchain P, Tournigand C, et al. Chemotherapy-free intervals (CFI) in patients with metastatic colorectal cancer (MRC). J Clin Oncol. 2006;24(18S):3581.
21. Maindrault-Goebel F, de Gramont A, Louvet C, et al. High-dose intensity oxaliplatin added to the simplified bimonthly leucovorin and 5-fluorouracil regimen as second-line therapy for metastatic colorectal cancer (FOLFOX 7). Eur J Cancer. 2001;37:1000–5.
22. de Gramont A, Buyse M, Abrahantes JC, et al. Reintroduction of oxaliplatin is associated with improved survival in advanced colorectal cancer. J Clin Oncol. 2007;25:3224–9.
23. Grothey A, Hart L, Rowland K, et al. Intermittent oxaliplatin administration improves time-to-treatment failure in metastatic colorectal cancer: final results of the Phase III of the CONcePT Trial. J Clin Oncol. 2008;26:4010.
24. Hejna M, Kornek GV, Raderer M, et al. Reinduction therapy with the same cytostatic regimen in patients with advanced colorectal cancer. Br J Cancer. 1998;78:760–4.
25. Maughan TS, James RD, Kerr DJ, et al. Comparison of intermittent and continuous palliative chemotherapy for advanced colorectal cancer: a multicentre randomised trial. Lancet. 2003;361:457–64.
26. Chibaudel B, Maindrault-Goebel F, Lledo G, et al. Can chemotherapy be discontinued in unresectable metastatic colorectal cancer? The GERCOR OPTIMOX2 study. J Clin Oncol. 2009;27:5727.
27. Maughan TS, Adams RA, Smith C, et al. COIN A three-arm randomised controlled trial comparing either COntinuous chemotherapy plus cetuximab or INtermittent chemotherapy with standard continuous palliative combination chemotherapy with oxaliplatin and a fluoropyrimidine in first line treatment of metastatic colorectal cancer. Eur J Cancer. 2009;7(6LBA):4–5.
28. Perez-Staub N, Chibaudel B, Figer A et al. Who can benefit from chemotherapy holidays after first-line therapy for advanced colorectal cancer? A GERCOR study. J Clin Oncol. 2008;26(Suppl):4037.
29. Saltz LB, Clarke S, Diaz-Rubio E, et al. Bevacizumab in combination with oxaliplatin-based chemotherapy as first-line therapy in metastatic colorectal cancer: a randomized phase III study. J Clin Oncol. 2008;26:2013–9.
30. Hurwitz H, Fehrenbacher L, Novotny W, et al. Bevacizumab plus irinotecan, fluorouracil, and leucovorin for metastatic colorectal cancer. N Engl J Med. 2004;350:2335–42.
31. Kabbinavar FF, Schulz J, McCleod M, et al. Addition of bevacizumab to bolus fluorouracil and leucovorin in first-line metastatic colorectal cancer. Results of a randomized phase II trial. J Clin Oncol. 2005;23:3697–705.
32. Giantonio BJ, Catalano PJ, Meropol NJ, et al. Bevacizumab in combination with oxaliplatin, fluorouracil, and leucovorin (FOLFOX4) for previously treated metastatic colorectal cancer: results from the Eastern Cooperative Oncology Group Study E3200. J Clin Oncol. 2007;25:1539–44.

33. Chen HX, Mooney M, Boron M, et al. Phase II multicenter trial of bevacizumab plus fluorouracil and leucovorin in patients with advanced refractory colorectal cancer: an NCI Treatment Referral Center Trial TRC-0301. J Clin Oncol. 2006;24:3354–60.
34. Van Cutsem E, Köhne CH, Hitre E, et al. Cetuximab and chemotherapy as initial treatment for metastatic colorectal cancer. N Engl J Med. 2009;360:1408–17.
35. Bokemeyer C, Bondarenko I, Makhson A, et al. Fluorouracil, leucovorin, and oxaliplatin with and without cetuximab in the first-line treatment of metastatic colorectal cancer. J Clin Oncol. 2009;27:663–71.
36. Jonker DJ, O'Callaghan CJ, Karapetis CS, et al. Cetuximab for the treatment of colorectal cancer. N Engl J Med. 2007;357:2040–8.
37. Cunningham D, Humblet Y, Siena S, et al. Cetuximab monotherapy and cetuximab plus irinotecan in irinotecan-refractory metastatic colorectal cancer. N Engl J Med. 2004;351:337–45.
38. Van Cutsem E, Peeters M, Siena S, et al. Open-label phase III trial of panitumumab plus best supportive care compared with best supportive care alone in patients with chemotherapy-refractory metastatic colorectal cancer. J Clin Oncol. 2007;25:1658–64.
39. Douillard JY, Siena S, Cassidy J, et al. Randomized phase 3 study of panitumumab with FOLFOX4 vs FOLFOX4 alone as first-line treatment in patients with metastatic colorectal cancer: the PRIME trial. Eur J Cancer. 2009;10LBA:6.
40. Peeters M, Price T, Hotko Y, et al. Randomized phase 3 study of panitumumab with FOLFIRI vs FOLFIRI alone as second-line treatment in patients with metastatic colorectal cancer. Eur J Cancer. 2009;14LBA:10.
41. Hecht JR, Mitchell E, Chidiac T, et al. A randomized phase IIIB trial of chemotherapy, bevacizumab, and panitumumab compared with chemotherapy and bevacizumab alone for metastatic colorectal cancer. J Clin Oncol. 2008;27:672–80.
42. Punt CJA, Tol J, Rodenburg CJ, et al. Randomized phase III study of capecitabine, oxaliplatin and bevacizumab with or without cetuximab in advanced colorectal cancer CAIRO2 study of the Dutch Colorectal Cancer Group (DCCG). J Clin Oncol. 2008;26:LBA4011.
43. Adam R, Delvart V, Pascal G, et al. Rescue surgery for unresectable colorectal liver metastases downstaged by chemotherapy. A model to predict long-term survival. Ann Surg. 2004;240:644–58.
44. Adam R. The importance of visceral metastasectomy in colorectal cancer. Ann Oncol. 2000;11 Suppl 3:29–36.
45. Folprecht G, Grothey A, Alberts S, Raab HR, Köhne CH. Neoadjuvant treatment of unresectable colorectal liver metastases: correlation between tumour response and resection rate. Ann Oncol. 2006;16:1311–9.
46. Colucci G, Gebbia V, Paoletti G, et al. Phase III randomized trial of FOLFIRI versus FOLFOX4 in the treatment of advanced colorectal cancer: a multicenter study of the Gruppo Oncologico Dell'Italia Meridionale. J Clin Oncol. 2005;23:4866–75.
47. Souglakos J, Androulakis N, Syrigos K, et al. FOLFOXIRI (folinic acid, 5-fluorouracil, oxaliplatin and irinotecan) vs FOLFIRI (folinic acid, 5-fluorouracil and irinotecan) as first-line treatment in metastatic colorectal cancer (MCC): a multicentre randomised phase III trial from the Hellenic Oncology Research Group (HORG). Br J Cancer. 2006;94:798–805.
48. Grothey A, Sargent D, Goldberg RM, et al. Survival of patients with advanced colorectal cancer improves with the availability of fluorouracil-leucovorin, irinotecan, and oxaliplatin in the course of treatment. J Clin Oncol. 2004;22:1209–14.
49. Inoue Y, Miki C, Watanabe H, et al. Schedule-dependent cytotoxicity of 5-fluorouracil and irinotecan in a colon cancer cell line. J Gastroenterol. 2006;41:1149–57.
50. Mabro M, Artru P, André T, et al. A phase II study of FOLFIRI-3 (double infusion of irinotecan combined with LV5FU) after FOLFOX in advanced colorectal cancer patients. B J Cancer. 2006;94:1287–92.
51. Bidard FC, Tournigand C, André T, et al. Efficacy of FOLFIRI-3 (irinotecan D1, D3 combined with LV5-FU) or other irinotecan-based regimens in oxaliplatin-pretreated metastatic colorectal cancer in the GERCOR OPTIMOX1 study. Ann Oncol. 2009;20:1042–7.
52. Grothey A, Sugrue MM, Purdie DM, et al. Bevacizumab beyond first progression is associated with prolonged overall survival in metastatic colorectal cancer: results from a large observational cohort study (BRiTE). J Clin Oncol. 2008;26:5326–34.
53. Kohne C, Bajetta E, Lin E, et al. Final results of CONFIRM 2: a multinational, randomized, double-blind, phase III study in 2nd line patients (pts) with metastatic colorectal cancer (mCRC) receiving FOLFOX4 and PTK787/ZK 222584 (PTK/ZK) or placebo. J Clin Oncol. 2007;18S:4033.
54. Sobrero AF, Maurel J, Fehrenbacher L, et al. EPIC: phase III trial of cetuximab plus irinotecan after fluoropyrimidine and oxaliplatin failure in patients with metastatic colorectal. Cancer J Clin Oncol. 2008;26:2311–9.
55. Langer C, Kopit J, Awad M, et al. Mutations in patients with metastatic colorectal cancer receiving cetuximab in combination with irinotecan: results from the EPIC trial. ESMO 2008, Abstract 385P. Ann Oncol. 2008;19(Suppl 8):viii133.

Targeted Therapy of Colorectal Cancer Liver Metastasis

17

Jun Zhou and Lin Shen

17.1 Introduction

The liver metastasis is the main death cause of the colorectal cancer. About 20 % of patients at first diagnosis have liver metastasis; besides, in the follow-up after colorectal cancer operation, there will be 20–45 % of patients with liver metastasis. This means that at least half of patients with colorectal cancer will have liver metastasis during the development of the colorectal cancer.

Surgical removal is the only radical means to completely treat the colorectal cancer liver metastasis. However, in patients who are first discovered with colorectal liver metastasis, only 20 % can accept liver surgery whose aim is completely treatment. There are some patients who belong to potential liver metastasis cutoff group. These patients can be carried on with the preoperative rational treatment to possibly achieve the removal purpose. Of course, there are some patients that had already lost the opportunity of radical resection surgery when founded, but if the drugs or other means can achieve apparent effects, then there is still 7–14 % who can transfer to liver metastasis which can be carried on with radical resection surgery.

For the patients with inoperable liver metastasis, the median survival is less than 20 months; the 5-year survival rate is less than 5 %. In contrast, according to current literature reports, the 5-year survival rate of the patients with resectable colorectal cancer liver metastases is up to 20–58 %. And, for the initial unresectable patients, if the adoption of new adjuvant therapy can achieve the resectable aim, then the 5-year survival rate of these patients can be close to that of the initial survival of resectable patients with the same level.

Therefore, the opportunity to access to curative liver resection is the most influential factor whether the patients with liver metastasis of colorectal cancer can be long-term survival. This aim has not only become a main problem in the comprehensive treatment of liver metastases of colorectal cancer but also is one of the major pursuing goals of neoadjuvant chemotherapy or targeted therapy.

17.2 The Neoadjuvant Chemotherapy of Colorectal Cancer Liver Metastasis

The meaning of neoadjuvant chemotherapy is that for colorectal cancer liver metastases which can be removed, we can reduce the metastatic

J. Zhou • L. Shen (✉)
Department of Gastroenterology, Beijing Cancer Hospital, Peking University School of Oncology, Beijing, China
e-mail: lin100@medmail.com.cn

X. Qin et al. (eds.), *Multidisciplinary Management of Liver Metastases in Colorectal Cancer*,
DOI 10.1007/978-94-017-7755-1_17

tumor burden and liver damage, prevent recurrence, and prolong the disease-free survival term. The initial state of inoperable colorectal cancer liver metastasis and the drug treatment before surgery can make some patients access the opportunity of surgery treatment and obtain long-term disease-free survival. Recent studies indicate that the higher the chemotherapy remission rate in patients with colorectal liver metastases, the higher the cut rate. In 2005, Folprecht et al. published an important review in Annals of Oncology. In the paper, the researchers conclude many period II/III clinical studies on the new adjuvant treatment of unresectable liver metastases. The results show that the remission rate and the cutoff rate of the unresectable liver metastasis of patients are significantly positively correlated ($r = 0.96$, $P = 0.002$). Not only that, the study also shows that even for patients with liver metastases without the initial choice, the remission rate and the cut off rate are also clearly related ($r = 0.74$, $P < 0.001$).

Therefore, a reasonable choice of neoadjuvant chemotherapy and the achievement of the chemotherapy remission rate as far as possible in a short time have become important therapeutic targets of the potentially resectable or unresectable liver metastasis of colorectal cancer. Combination of three drugs in the program, FOLFOXIRI program (5-FU + oxaliplatin + irinotecan), has higher performance and higher operation resection rate in the treatment of colorectal liver metastasis than those of two-drug combination rate but higher side effects, so that people have some worries about their clinical application. So what kind of programs can further improve the remission rate on the base of the existing chemotherapy?

In recent years, *targeted drugs are generally the epidermal growth factor receptor (EGFR) monoclonal antibody and vascular endothelial growth factor monoclonal antibody and chemotherapy, which are used in advanced colorectal cancer and significantly improve the patient's chemotherapy benefit*. At the same time, because the adverse effects of EGFR monoclonal antibody are particular mild, this accordingly makes the drugs in combination of two targeted chemotherapy drugs becomes a new direction in new adjuvant treatment of colorectal cancer liver metastases.

17.3 Epidermal Growth Factor Receptor (EGFR) Monoclonal Antibody

Currently, the recommended EGFR monoclonal antibodies for advanced colorectal cancer include cetuximab and Jesper monoclonal antibodies. A large number of clinical studies approve that only the KRAS wild-type tumor tissue patient can benefit from the EGFR monoclonal antibody treatment. Currently, it is only recommended for this type of patients. Among all kinds of treatments, the efficiency of combination of the antibody with the chemotherapy is 10 % higher than that of the chemotherapy alone. Especially the efficiency of the first-line treatment with the chemotherapy can reach 65 % and efficacy in patients with liver metastasis is up to 77 %. It is reasonable to expect such a high remission rate in patients with colorectal cancer can bring high removal rate.

17.3.1 Cetuximab Monoclonal Antibody

17.3.1.1 The Study on the Irinotecan Combination

In 2005, Peeters et al. published a clinical study result. In forty-two cases of unselected patients with advanced colorectal cancer who received FOLFIRI + cetuximab combined chemotherapy, the effective rate is 45 %, eight of them received R0 resection of liver metastasis after chemotherapy, and the resection rate is19 % [3].

In 2006, Folprecht et al. published a phase I/II clinical study result. In twenty-one unselected advanced colorectal cancer (liver metastasis or extrahepatic metastasis) patients who received irinotecan weekly programs (AIO) + cetuximab combined chemotherapy, the effective rate was 67 % (14/21), four of them received R0 resection of liver metastasis, and the resection rate is 24 % [2].

In 2007, Min et al. published a phase II clinical study result. In twenty-three patients with initial unresectable liver metastasis of colorectal cancer who received FOLFIRI + cetuximab combined chemotherapy, the effective rate is 39.1 % (9/23), seven of them received radical resection of liver metastasis, and the resection rate is 30.4 % [1].

CRYSTAL study is a phase III clinical experiment aiming to the first-line treatment for advanced colorectal cancer. The results are published in the New England Journal of Medicine in April of 2009. 1217 patients with positive expression of EGFR who have lost opportunities for radical surgery were randomly enrolled into the FOLFIRI + cetuximab combined chemotherapy group or FOLFIRI chemotherapy-alone group. The proportion of patients receiving follow-up surgery after chemotherapy in united targeted drug group and the chemotherapy group are 6 % and 2.5 %, respectively. And the difference between R0 resection rate is three times (4.3 % and 1.5 %). Further analysis revealed that among the K-ras wild-type-alone liver metastasis patients, the efficiency of the combined targeting drug therapy group can be up to 77 %, far higher than 50 % of the chemotherapy-alone group. And the joint targeting group's R0 resection rate of liver metastasis is 9.8 %, while the resection rate of the chemotherapy-alone group is only 4.5 % [4]. CRYSTAL study is a phase III randomized controlled clinical study; from a more advanced level of proven evidence-based medicine, it is approved that improvement of the remission rate of tumor can increase the resection rate; even in the patients whose initial judge is unresectable, we also should make each effort to get re-excision opportunities for patients.

17.3.1.2 The Study in Oxaliplatin Combination

ACROBAT study is a phase II clinical trial aiming to first-line treatment for advanced colorectal cancer. Forty-three cases of unselected patients have received the FOLFOX + cetuximab combined chemotherapy. The efficiency rate is up to 72 %, ten of them received radical resection of liver metastasis after chemotherapy, and the resection rate is up to 23 % [5].

OPUS study is a phase II randomized open clinical trial aiming to first-line treatment for advanced colorectal cancer. Three hundred thirty-eight cases of unselected patients whose EGFR expressions were positive were randomized into the FOLFOX4 + cetuximab group or FOLFOX chemotherapy-alone group. After treatment, respectively, there are 4.7 % and 2.4 % patients who had radical surgery and achieved R0 resection. Because of case number limit, there is no liver resection rate data of liver metastasis patients, but the result is very similar to that of CRYSTAL study, which approves that cetuximab can improve the R0 resection rate in patients with advanced colorectal cancer.

In addition, OPUS study makes a retrospective analysis on the tumor's K-ras gene status. For K-ras wild-type patients, comparing the combination treatment group with chemotherapy-alone group, at the same time that the efficient rate (61 % vs. 37 % $P=0.011$) increases, R0 resection rate also increases (9.8 % vs. 4.1 %).

Because the chemotherapy + EGFR antibody therapy has up to 60 % of remission rate for the wild-type K-ras gene patients, the results of the OPUS study suggest the K-ras wild-type patients with liver metastasis may obtain higher resection rate from the united targeted drug therapy. CELIM study is aiming to evaluate the healing effect of the cetuximab combined with FOLFOX (53 cases)/FOLFIRI (53 cases) in first-line treatment of unresectable liver metastasis of colorectal cancer, 67 patients with KRAS wild-type have been evaluated, combination therapy group's tumor efficient rate (CR/PR) is up to 79 %, and R0 resection rate is 33 % (22/67). According to seven surgeons' judgment with blind method on 180 pieces of CT or MRI scans at baseline and after 4 months' treatment of 75 patients (68 %), the resectability rate of liver metastasis has increased to 60.3 % after cetuximab combination therapy comparing with 32 % before the treatment, the net effect increases 28 %, efficiency is improved by 87.5 % ($P<0.01$), and the doctors have high degree of consistency in determination of the surgical resectability [11].

This test showed that cetuximab combined with FOLFOX/FOLFIRI can significantly improve the liver metastasis resection rate, which would place the treatment of colorectal liver metastasis a particularly significant impact, mainly using the high performance of cetuximab combination chemotherapy in wild-type KRAS gene patients, screening the patients who can benefit in the targeted drug therapy.

17.3.1.3 Cetuximab Being Used After Second-Line Treatment for Patients with Liver Metastasis

Adam et al. have report a multi-center clinical study. 151 cases of first-line treatment failure patients with colorectal liver metastasis have received cetuximab chemotherapy, averagely for six periods. Twenty-seven patients received liver surgeries, 13 patients received R0 liver resection, and finally 12 cases received R1 Resection. One patient died in 60 days after surgery; the procedure-related mortality rate is 3.7 %. Sixteen patients were followed up each month, all survived, including ten cases of disease-free survival [6]. This also shows that even in patients who failed first-line chemotherapy, the opportunities through joint targeted drug treatment should not be given up.

17.3.2 Panitumumab

Panitumumab combined with chemotherapy in patients with advanced colorectal cancer is similar to cetuximab, also only fits for K-ras wild-type patients. In 2009 at ESMO meeting, the PRIME study results of panitumumab combined with FOLFOX4 for first-line treatment studies are reported. The study enrolled a total of 1,183 patients with a median age of 62 years old. The results showed that in patients with K-ras wild type (60 %), the combination group and the chemotherapy-alone group's median progression-free survival periods were 9.6 months and 8.0 months ($P = 0.0234$); treatment-effective rates were 55 % and 48 %. In K-ras mutant-type patients, PFS were 7.3 months and 8.8 months ($P = 0.0227$), respectively. Incidence rates of adverse events are similar in the two groups. However, there is no data of effective rate among patients with liver metastasis and resection rate in the PRIME study.

There is a PLANET phase II clinical study in progress which is similar to CELIM study aiming to panitumumab. The study plans to enroll 80 patients with unresectable colorectal liver metastasis who are randomized into panitumumab + FOLFOX4 treatment and panitumumab + FOLFIRI treatment. The main objective is response rate; the secondary objective includes the resection rate. It has not been reported if the results are similar to CELIM study.

17.4 Vascular Endothelial Growth Factor Antibody: Bevacizumab

Brigit et al. in 2008 published a single-center, non-randomized phase II clinical study result aiming at potential curable colorectal cancer liver metastasis patients. Fifty-six cases of first-line treatment patients all received Xeloda + oxaliplatin + bevacizumab joint program preoperatively and postoperatively for 12 weeks, and within 5 weeks before and after surgery bevacizumab cannot be used. Effective rate is 73 % (41/56); three patients enter into the second-line treatment during neoadjuvant chemotherapy progress, one patient has extrahepatic metastasis, and the remaining 52 patients underwent liver resection, while 11 cases carry on primary tumor resection at the same time. There was no significant blood loss and postoperative poor wound healing, there is no surgical complication in 42 patients, and only 1 patient required reoperation [7].

First BEAT is a phase IV, open clinical study. The purpose is to evaluate the safety and effectiveness of the surgery after first-line bevacizumab combined with chemotherapy in patients with metastatic colorectal cancer under the state without choice. The chemotherapy programs included FOLFOX, FOLFIRI, XELOX, and 5-FU/capecitabine monotherapy. 1914 cases of unselected patients with untreated advanced colorectal were enrolled into the group and can be evaluated; 215 patients (11.2 %) received surgery with curative intent, 79 % of which achieved R0 resection. The postoperative mortality within 60 days is 2.5 %; 3° or more adverse events were bleeding (3.2 %), gastrointestinal perforation (1.8 %), arterial thrombosis (1.3 %), hypertension (5.1 %), proteinuria (1.0 %), and wound complications (1.0 %). It is noteworthy that there are two points: first is that among 704 cases of patients with liver metastasis alone, 102 cases (14.5 %) received radical surgery and 81 patients (81.4 %) received R0 resection [8, 9]. Second is that 82 % patients with R0 resection survive more than 2 years, far higher than 40 % of ITT population.

XELOX 1/NO16966 is a phase III open study (two treatment groups); initially it was to assess the safety and effectiveness of the FOLFOX4 program and XELOX program as first-line treatment of metastatic colorectal cancer. Improvement was made in this pilot program; bevacizumab was used. And the trial becomes a randomized, 2×2 partly blinded, placebo-controlled trial. Although the purpose of this study does not aim to evaluate the treatment of patients with liver metastasis, in ASCO of 2008, Cassidy et al. summarized in the study that in liver metastasis patients and bevacizumab-alone group, R0 resection rate was 12.3 %, and it is 11.5 % in the chemotherapy group. The two groups were not significantly different; both groups of patients' bleeding and wound complications were also not significantly different [10]. Therefore, there must be further clinical studies in bevacizumab for colorectal surgery for improving the rate of radical resection.

17.5 Small Molecular Targeted Drugs

In 2004 Fisher et al. issued a phase II clinical study; in the study, 27 patients with advanced colorectal cancer received first-line gefitinib combined regimen FOLFOX4 program; efficiency rate reaches 78 % (21/27), of which nine patients received curative liver resection, among which five patients are initially unresectable. Nevertheless, as from 2006 to 2008, there were a number of clinical studies issued that small molecular targeted drugs, including erlotinib and gefitinib, do no good in advanced colorectal cancer; therefore, application of small molecule drugs targeted in the treatment of colorectal cancer is clearly not the focus of the study. There are still studies in progress on imatinib combined with panitumumab chemotherapy.

17.6 Three-Drug Chemotherapy Combined with Targeted Drugs

For a long time, the standard chemotherapy program of advanced colorectal cancer is FOLFOX and FOLFIRI representing two-drug combination program. Therefore, in the attempts to improve chemotherapy remission rates, oxaliplatin, irinotecan, and fluorouracil/leucovorin are combined to form a three-drug program which is a necessary research direction to consider. In 2006 ASCO-GI reported a phase III clinical study, which shows that, comparing FOLFOXIRI with FOLFIRI, the remission rate significantly increased (66 % vs. 41 %); R0 resection rate was also significantly increased (15 % vs. 6 %). The incidence rate of three-drug group's 3–4° adverse effects including diarrhea, vomiting, and neurological toxicity has increased, and neutropenia decreases by 50 %. But the authors conclude that the increase of adverse effects is acceptable.

Although thinking of the oxaliplatin's sinusoidal damage and steatosis caused by irinotecan, clinicians still have concerns about the use of three-drug joint programs, but the phase III clinical results also suggest that the three-drug chemotherapy combined with targeted drugs is not completely impossible to explore.

In ASCO of 2009, Folprecht et al. published a phase I clinical study which studies the application of cetuximab combined FOLFOXIRI program in first-line treatment of a good general condition (ECOG 0-1) advanced colorectal carcinoma. One of the aims of the study is to explore that, if the general condition of the liver metastasis colorectal cancer patients is good, it is feasible of three-drug combination combined targeted drugs. In research programs, FOLFOX program is fixed, but irinotecan dose increases (cetuximab 500 mg/m^2, 2 h, OXA 85 mg/m^2, 2 h, FA 400 mg/m^2, 2 h, 5-FU 3,200 mg/m^2, 46 h; CPT-11 95,125, 165 mg/m^2, 1 h, q2w). The results showed that the remission rate in all patients is 75 %. Recommended dose group was 125 mg/m^2.

Subsequently, in this year's ESMO, C. Garufi et al. published the preliminary results of POCHER study. The main objective of the study is the resection rate of the patients with liver metastases. Forty-three cases of patients with unresectable liver metastases were selected, not considering K-ras status. The retrospective study showed that 75 % of patients are wild type. Apply Cmab + CPT-11-FFL (CPT-11/5-FU/FA/L-OHP, Falcone 2007) chemotherapy. The results are that the effective rate is 79 % (34/43 cases); there are already 58 % (25 cases) patients who had radical resection, and two cases are ready for resection. Average preoperative chemotherapy is five periods (10 weeks), and average postoperative chemotherapy is six periods. The median progression-free survival is 13 months; 2-year survival rate is 63 %. Main adverse reactions are diarrhea (G3/4 80 %, after dose adjusting 36 %) and abdominal pain but will not delay surgery.

These studies showed that for patients in general good condition and with good tolerability of chemotherapy, a reasonable choice of dose intensity of three-drug chemotherapy combined with targeted drugs is possible to further improve the remission rate and resection rate. Of course, this requires further clinical study of a large sample size.

17.7 Perioperative Treatment of Patients with Initially Resectable Liver Metastases

The above studies aim to the patients with initial unresectable or unselected metastatic colorectal cancer. And the study mainly focuses on improvement of the resection rate of new adjuvant therapy. So, for patients with resectable liver metastases, relevant research's aim is mainly whether perioperative chemotherapy improves survival.

For the patients with initial resectable liver metastases of colorectal cancer, EORTC 40983 study has confirmed that perioperative FOLFOX4 chemotherapy improved the 3-year disease-free survival and does not increase the procedure-related mortality. And patients who do not benefit from the operation can be filtered out. However, there is no study on the effect of targeted drugs on patients with resectable liver metastases of new adjuvant therapy. Although there is a lack of targeted drugs used in adjuvant treatment of liver metastasis of information, these have yet to be explored in further clinical studies.

In summary, for the EGFR monoclonal antibody, because of its high remission rate on the wild-type K-ras patients, for such patients with liver metastases, chemotherapy combined with EGFR monoclonal antibody as a new adjuvant therapy program can significantly increase the resectable rate and R0 resection rate, which may become the first choice in the preoperative treatment of this kind of patient. And for preoperative targeted drug therapy, because the medication is shorter, but the benefit is larger, from the aspects of the drugs economics, it is more conducive to China's status quo. It is believed that with the future more molecular markers appeared, EGFR monoclonal antibody's application populations may be more specific, and efficacy may be further improved, which results in higher removal rate.

For bevacizumab, from the existing clinical studies, the initial fears are to increase the surgical complications, but the clinical results of view show no significant increase, which may be two reasons, First, in clinical study, the preoperative discontinuation of bevacizumab occurs 5–6 weeks before the operation, and, second, the worries on such issues have led to concerns that they are very vigilant. However, despite no increase in adverse reactions, because of the negative phase III results, its curative effect, especially for patients with colorectal cancer liver metastases in the preoperative treatment, remains to be confirmed by further clinical studies.

References

1. Min BS, Kim NK, Ahn JB, Roh JK, Kim KS, Choi JS, Cha SH, Kim H. Cetuximab in combination with 5-fluorouracil, leucovorin and irinotecan as a neoadjuvant chemotherapy in patients with initially unresectable colorectal liver metastasis. Onkologie 2007;30: 637–43.
2. Folprecht G, Lutz MP, Schöffski P, Seufferlein T, Nolting A, Pollert P, Köhne CH. Cetuximab and irinotecan/5-fluorouracil/folinic acid is a safe combination for the first-line treatment of patients with cetuximab/FOLFOX-4 in the treatment of mCRC epidermal growth factor receptor expressing metastatic colorectal carcinoma. Ann Oncol. 2006;17: 450–6.
3. Peeters M, Raoul JL, van Laethem JL, Rougier P, Brezault C, Husseini F, Cals L, Zubel A, Vedovato JC. Cetuximab in combination with irinotecan/5-fluorouracil (5-FU)/folinic acid (FA) (FOLFIRI) in the first-line treatment of metastatic colorectal cancer (mCRC). Eur J Cancer (Suppl). 2005;3:188.
4. van Cutsem E, Nowacki M, Lang I. Randomized phase III study of irinotecan and 5-FU/FA with or without cetuximab in the first-line treatment of patients with metastatic colorectal cancer (mCRC): the CRYSTAL trial. Slides presented at ASCO 2007 annual meeting, Chicago, 15 Jun 2007. Abstract 4000.
5. Tabernero J, van Cutsem E, Díaz-Rubio E, Cervantes A, Humblet Y, André T, van Laethem JL, Soulié P, Casado E, Verslype C, Sastre J, Tortora G, Ciardiello F, Kisker O, de Gramont A. Phase II trial of cetuximab in combination with fluorouracil, leucovorin, and oxaliplatin in the first-line treatment of metastatic colorectal cancer. J Clin Oncol. 2007;33:5225–32.
6. Adam R, Aloia T, Levi F. Hepatic resection after rescue cetuximab treatment for colorectal liver metastases previously refractory to conventional systemic therapy. J Clin Oncol. 2007;25(29):4593–602.
7. Gruenberger B, Tamandl D, Schueller J. Bevacizumab, capecitabine, and oxaliplatin as neoadjuvant therapy for patients with potentially curable metastatic colorectal cancer. J Clin Oncol. 2008;26(11):1830–5.
8. Okines A, Puerto OD, Cunningham D, Chau I, Van Cutsem E, Saltz L, Cassidy J. Surgery with curative-intent in patients treated with first-line chemotherapy plus bevacizumab for metastatic colorectal cancer First BEAT and the randomised phase-III NO16966 trial. Br J Cancer. 2009;7:1033–8
9. Berry SR, Van Cutsem E, Kretzschmar A. Final efficacy results for bevacizumab plus standard first-line chemotherapies in patients with metastatic colorectal cancer: first BEAT. J Clin Oncol. 2008;26(Suppl; abstr 4025).
10. Cassidy J, Cunningham D, Berry SR. Surgery with curative intent in patients (pts) treated with first-line chemotherapy (CT) + bevacizumab (BEV) for metastatic colorectal cancer (mCRC): first BEAT and NO16966. J Clin Oncol. 2008;26(Suppl; abstr 4022).
11. Bechstein WO, Lang H, Köhne C, et al. Resectability and agreement between surgeons: review of CT and MR scan of the CELIM study: (multicenter randomized trial of cetuximab/FOLFOX versus cetuximab/FOLFIRI in unresectable liver metastases. J Clin Oncol. 2009;27:15s(Suppl; abstr 4091).

18 Interventional Treatment of Liver Metastasis of Colorectal Cancer

Jianhua Wang and Yi Chen

18.1 Arterial Infusion Chemotherapy and Arterial Embolism

The transcatheter arterial infusion (TAI) and transcatheter arterial embolization (TAE) have good effects on a variety of solid tumors. In the treatment of liver cancer, they are more effective, especially. Currently, TAI and TAE not only are main methods in the treatment of unresectable colorectal cancer liver metastases but also play important roles in the adjuvant treatment and new adjuvant therapy of colorectal cancer liver metastases [1–4].

18.1.1 Theoretical Basis

(1) In the treatment of TAI, the local chemotherapeutic drug concentration is significantly increased comparing with intravenous chemotherapy, and the cancer treatment effect is also significantly increased. The total amount of drug entering into the systemic circulation is decreased, so the side effects are reduced comparing with intravenous chemotherapy. The previous studies show that when floxuridine (FUDR) was perfused via hepatic artery, the liver uptake rate was up to 95 %, and the drug concentration in the liver tumor was 16 times that of the intravenous infusion. (2) Ninety-five percent of the blood supply of the colorectal cancer liver metastases whose diameter is greater than 3 mm is from hepatic artery. However, about 75 % of the blood supply of the normal liver tissue is from the portal vein. TAI and TAE can effectively kill tumor cells and protect the normal liver cells. (3) TAE can block the arteries feeding the tumor, make the tumor hypoxia-ischemia and necrosis, and increase its sensitivity to chemotherapeutic drugs. In previous opinions, the liver metastatic tumors had poor blood supply, only suitable for the treatment of TAI. Since the development of digital subtraction angiography (DSA), we find that the gastrointestinal source tumors, especially colorectal cancer liver metastases, are more likely to be moderate or even to have rich blood supply in a small amount. Thus, TAE is very important in the treatment of these metastases (Fig. 18.1). (4) Some kind of the embolic materials can carry chemotherapeutic drugs, which would slowly release to kill the tumor continuously. This method is also known as transcatheter arterial chemoembolization (TACE).

J. Wang (✉) • Y. Chen
Zhongshan Hospital, Fudan University, 180 Fenglin Road, Xuhui District, Shanghai 200032, China
e-mail: wang.jianhua@zs-hospital.sh.cn

X. Qin et al. (eds.), *Multidisciplinary Management of Liver Metastases in Colorectal Cancer*, DOI 10.1007/978-94-017-7755-1_18

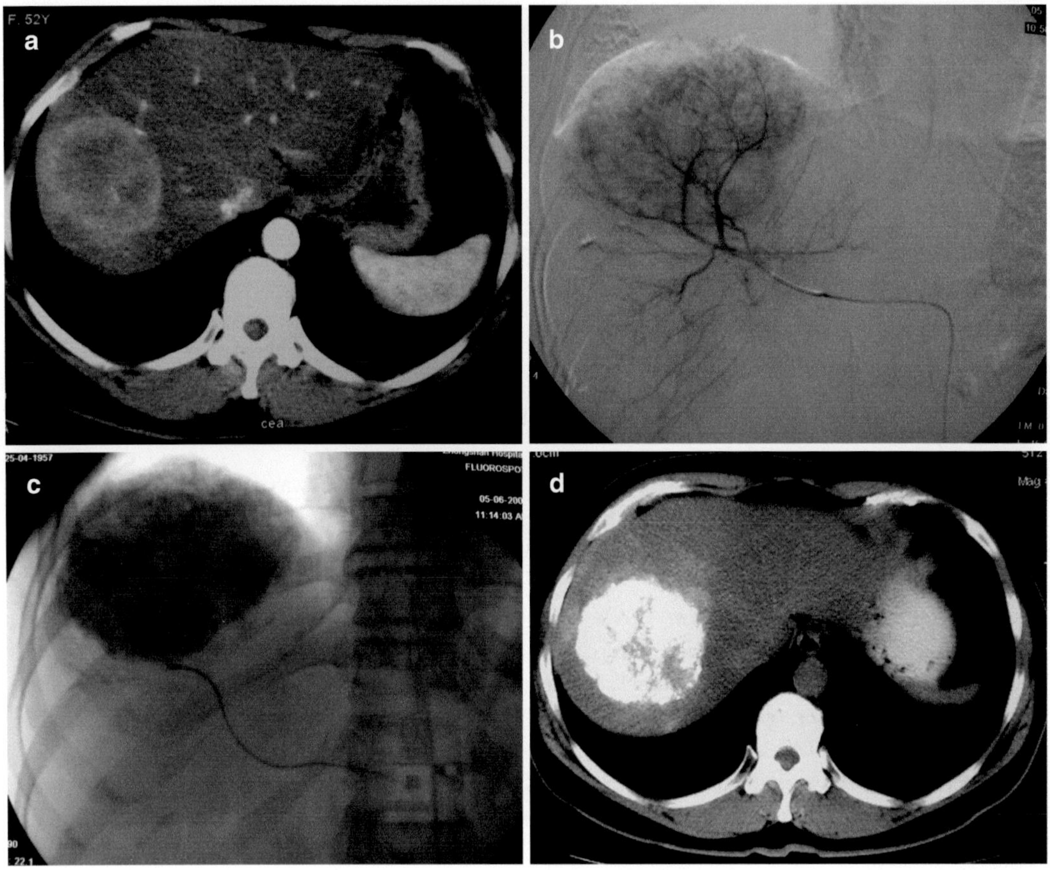

Fig. 18.1 Affluent blood supply of colorectal cancer liver metastases. (**a**) Female, 52-year-old patients with liver metastasis of colon cancer; enhanced arterial lesions advanced the top right lobe diaphragm. (**b**) Hepatic artery angiography showed the lesion with affluent blood supply. (**c**) Lipiodol chemoembolization epirubicin emulsion; the lipiodol deposited well. (**d**) Postoperative CT scan shows lipiodol deposition

18.1.2 Indications and Contraindications

18.1.2.1 Indications

- Unresectable colorectal cancer liver metastases
- Neoadjuvant chemotherapy before surgical procedures for colorectal cancer liver metastases
- Prevention of colorectal cancer recurrence after liver metastasis surgery
- Rupture of colorectal cancer liver metastases

18.1.2.2 Contraindications

- Contraindications for vascular imaging.
- Tumor/liver ratio is greater than 75 %.
- Liver and kidney dysfunction.
- Severe bone marrow suppression.
- Uncorrected coagulopathy.
- Uncontrolled severe infection.
- Intracranial metastasis.
- Terminal-stage patient.

18.1.3 Preoperative Preparation

18.1.3.1 Preoperative Check

During 3 days before intervention surgery, examinations should be taken including blood/urine/stool routine test, liver and kidney function test, coagulation function, electrolyte test, and tumor markers (CEA). Liver MRI or CT scanning should be carried on within 2 weeks before surgery. If being accompanied with other distant metastasis, the appropriate imaging should also be carried on.

18.1.3.2 Patient Preparation

Inform patients and their families of the surgery process, postoperative reaction, and possible complications. Let the patients sign the consent and fast 4 h before surgery. Administer 10 mg intramuscular injection of diazepam 30 min before surgery. Prepare the skin puncture site.

18.1.3.3 Drug Preparation

- Conventional drugs
  Conventional drugs include local anesthetics (such as 1 % lidocaine), heparin, saline, nonionic contrast agent, and so on.
- Emergency drugs
  Operating rooms for interventional procedure should be equipped with emergency rescue drugs such as epinephrine, atropine, nikethamide, dopamine, hydrocortisone, dexamethasone, nitroglycerin, cedilanid, and so on.
- Chemotherapeutics
  Drugs in TAI treatment are commonly used as floxuridine (FUDR)/fluorouracil (5-FU), cisplatin/carboplatin/oxaliplatin, irinotecan, epirubicin (EADM)/pirarubicin (THP), mitomycin C (MMC), and so on. Usually two to three kinds of drugs are combined to carry on perfusion. For hypervascular lesions, part of the drugs and lipiodol are mixed into emulsion to carry on transcatheter arterial chemoembolization (TACE).
- Embolics
  - Lipiodol: Peripheral embolic agent having a special affinity with tumor. The tumor tissue cannot easily remove it. It is a commonly used embolization agent for the hypervascular tumor. In general, the mechanism of lipiodol "orientation" thrombosis is that the tumor tissues are rich of new vessels, with great blood flow, and the lipiodol can flow to tumors due to the syphonage. The tumor vessel is distorted and irregular, lacking muscular and elastic layers and neural regulation. So the blood flow out is slow, which cannot effectively flush the attached lipiodol. Also, the tumor tissue lacks reticuloendothelial system which can remove the lipiodol. The lipiodol and chemotherapeutic agents are often mixed into emulsion to carry on embolization chemotherapy, which can not only make the tumor ischemia and hypoxia but also slowly release the chemotherapy drugs to kill the tumor continuously.
  - Gelatin sponge: Safe, nontoxic, low cost, and most commonly used as embolic agent in TAE. It can be cut into different sizes of strips or granulars according to the need and adds the contrast agent to carry on injections. When used in the embolization of part of vascular cavity, it can be absorbed completely within 7–12 days. Then the blood vessel will reopen. The complete embolization can lead to permanent embolism, which is commonly used in the reduction of tumor blood supply or tumor hemorrhage.
  - Other embolics: stainless steel rings, beads, glue, and Baiji, which are less used.

18.1.3.4 Equipment Preparation

18G needle, 4F or 5F vascular sheath, 0.035 or 0.038 smooth guide wire, 4F or 5F varieties of preforming catheter, such as the celiac artery, hepatic artery, and left gastric artery catheters, the 3F microcatheter, etc. (cobra, RH, RLG, Simmons I, Simmons II, multipurpose, etc.).

18.1.4 Treatment Method

The Seldinger method is used to puncture the femoral artery and place the intravascular sheath. Usually RH catheter is selected to selectively enter into the hepatic artery for angiography, which can make sure the metastatic lesion's number, size, location, blood supply, arteriovenous fistula, and so on. If there is hepatic artery variation or other arteries (superior mesenteric artery, left gastric artery, inferior phrenic artery) taking part in the liver blood supply, the corresponding catheter should be chosen to selectively enter into these arteries to carry on angiography. The catheter tip is placed in the hepatic artery and dilutes the chemotherapy drug to carry on perfusion. There are two drug administration methods: once-shock perfusion and continuous perfusion. The former fits for the nonspecific cell period chemotherapy drug administration. After perfusion, the catheter and vascular sheath are removed; the operation is relatively convenient. The latter fits for specific cell period chemotherapy drug administration, which needs indwelling catheters and vascular sheath. The patients had to stay in bed for several days, which will increase the incidence of thrombosis and other complications. For the metastases of rich blood supply, some of the chemotherapy drugs and lipiodol are mixed into the emulsion to carry on embolization. If you can carry on superselective catheterization, make the catheter tip as close as possible to lesions to reduce the damage to normal liver tissue. It should be noted before embolization to avoid the right gastric artery, cystic artery, and other feeding arteries of the hollow organs to prevent ectopic embolism. The whole embolization process should be completed under the fluoroscopic monitoring, which can not only observe the deposition of lipiodol in the lesion but also detect lipiodol reflux in time. After using the lipiodol emulsion to carry on chemotherapy embolization, if the blood flow of the lesion's blood supply artery is still fast, use thin strips or particles of gelatin sponge to enhance the embolization according to the circumstances to further reduce the tumor blood supply. Use the cases of the lipiodol emulsion chemotherapy embolization; the liver area plain film is shot to record lipiodol deposition.

18.1.5 Postoperative Management

- The patient is supine, with the puncture side limb braking for at least 6 h to observe bleeding and hematoma formation at the puncture site, dorsalis pedis arterial pulse, body skin color, temperature, feeling, and so on.
- Monitor the vital signs; ECG monitoring is used for high-risk patients.
- In 3–5 days after liver surgery, carry on liver protection, acid suppression, antiemetics, antibiotics, and symptomatic and supportive treatments.
- The embolism syndrome is a common reaction after TAE, including a series of clinical syndromes such as nausea, vomiting, upper abdominal pain, gastrointestinal motility decrease, and liver dysfunction, mostly transient. The fever is often led by the metabolites of tumor necrosis affecting body temperature regulation center and can last for several days to several weeks. The nonsteroidal anti-inflammatory drugs can be used to carry on symptomatic treatment. Abdominal pain is often caused by visceral ischemia after embolization, the tumor near the liver capsule and other factors. The treatment objectives of modern medicine for cancer pain or pain associated with cancer are to sustainably and effectively eliminate the pain and maximally improve the patient's life quality. Therefore, we should correctly grasp the principle of three-step analgesic to relieve pain in patients in a timely manner. But during the treatment process, we should pay attention to identify the acute abdominal pain. Gastrointestinal motility decrease should be properly administrated with gastrointestinal motility drugs. Encourage patients to get out of bed and carry on eating.
- In 3–5 days after the surgery, review the liver and kidney function and blood routine to decide whether to continue to carry on liver protection and support and symptomatic treatment. In 6–8 weeks, carry on follow-up with CT/MRI and CEA to observe the healing effects.

18.1.6 Healing Effect

18.1.6.1 Unresectable Colorectal Cancer Liver Metastases

Similar to the history of intravenous chemotherapy for colorectal cancer liver metastasis, 5-FU/FUDR + LV is the most widely and deeply studied drug in the arterial treatment. Since the 1980s, many institutions have carried on a large number of random control studies on 5-FU/FUDR + LV through arterial and intravenous administration. Some scholars [5, 6] summarized seven groups of the classic studies. The results showed that the effective rates of arterial and intravenous administrations were 41 and 14 %, with a significant difference, but the survival terms of the two had no significant difference. They thought the reason that the survival terms of the two were similar was that some patients in the intravenous administration group crossed over to the arterial treatment group after lesion progress, while some patients in the arterial administration group crossed over to the intravenous administration group due to port catheter system (PCS) implantation failure or complications or other factors. The arterial administration group's extrahepatic metastasis lesion has not been well controlled. Kemeny et al. [7] randomly divided 135 patients with colorectal cancer liver metastasis into two groups, arterially and intravenously administered with FUDR and LV. The effective rate of the arterial administration group was 47 %, significantly higher than 24 % of the intravenous group ($P=0.012$). The former's median survival term ($P=0.0034$) and median progress time ($P=0.034$) were significantly longer than the latter.

In the 1990s, the appearance of oxaliplatin and irinotecan makes the colorectal cancer chemotherapy embark on a new level and makes the effective rate of the colorectal cancer liver metastasis remarkably increased, and the survival term is significantly prolonged. Many scholars studied the two drugs' arterial administration. Dzodica et al. [8] studied the arterial and intravenous administration of oxaliplatin in VX2 rabbit model. The peripheral peak concentration of arterial administration was significantly lower than that of intravenous administration, which indicated that the arterial administration had a relatively higher therapeutic index. Irinotecan is a kind of prodrug, which must be catalyzed into active product 7-ethyl-10-hydroxycamptothecin (SN-38) by the carboxylesterase in the human body to play a pharmacological effect. Because the liver carboxylesterase concentration was higher than that in other organs, the conversion rate of SN-38 by the hepatic artery administration was significantly higher than that by intravenous administration ($P=0.015$) so that the former's hepatic SN-38 concentration was higher than that of the latter [9]. Irinotecan, oxaliplatin, and FUDR all have good effects on the colorectal cancer liver metastases, and the action mechanisms and dose-limiting toxicities of three chemotherapy drugs are different, which makes the combination of three drugs have theoretical basis. Currently, a number of in vitro drug sensitivity tests have confirmed that these three drugs have synergistic effect between each other, for example, oxaliplatin and irinotecan active metabolite SN-38 could synergistically inhibit human HT29 colon cancer cell lines. Oxaliplatin and fluorouracil could synergistically inhibit human LoVo colon cancer cell lines. SN-38 and 5-FU could synergistically inhibit varieties of human colon cancer cell lines. Falcone et al. [10] reported the random control study results of irinotecan, oxaliplatin, and FUDR's FOLFOXIRI program and FOLFOX program, which approved that the effective rate of FOLFOXIRI group was significantly higher than that of the latter. The median survival term and median progress time were significantly longer than the latter. Therefore, FOLFOXIRI program becomes a hot spot in colorectal cancer chemotherapy study. Intervention Division, Zhongshan Hospital, used irinotecan, oxaliplatin, and FUDR as first-line or second-line program to treat 32 patients through arterial perfusion with unresectable colorectal cancer liver metastases. The total efficiency rate was 46.9 %, median survival term was 17.7 months, and it achieved good results (Fig. 18.2).

18.1.6.2 The Adjuvant Treatment of Colorectal Cancer Liver Metastases

After resection of liver lesions, implementation of TAI can not only control the small undiscovered intrahepatic metastasis lesions but also prevent intrahepatic recurrence. Kermeny et al. [11] carried on a control study between the patients who received arterial perfusion chemotherapy after the operation of colorectal cancer liver metastases and the patients who do not receive

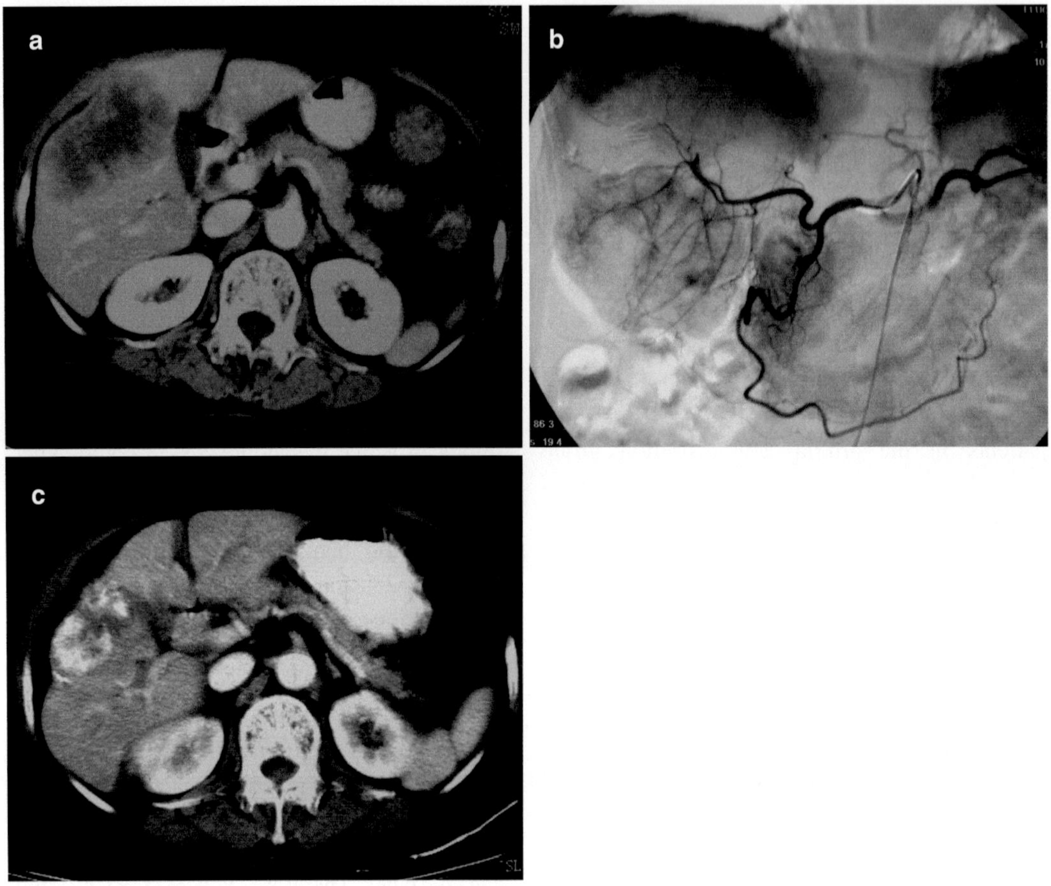

Fig. 18.2 Irinotecan, oxaliplatin, and FUDR combined arterial treatment for colorectal cancer liver metastases. (**a**) Female, 74-year-old patients with liver metastasis of colon cancer. (**b**) Adopt irinotecan, oxaliplatin,, and FUDR programs; carry on TAI and TAE. (**c**) After two treatments, the lesion was significantly reduced to PR

the treatment. The 4-year intrahepatic recurrence free rates were 67 % and 43 %, respectively, with a significant difference. In another study, 156 patients who received the colorectal cancer liver metastasis resection were randomly divided into two groups [12]: one was given arterial administration of FUDR and intravenous administration of 5-FU and LV; the other was given intravenous administration of 5-FU And LV. Both treatment periods were six cycles. The 2-year survival rates of intravenous administration group and the artery and vein combined administration group were 72 and 86 % ($P=0.03$). The two groups' median survival term was 62.7 and 72.2 months. The death risk of the intravenous administration group was 2.34 times of the artery and vein combined administration group.

18.1.6.3 The Neoadjuvant Treatment of Colorectal Cancer Liver Metastases

The advantages of arterial neoadjuvant treatment are as follows: (1) control and reduce intrahepatic metastasis lesions, decrease tumor stage, make the unresectable tumor resectable, improve the curative resection rate, and reduce the relapse rate; (2) control preoperatively existing small lesions and reduce the postoperative recurrence; (3) prevent postoperative changes in tumor blood supply and influence the effects of chemotherapy; (4) prevent the tumor proliferation stimulation induced by the primary tumors and control the iatrogenic transfer; (5) as a chemotherapy-sensitive test, rationally select the sensitive drug and help to determine prognosis; and (6) screen the patients who cannot receive the surgical treatment.

There are a lot of reports about radical resection of inoperable colorectal cancer after receiving intravenous chemotherapy [13], but there is still less experience in the arterial neoadjuvant therapy of the colorectal cancer liver metastases. Zelek et al. [14] treated 31 patients with unresectable liver metastases of colorectal cancer, among which 11 patients received the radical resection through the method of intravenous administration of irinotecan and 5-FU, combining with artery epirubicin.

18.1.7 Complications

18.1.7.1 Puncture- and Catheterization-Related Complications

- Puncture site hematoma and pseudoaneurysm formation
  Poor blood coagulation and improper hemostasis can cause puncture site bleeding, hematoma, or even formation of pseudoaneurysm. After the formation of hematoma, it should be noted whether there is expansion of the scope of hematoma or local swelling throb. If there is progressive expansion of the hematoma, it is needed to carry on repressure dressing and use hemostatic. In early hematoma formation period, we can puncture with a big syringe needle into the thick hematoma to carry on the aspiration to relieve the congestion as much as possible. If there is local swelling throb near the puncture site, the color Doppler imaging should be carried on to make clear whether there is pseudoaneurysm formation. If pseudoaneurysm is found, mark the position of the orificium fistulae by the color Doppler imaging and carry on pressure dressing. If these measures are ineffective, according to the situation, inject the prothrombin complex under the guidance of the ultrasound or carry on surgical intervention.
- Arterial dissection
  This is caused by entering into the arterial intima through the guide wire or catheter and lifting the intima. It is common in the cases with the basis of atherosclerosis or tortuous blood vessels. The symptom is that the blood flow cannot reach the remote artery, and local contrast agent takes on stasis strip. Try to use soft head leaned over the guide wire sandwich. But in most cases the intervention operation must be terminated.
- Arterial spasm
  It is related with the stimulation of the catheter, guide wire, and chemotherapy drugs on the arterial wall. It often occurs in cases with fine and tortuous-shaped arteries. Minor seizures generally do not affect further operations. More severe spasm makes the artery canal narrower, apparently decreasing the blood flowing into the spastic distal segment, which will affect the follow-up treatment. In the operation, gently operate the guide wire and catheter and slowly perfuse the chemotherapy drugs. The micro-catheters are used for patients with arterial spasm to avoid the incidence of this complication. In case of spasm, immediately stop the guide wire and catheter manipulation and slowly inject with 2 % lidocaine. If it's void, we can dilute 30 mg papaverine with 10 ml normal saline to inject slowly. If all above treatment methods are ineffective to severe spasm, the operation should be terminated.
- Arterial injury or perforation
  If the guide wire operation injures the arterial wall or the contrast agent rate is too large, it will lead to the arterial wall perforation, which shows as contrast agent extravasation. The minor injury can be treated with local and systemic hemostatic agents. Serious injury and perforation require gelatin sponge, stainless steel embolization, or even surgical repair.
- Vagal reflex
  This may be related with the guide wire and catheter's stimulation of the receptors on artery walls. The heart rate and blood pressure decrease at the same time. In severe cases, loss of consciousness occurs. Intravenous injection of atropine must be carried on immediately. If necessary, repeat the injection. And at the same time, give other treatments accordingly.

- Bend or rupture of the guide wire and catheter
  This may be related with vascular distortion, unskilled surgeon operation, operation not under the fluoroscopic monitoring, or other factors. The guide wire bend can be taken out carefully through the catheter under the fluoroscopic monitoring. The catheter bend segment should be withdrawn within the blood vessels with wider diameter (such as abdominal aorta). After probing with the guide wire soft head, take it out under the fluoroscopic monitoring. Guide wire and catheter's rupture should be firstly disposed with the capture device. If not successful, the surgery is needed.

18.1.7.2 Drug-Related Complications

During arterial perfusion chemotherapy and chemoembolization, the liver and gastrointestinal blood concentrations are significantly higher than peripheral blood drug concentrations. So the liver and upper gastrointestinal local adverse reactions are obvious. The incidence rates of the bone marrow suppression, alopecia, diarrhea, and other systemic adverse reactions are lower than those in the intravenous chemotherapy. In addition to chemotherapy drug adverse reactions, the common complications are as follows:

- Liver failure
  Poor liver function reservation and portal vein involvement are high-risk factors for postoperative liver failure. This complication can be prevented by a comprehensive assessment of preoperative liver function of patients, attention for intraoperative superselective catheterization, and reduction in the high-risk cases.
- Renal failure
  Renal failure is not only related with renal toxicity of chemotherapy drugs but also related with the metabolite injury and renal tubular blockage caused by the necrosis of a large number of tumor cells in short term after the chemotherapy embolization. Preventive measures can be taken by avoiding using chemotherapy drugs with greater renal toxicity as possible as you can and full hydration and alkalinization of urine after surgery.
- Ectopic embolization
  Ectopic embolization generally refers to the liquid embolic agent flowing back into the cystic artery, right gastric artery, and gastroduodenal artery during TAE, causing damage or perforation of the gallbladder or stomach. During the surgery, the catheter head should avoid the abovementioned artery, and avoidance of regurgitation during the chemotherapy embolization can play a preventive role.
- Bile duct sclerosis and biloma
  Because the blood supply of bile duct system is from the liver artery, hepatic artery administration can cause bile duct complications. There are many reports about bile duct sclerosis in western countries, which mostly appears in cases with FUDR administration through the artery. The occurrence rate is up to 3–26 %; the clinical symptoms are similar to primary sclerosing cholangitis. At the same time of the administration, the arterial administration of dexamethasone or switch to 5-FU can reduce the incidence rate of this complication. Biloma formation may be related to bile leakage after the local bile duct wall ischemic necrosis. Small-volume bile tumor need not be treated. If the volume is great and produces symptoms of oppression, puncture and drainage can be carried on.
- Liver abscess
  The biliary tract surgery history is the high-risk factor for the formation of liver abscess after TAI or TAE. The biliary tract surgery can lead to intestinal bacteria retrograding into the liver. The cytotoxic effect of chemotherapy drug and liver tissue local ischemia after the embolization can both cause decrease of anti-infection immunity and lead to liver abscess. After the formation of abscess, the combination administration of sensitive antibiotics is needed, and puncture and drainage should be carried on after the abscess grows mature.

18.1.8 Prospect

In recent years, the targeted therapy drug develops very fast and has achieved good clinical healing effects. The colorectal cancer targeted therapy drugs with clear healing effects are cetuximab targeting epidermal growth factor receptor and bevacizumab targeting vascular endothelial growth factor [15, 16]. Therefore, it is a new direction of the treatment of colorectal cancer liver metastases to combine the molecular biology and the traditional chemotherapy drugs. TAI can increase the tumor's local blood drug concentrations and reduce the side effects of drugs on the systematic circulation, playing a role in organ targeting. In this way, TAI can enhance the efficacy of molecular targeted drugs, and it is worthy of further study.

18.2 Percutaneous Port Catheter System Implantation

Port catheter system (PCS) implantation is to percutaneously make the indwelling catheter into the target vessel. Its end is connected with the kit indwelled under the skin to establish the long-term intravascular drug delivery pathway involvement technology. PCS implantation has the following advantages: it is a simple delivery method through an operation; it can establish a long-term use vascular access for the TAI to avoid repeated intubation; it can, with just a puncture into the kit, administer drugs; it can be carried on at outpatient service; and it can decrease the average cost of treatment. In 1981, percutaneous PCS implantation appeared in the United States. The first Chinese percutaneous PCS implantation via subclavian artery was reported in 1994. And then it is carried on in the domestic field extensively. Comparing with the surgical implantation, the percutaneous PCS implantation has less damage and fewer complications, no destruction of the arterial anatomy, and long patency [17]. If necessary, PCS can be adjusted or removed [18]. PCS only provides a therapeutic method with no tumor treatment effect itself. The main effects of TAI through PCS are related with the chemotherapy regimens, tumor differentiation degree, catheter indwelling position, patient's physical conditions, and other factors [19, 20].

18.2.1 Indications and Contraindications

18.2.1.1 Indications

- The metastasis lesions needing multiple TAI administrations.
- The hepatic artery as the only blood supply artery for the hepatic lesion. If there are other visceral arteries participating in the blood supply, embolization on these vessels should be carried on.

18.2.1.2 Contraindications: In Addition to TAI and TAE Contraindications, There Are

- The kit implementation site may be carried on hyperthermia or radiotherapy.
- There is infection or scarring or swelling lymph nodes in PCS kit implantation site.

18.2.2 Preoperative Preparation

- Preoperative check
  During 3 days before intervention surgery, examinations should be taken including blood/urine/stool routine test, liver and kidney function test, coagulation function, electrolyte test, and tumor markers (CEA). Liver MRI or CT scanning should be carried on within 1 week before surgery. If being accompanied with other distant metastasis, the appropriate imaging should also be carried on.
- Patient preparation
  Inform patients and their families of the surgery process, postoperative reaction, and possible complications. Let the patients sign the consent. In addition, patients should be informed of the implanted chemotherapy kit's size, shape, implant position, influence on the daily life, and nursing kit, so that patients can have adequate psychological preparation.
- Drug preparation
  The same as "Section I."
- Equipment preparation
  - Conventional interventional devices
    These include 21G puncture kit (including the 21G puncture needle, 0.018 in. thin

guide wire, and 4F trocar) or 18G puncture needle, 180 cm long and 0.035 or 0.038 in. smooth guide wire, and 4F or 5F catheter various preformed catheter (cobra and RH are the most commonly used).

- Port catheter system

  This is composed of the kit, interface nut, indwelling catheter, and tunnel needle. PCS kit shell is made by hard plastics or metal. Puncture membrane is made by the high-density silicone, which is located in the upper shell, can bear hundreds of puncture, and will not leak. In one side of the kit, there is OD 0.038 in. stainless steel pipe. After setting into the indwelling tube, screw the interface nut on and fix the indwelling catheter and the shell closely. The indwelling catheter's outer diameter is usually 5F, and the inner diameter can pass the 0.038 in. guide wire.
- Other instruments

  These include the commonly used surgical instruments, such as scalpels, forceps, surgical forceps, needle holder, needle and suture, and so on.

18.2.3 Operative Technique

18.2.3.1 Angiography

Angiography usually starts from the femoral artery way to carry on catheter digital subtraction angiography. Through angiography, tumor arterial blood supply conditions are known to determine suitability for PCS implantation. TAI and TAE are also carried on through this pathway.

18.2.3.2 Approach Choice

When carrying on PCS implantation, the blood vessel approach can be the left subclavian artery or the femoral artery [21, 22]. The corresponding kit implantation sites are the left anterior chest wall, the lower abdominal wall, or the groin inner thigh. Generally, it is preferred to select the approach of the left subclavian artery so that the kit implantation's influence on the patient's postoperative life is relatively slight, easy care, and the indwelling tube in the aorta is along the direction of the blood flow, not easy to be shifted. But it is difficult to carry on the left subclavian artery puncture and catheter manipulation. The operators are required to have appropriate experience. Femoral artery puncture and catheter manipulation approaches are more convenient, but the indwelling tube in the aorta is in the reverse direction of blood flow, relatively easy to be shifted. Because PCS kit is close to the groin, the care requirements are higher; otherwise, it easily leads to infection.

18.2.3.3 The Left Subclavian Artery Puncture Technique

The left subclavian artery directly starts from the aortic arch, along the inside apex, from the apertura thoracis superior to the root of the neck chest, passing the scalenus gap through the top of the first rib to the outer edge of the first rib, transitional the axillary artery. Usually the sites of puncture are the outside segment of the left subclavian artery and the outer edge of the first rib 1–2 cm at the initial segment of the axillary artery. The needle point usually selects at the subclavian fossa 3–4 cm below the top. Slim patient may be touched at the axillary artery pulse. The depth of puncture at the midpoint of the clavicle with 21G needle is about 4–5 cm, and then the end of needle is connected to the syringe. Take back the needle when withdrawing. Remove the syringe when there is blood return. If the needle tip is located in the left subclavian artery, we can see the bright red blood drop out quickly at the end of needle. If the puncture is not successful, move the needle 0.5 cm downward every time, until the needle parallels with the cross section of the body. During the puncture, if the patients feel numbness in the left upper extremity, which means the axillary plexus is hit, the needle tip is in upper direction. If the subclavian vein is hit, it indicates the needle tip is in lower direction. If the pleural cavity is hit, it proves too deep and low puncture. During the puncture process, remove the pillows to relax the patient's shoulders, which can improve the success rate of puncture. After hitting, send the 0.018 in. guide wire into the ascending aorta under fluoroscopic monitoring, along the guide wire sent into the 4F stent. After removal of the core and the 0.018 in. guide wire, send the 0.038 in. or 0.035 in. after smooth guide wire. Then set up the puncture channel.

Another way is through the established femoral artery approach to send 0.035 in. guide wire into the left subclavian lower artery as the guidance. Under fluoroscopic monitoring, aim at the 0.035 in. guide wire to carry on puncture. During PCS implantation, TAI is usually carried on through the femoral artery approach, and this method's puncture success rate is high with few complications. Thus, it becomes the most commonly used method of left subclavian artery puncture.

18.2.3.4 Indwelling Catheter Placement

Along the guide wire sent into the catheter (cobra catheter is most commonly used), avoid using the vascular sheath to prevent bleeding after the exchange of indwelling catheters. With the help of the guide wire, make the catheter selectively enter into the hepatic artery. If the catheter cannot cross the gastroduodenal artery, you can use stainless steel ring to close the gastroduodenal artery and place the catheter head in the hepatic artery. After angiography approves the catheter position, send the guide wire and make the guide wire tip reach the distal arterial branches to provide good support. Under fluoroscopic monitoring, fix the guide wire, withdraw the catheter until the catheter exits out of the body, and at the same time, press the puncture point to prevent bleeding. Along the guide wire, send the indwelling catheter into the desired location. The fluoroscopic imaging of the indwelling catheter is poor under fluoroscopic monitoring. If necessary, enlarge the image to identify catheter tip position and carry on confirmation by contrast agent injection. After the indwelling catheter is in place, patients should be told to take a deep breath or cough to increase range of organ position movement to observe whether the catheter tip position is shifting. If there is shift, the indwelling catheter should be readjusted.

18.2.3.5 Kit Access and Implantation

In the left anterior chest wall, 2–3 cm under the puncture point, carry on local anesthesia and cut off about 3 cm skin to isolate the subcutaneous tissue. Subcutaneous tissues are bluntly dissected to make a subcutaneous cyst. The size to accommodate the kit can prevail. The tunnel needle puncture gets through the subcutaneous tissue to the cavity. The needle ends at the catheter connection, which would lead to the catheter lumen outside the incision. Cut off the excess catheter with a metal pipe connection kit and tighten the nut and the interface. Scalp needle with heparin saline is injected into the kit as a test to observe any leaks in the interface. Further injection of contrast agent is done to confirm that the catheter tip will not shift into the skin or into the cavity inside the kit. Contrast agent is injected again to confirm that there is no folding of the part out of the catheter and then suture the subcutaneous tissue and skin. Bolus injection of heparin saline is performed to fill the kit and indwelling catheter to prevent thrombosis within the catheter system kit.

In the femoral artery indwelling, the puncture kit can also be implanted 3–4 cm at the bottom of the ipsilateral abdominal wall. Pitch location of the puncture kit is far from the indwelling. The indwelling catheter in the act of making a small incision through the skin with a needle for fractional tunnel will lead to cyst catheter incision.

18.2.3.6 Delivery Method

Expose the site of the kit and conventional disinfection. With the left thumb, index finger, and middle finger, touch the edge of PCS. Clear the center of PCS. Puncture the kit vertical penetration film with a scalp needle until the tip touches the bottom of the kit. During first injection with heparin saline, observation is smooth, with or without leakage. And then inject chemotherapy drugs to PCS. After the end of injection, make a sealed tube with heparin saline. The kit of chemotherapy should be the first in a small amount of contrast agent injection under fluoroscopy to confirm the catheter tip position. Monthly PCS system should be flushed with heparin saline.

18.2.4 Postoperative Treatment

- The patient is supine, with the left upper and/ or puncture side limb braking to observe the puncture site and the kit with indwelling bleeding, hematoma formation, the pulse of puncture artery and the left radial artery, body skin color, temperature, feeling, and so on.
- In 3–5 days after liver surgery, carry on liver protection, acid suppression, antiemetic, antibiotics, and symptomatic and supportive treatments.
- Remove sutures 7 days after surgery. For patients with poor wound healing or high tension, prolong the suture time or add interrupted sutures. If necessary, fix the incision with butterfly tape to reduce the tension. Minimize the activity of the left upper limb. Maintain the kit clean and dry the skin at the implant, especially for patients with implants through the femoral artery.

18.2.5 Complications

Puncture-related complications are the same as those in "Section I." The short-term PCS implantation-related complications are pneumothorax, wound infection, hematoma formation, and delayed healing. Long-term complications include catheter displacement, obstruction, hepatic artery occlusion, and skin necrosis.

- *Pneumothorax*
  Pneumothorax is usually caused by puncture of deeper or lower subclavian artery and puncture of parietal pleura. Slight pneumothorax is usually self-absorbed without special treatment. Severe pneumothorax needs thoracic close drainage. This complication can be avoided by the puncture of the left subclavian artery aimed at the guide wire indwelled through the femoral artery. Without the help of the guide wire, the anatomy of the left subclavian artery should be more familiar before the surgery. Of course, it is important to identify the adjacent structure and the surface projection to avoid too-deep puncture of the needle (no deeper than the edge of the first rib under fluoroscopy).
- *Hematoma formation*
  Poor blood coagulation can cause puncture site bleeding, local swelling, ecchymosis, and fluctuation feeling. For high-risk patients, coagulation function should be corrected before the surgery, and hemostatics should be use after the surgery. During the surgery, more attention should be paid to prevent the bleeding of small vessels. Minimize the residual cavity space. For wound bleeding heavily, indwell subcutaneous intracavitary drainage to prevent hematoma formation. If hematoma has formed, rough needle can be taken for puncture and aspiration. Take incision and drainage if necessary.
- *Wound infection*
  PCS is a sterile implant incision and usually has no infection. The keys to prevent infection are strict aseptic technique, removing sutures before the accumulation of blood within the wound, and routine use of antibiotics. Once infection occurred, it is important to use effective antibiotics in time. If necessary, take local treatment appropriately. For prolonged unhealed wound, PCS should be removed.
- *Wound delayed healing or cracking*
  It is often associated with poor nutritional status of patients and greater tension on the incision. The subcutaneous PCS kit can often cause greater tension of the incision. The kit should be buried between the deep fasciae, just under the smooth skin. For incision with greater tension, suture removal should be delayed or interrupted to improve the nutritional status of patients and promote wound healing. If wounds would not heal, the PCS system should be removed.
- *Catheter displacement*
  Catheter displacement can be divided into the proximal displacement and the distal displacement. The proximal displacement is more common as the catheter tip shifts to the proximal opening of the gastroduodenal

artery or celiac trunk. The chemotherapy drug concentration decreases in hepatic perfusion, and the gastrointestinal adverse reactions increase. In the distal displacement, the catheter tip shifts to the hepatic artery bifurcation, causing some lesions. The following measures can prevent catheter displacement: The catheter should retain a certain length within the target vessel; the catheter should not be stretched too tight or too loose; before connecting the kit, let the patient take a deep breath or cough to observe the movement of the catheter tip; and make appropriate adjustment. Catheter can be fixed through a variety of techniques to prevent displacement, but the operation is more complex and time-consuming [23]. Once the catheter displacement occurs after surgery, separate the catheter from the kit, and replace the indwelling catheter.

- *Catheter obstruction*
  It usually occurs in patients without heparin saline flush for a long time. Some obstructions can get repass by 2 ml syringe injection with urokinase solution.
- *Hepatic artery occlusion*
  This is related to stimulation to endangium by chemotherapy drugs or catheter tip. The vessel wall cannot withstand the catheter tip of PCS and is easily injured [24].
- *Leakage of chemotherapy drugs*
  Needle failing to puncture into the kit completely or the catheter failing to connect with the kit tightly will lead to the leakage of chemotherapy drugs during chemotherapy infusion. The needle can puncture into the kit through the membrane only when the injection pressure is high, and sometimes the needle will be withdraw so that the needle will retreat out of the film, leading to the leakage. Therefore, the needle should come into contact with the posterior wall of the kit and then inject chemotherapy drugs. In the event of leakage, cryoablation or procaine can be used for local blocking. For drugs with serious local stimulation (such as mitomycin C), the kit often needs to be removed.

18.3 Radio-Frequency Ablation

Over the last decade, the local treatment of liver tumors developed rapidly and achieved good clinical efficacy. The local treatments include radio-frequency ablation (RFA), microwave treatment, laser-induced thermotherapy (LITT), high-intensity focused ultrasound (HIFU), cryoablation, and so on. In the treatment of colorectal cancer liver metastases, the RFA is reported by more researches and clinical trials. Here is a brief introduction of the RFA for colorectal cancer liver metastases.

18.3.1 Mechanism

RFA system consists of RF generator, needle electrode, and skin electrodes. During the treatment, CT and other imaging methods guide the needle electrode into the tumor. Skin electrode is one or two large electrodes placed at the body surface with relatively good electrical and thermal conductivity, such as the thighs or back. Thus, the RF generator, the needle electrode, the skin electrodes, and the body form a circular path. When the RF generator works, the needle electrode and the skin electrodes produce the RF current in the patient's body. Under the action of the needle electrodes, the surrounding tissues appear with ion oscillation, heat, and tissue-temperature rise [25]. According to the literature [26], cells can still maintain a steady state at 40 °C; when the temperature rises to 42–45 °C, external stimulus easily causes damage; when the temperature rises to >46 °C, cells began to appear with irreversible damage; at 60–100 °C, coagulation necrosis occurs; when the temperature exceeds 105 °C, carbonization occurs and then the carbonized tissues will inhibit the heat conduction. Therefore, 60–100 °C is the best temperature range for RFA treatment of cancer. Heat inactivation of tumor necrosis in vivo is different from the tumor tissue, the tumor cell antigen of which rapidly liquefied and degraded. After RFA treatment, the temperature of tumor tissue can be fixed and retained in the body. The inactivation of tumor tissues lasts quite a long time, and the interaction between the tumor tissues and the immune system can produce long-term immune effect, which may facilitate the killing of tumor cells and tiny metastases, thus playing ectopic antitumor effect [27].

18.3.2 Indications [28, 29]

Lesion diameter ≤4 cm, no more than 3 cm, and no extrahepatic metastases are the best indications for RFA, which can achieve radical results. If the diameter or number of lesions fails to meet the above standard or extrahepatic metastasis has occurred, appropriate palliative treatment may be conducted.

18.3.3 Contraindications [30]

- Contraindications of liver biopsy, such as severe coagulation disorders, sepsis, and so on.
- Hilar tumors. The hepatic artery and portal vein blood can take away the heat so that the hepatic artery and portal vein avoid heat damage. But bile flows very slowly and could not take away the heat. If the effect of hepatic RFA of tumors damages the large bile duct, there may be biliary fistula, or bile duct stricture.
- Tumors near the gallbladder, stomach, intestine, and other hollow organs as a relative contraindication to RFA treatment by laparotomy.
- Liver function Child-Pugh classification, grade C.
- End-stage patients.

18.3.4 Preoperative Preparation

18.3.4.1 Preoperative

During 3 days before intervention surgery, examinations should be taken including blood/urine/stool routine test, liver and kidney function test, coagulation function, electrolyte test, and tumor markers (CEA). Liver MRI or CT scanning should be carried on within 1 week before surgery. If being accompanied with other distant metastasis, the appropriate imaging should also be carried on.

18.3.4.2 Patient Preparation

Inform patients and their families of the surgery process, postoperative reaction, and possible complications. Let the patients sign the consent and fast four hours before surgery. Administer preoperative sedation with 10 mg intramuscular injection of diazepam 30 min before surgery.

18.3.4.3 Drug Preparation

- Conventional drugs
  Local anesthetics, analgesics, saline, and so on
- Emergency drugs
  The same as "Section 1"

18.3.4.4 Equipments

Radio-Frequency Ablation Instrument

RFA instrument consists of needle electrode, RF generators, wires, and the skin electrode. Different manufacturers of radio-frequency catheter ablations mainly differ in needle electrode. Commonly used needle electrodes include:

- *Umbrella needle electrode* [31]. The insulations of the needle electrode, bevel needle, and bar electrode within the arc consist a number of pieces of wires. According to the different manufacturers and device models, the number of wire inside the needle electrode ranges from 4 to 12. After the needle electrode was inserted into the tumor, the electrode wire out of the needle bar was umbrella-like open, increasing the scope of RFA treatment.
- *Bipolar needle electrode* [32]. It is a two-parallel-needle electrode enhancing radio-frequency current work that is created between two electrodes, without the use of skin electrodes. Its effect is equivalent to the effect that two single-needle electrodes work at the same time.

- *Self-cooling needle electrode* [33]. There are two parallel needle hollow lumens; the lumen in the flow of liquid can take the heat around the needle electrode to prevent over-high temperature around the needle electrodes and subsequent carbonization, thereby enhancing the radio-frequency current and heat conduction.
- *Saline-enhanced needle electrode* [34]. On the needle electrode tip, there is a side hole, and the injection holes at the needle end are connected. During treatment, normal saline is injected from the pin end and can disperse in the treatment area through the side hole. Organizations can increase the electrical conductivity, thereby enhancing the RF current and thermal effects; liquid thermal conductivity is better than solid since it can prevent tissue charring near the needle electrode.

18.3.4.5 CT or Ultrasound Image Guidance Equipment

Ultrasound and CT imaging are commonly used in guiding RFA therapy, both having advantages and disadvantages. The spatial resolution and density resolution of CT are much higher than ultrasound. But ultrasound shows a more clear and precise image between the human tissue and the needle electrode. During RF treatment, large quantities of microbubbles will form a lot of acoustic interface, interfering with observation of ultrasound treatment of lesions. However, ultrasound guidance is simple and can real-time display puncture procedure to adjust the direction and depth of the needle electrodes. CT guidance is a more complicated operation; image acquisition and needle insertion are conducted separately, and the patients are affected by X-ray radiation dose.

18.3.5 Operation Method

- According to the lesion location and operation need, the patients shall be in supine position, prone position, or lateral position, with the skin electrodes placed and fixed on the thigh or back, and then by virtue of ECG, the course of treatment shall be observed.
- Make 2–3 mm skin incision over the puncture point and carry on lidocaine as local anesthesia. With ultrasound or CT guidance, the needle electrode is inserted into the liver capsule. Let the patient calm his breathing and hold it to reduce liver capsule injury. Real-time ultrasound guidance should be used to monitor the whole course from the needle electrode's insertion into the body to reach lesions. Pay attention to avoiding the large blood vessels. When guided by CT, it is required to precalculate the needle's insertion angle and depth based on CT or MRI images. If necessary, use CT scans intermittently so as to confirm tip location, until the tips reach the intended site.
- Turn on the radio-frequency generator to start the radio-frequency treatment and determine treatment time according to treatment parameters set by different machines. Currently, the most commonly used umbrella needle electrode is required to open a sub-diameter needle before treatment to make the edge of ablation lesions beyond the scope of 0.5 cm. During the course of treatment, inject a small amount of cold water between the skin and electrodes from time to time to prevent skin burns. If patient has more severe pain, the pain can be alleviated with morphine or strong analgesia. For patients with vagal reflex, atropine can be used.
- After radio-frequency ablation, use the coagulation function. Have the patient hold his breath and then slowly withdraw the needle electrode. Note that before the withdrawal of the needle, ensure the complete close of minor needle. Cover a layer of gauze over the puncture point and bandage with bellyband.

18.3.6 Postoperative Management

- Maintain the supine position on the day of surgery, monitor vital signs, and observe whether there are such complications as bleeding and pneumothorax.
- Administer hemostatic agents as appropriate to prevent bleeding; give liver protection, antibiotics, and symptomatic treatment for 3 days.

- One week after operation, reexamine liver function and conduct blood routine examination; 4–6 weeks after operation, conduct CT or MRI; according to the tumor necrosis, decide whether to give RFA again or to give other treatments.

18.3.7 Complications

RFA complications are mainly related to the puncture operation or heat damage. Some scholars have summed up 41 groups of percutaneous RFA cases with a total of 2,320 cases of patients. Complications of RFA treatment of liver tumors are as follows [35]:

- *Minor complications*
  - Liver pain: usually occurs within a few days during and after operation; mostly occurs to lesions on the liver capsule
  - Fever: related to absorption and removal of necrotic tumor tissues
  - Pleural effusion: in the puncture tract through the diaphragm into the pleural cavity and the lesions seen in cases of the top, 1–2 weeks after surgery itself absorbed
  - Skin burns: caused by a skin electrode
  - Branch duct stenosis: a thermal burn of small bile duct branches, showing injured remote branch expansion, generally does not cause clinical symptoms
- *Serious complications*
  - Puncture tract cultivation: 0.5 %.
  - Abdominal bleeding: 0.5 % and more lesions in the liver capsule; in case of large amount of bleeding, transfusion and hepatic artery embolizations are required.
  - Liver abscess: 0.3 %.
  - Gastrointestinal perforation (not including the latter deaths): 0.2 %, the vast majority have the history of abdominal surgery and cause gastrointestinal tract fixed adhesion.
  - Blood pneumothorax: 0.1 %.
  - Others: myoglobin hyperlipidemia, diaphragm perforation, acute renal failure, etc. can only be seen in very few cases [18, 20].

18.3.7.1 Mortality

RFA mortality rate was 0.3 %. About half of the deaths are due to serious complications from thermal injury of normal tissues and organs (such as the colon, the large bile duct branches, etc.).

18.3.8 Healing Effect

18.3.8.1 For the Lesion Cannot Be Removed

Currently, RFA treatment of unresectable colorectal cancer liver metastases has been widely used [36, 37]. However, the treatment effect reported in the literature is quite different; 1-, 2-, and 3-year survival rates were 80–93, 50–75, and 21–53 %. This is because there are (1) different inclusion criteria of different cases, (2) different RFA devices, and (3) different degrees of acceptance of other palliative treatments. Many scholars analyzed that the factors for RFA treatment fail to resect colorectal cancer and affect the liver metastasis' curative effect and provided the basis for judging the prognosis. Siperstein et al. [38] treated 234 cases of colorectal cancer liver metastases, in patients with lesions less than or equal to three; the median survival term was 27 months, significantly longer than 17 months in patients with the number of lesions greater than three ($P=0.0018$); The median survival term (26 months) for CEA less than 200 ng/ml compared with that for CEA above 200 ng/ml (16 months) was significantly long ($P=0.003$). Veltri [39] has shown that for RFA lesions after treatment, the maximum diameter less than or equal to 3 cm has the complete necrosis rate of 66.7 % and the maximum lesion diameter greater than 3 cm has the complete necrosis rate of 33.3 % ($P<0.0001$); the average survival term was 36.2 months and 23.2 months, respectively, with a significant difference. In short-term outcomes, the greater the tumor burden is, the more reduced the RFA's effects are. RFA in inoperable liver metastases of colorectal cancer also holds an important position in comprehensive treatment. Siperstein's study results suggested that [38] in RFA combined with systemic chemotherapy group, the median survival term was 28 months compared with

19 months of median survival term in chemotherapy group alone. Recent EORTC (European Organisation for Research and Treatment of Cancer)-CLOCC Trial (Chemotherapy + Local Ablation Versus Chemotherapy) phase II clinical studies have shown that in RFA combined with systemic chemotherapy group, NED progression was 16.8 months, better than 10 months in chemotherapy group alone [40].

18.3.8.2 For the Resectable Lesions

For resectable colorectal cancer liver metastases, whether RFA can be used instead of surgery is still controversial. RFA involves small damage, fewer complications, and shorter hospital stay, which are far beyond the surgery. But in terms of comparing the RFA and surgical treatment for resectable liver metastases of colorectal cancer, different scholars have different views. First is the higher local recurrence rate of RFA. Livraghi et al. [41] reported 88 cases receiving RFA in patients with resectable colorectal cancer by 33 months (median) of follow-up, with recurrence rate as high as 40 %. For patients with 29 months of follow-up after surgical resection, intrahepatic recurrence was only 3.8–10.4 % [42, 43]. Surgery can find the small lesions which preoperative imaging examinations missed, such as peritoneal and lymph node metastases, and then promptly change the treatment program [43, 44]. But the surgery will affect the body's immune function and reduce the immune response to tumor [45]. Both experimental and clinical studies showed that after RFA treatment, T-cells' response to tumor got enhanced [46, 47].

Currently, the vast majority of patients with liver metastases are resectable and receive surgery. There is still no prospective controlled study comparing RFA and surgical resection. Some researchers conducted retrospective studies, but the results are not consistent. Oshowo et al. [48] retrospectively analyzed 45 patients with single liver metastases, 20 patients who received surgical resection, and 25 patients who received RFA as the great vessels are near the lesion or there is high risk for surgery or there are other factors associated with extrahepatic metastases. For the surgery group and the RFA group, the median survival term was 41 months and 37 months, respectively; 3-year survival rates were 55.4 and 52.6 %, both having no significant difference. Abdalla et al. [49] compared three groups as surgical resection, RFA combined with surgical resection, and RFA alone. Except the tumor site, there was no significant difference in clinical conditions. The 4-year survival rates of surgery group, RFA combined with surgical group, and RFA group alone were 65 %, 35 %, and 22 %, respectively, with significant differences. Therefore, RFA has comparable efficacy for resectable liver metastases of colorectal cancer. Strict prospective randomized studies are still needed for further evidence [50].

References

1. Kelly RJ, Kemeny NE, Leonard GD. Current strategies using hepatic arterial infusion chemotherapy for the treatment of colorectal cancer. Clin Colorectal Cancer. 2005;5(3):166–74.
2. Pasetto LM, Merenda R, Pilati P, et al. Hepatic metastases of colorectal cancer: locoregional intra-arterial treatment. Anticancer Res. 2006;26(6C):4785–92.
3. Dizon DS, Schwartz J, Kemeny N. Chemotherapy: a focus on hepatic artery infusion for colorectal cancer liver metastases. Surg Oncol Clin N Am. 2008;17(4):759–71.
4. Tsutsumi S, Yamaguchi S, Tsuboi K, et al. Hepatic arterial infusion combined with oral UFT/UZEL systemic chemotherapy for unresectable liver metastasis of colorectal cancer. Hepatogastroenterology. 2008;55(85):1419–22.
5. Meta-Analysis Group in Cancer. Reappraisal of hepatic arterial infusion in the treatment of nonresectable liver metastases from colorectal cancer. J Natl Cancer Inst. 1996;88(5):252–8.
6. Harmantas A, Rotstein LE, Langer B. Regional versus systemic chemotherapy in the treatment of colorectal carcinoma metastatic to the liver. Is there a survival difference? Meta-analysis of the published literature. Cancer. 1996;78(8):1639–45.
7. Kemeny NE, Niedzwiecki D, Hollis DR, et al. Hepatic arterial infusion versus systemic therapy for hepatic metastases from colorectal cancer: a randomized trial of efficacy, quality of life, and molecular markers (CALGB 9481). J Clin Oncol. 2006;24(9):1395–403.
8. Dzodic R, Gomez-Abuin G, Rougier P, et al. Pharmacokinetic advantage of intra-arterial hepatic oxaliplatin administration: comparative results with

cisplatin using a rabbit VX2 tumor model. Anticancer Drugs. 2004;15(6):647–50.
9. van Riel JM, van Groeningen CJ, Kedde MA, et al. Continuous administration of irinotecan by hepatic arterial infusion: a phase I and pharmacokinetic study. Clin Cancer Res. 2002;8(2):405–12.
10. Falcone A, Ricci S, Brunetti I, et al. Phase III trial of infusional fluorouracil, leucovorin, oxaliplatin, and irinotecan (FOLFOXIRI) compared with infusional fluorouracil, leucovorin, and irinotecan (FOLFIRI) as first-line treatment for metastatic colorectal cancer: the Gruppo Oncologico Nord Ovest. J Clin Oncol. 2007;25(13):1670–6.
11. Kemeny MM, Adak S, Gray B, Macdonald JS, et al. Combined-modality treatment for resectable metastatic colorectal carcinoma to the liver: surgical resection of hepatic metastases in combination with continuous infusion of chemotherapy – an intergroup study. J Clin Oncol. 2002;20(6):1499–505.
12. Kemeny N, Huang Y, Cohen AM, et al. Hepatic arterial infusion of chemotherapy after resection of hepatic metastases from colorectal cancer. N Engl J Med. 1999;341(27):2039–48.
13. Ychou M, Viret F, Kramar A, et al. Tritherapy with fluorouracil/leucovorin, irinotecan and oxaliplatin (FOLFIRINOX): a phase II study in colorectal cancer patients with non-resectable liver metastases. Cancer Chemother Pharmacol. 2008;62(2):195–201.
14. Zelek L, Bugat R, Cherqui D, et al. Multimodal therapy with intravenous biweekly leucovorin, 5-fluorouracil and irinotecan combined with hepatic arterial infusion pirarubicin in non-resectable hepatic metastases from colorectal cancer (a European Association for Research in Oncology trial). Ann Oncol. 2003;14(10):1537–42.
15. Van Cutsem E, Köhne CH, Hitre E, et al. Cetuximab and chemotherapy as initial treatment for metastatic colorectal cancer. N Engl J Med. 2009;360(14):1408–17.
16. Kabbinavar FF, Hurwitz HI, Yi J, et al. Addition of bevacizumab to fluorouracil-based first-line treatment of metastatic colorectal cancer: pooled analysis of cohorts of older patients from two randomized clinical trials. J Clin Oncol. 2009;27(2):199–205.
17. Ricke J, Hildebrandt B, Miersch A, et al. Hepatic arterial port systems for treatment of liver metastases: factors affecting patency and adverse events. J Vasc Interv Radiol. 2004;15(8):825–33.
18. Iguchi T, Inaba Y, Arai Y, et al. Radiologic removal and replacement of port-catheter systems for hepatic arterial infusion chemotherapy. AJR Am J Roentgenol. 2006;187(6):1579–84.
19. Tono T, Ukei T, Masutani S. Management of hepatic arterial infusion port following prophylactic regional chemotherapy in patients who have undergone curative resection of colorectal liver metastases. Surg Today. 2003;33(9):679–83.
20. Sameshima S, Horikoshi H, Motegi K, et al. Outcomes of hepatic artery infusion therapy for hepatic metastases from colorectal carcinoma after radiological placement of infusion catheters. Eur J Surg Oncol. 2007;33(6):741–5.
21. Zanon C, Grosso M, Clara R, et al. Percutaneous implantation of arterial Port-a-cath via transsubclavian access. Anticancer Res. 1999;19: 5667–71.
22. Herrmann KA, Waggershauser T, Sittek H, et al. Liver intraarterial chemotherapy: use of the femoral artery for percutaneous implantation of catheter-port systems. Radiology. 2000;215:294–9.
23. Yamagami T, Terayama K, Yoshimatsu R, et al. Use of N-butyl cyanoacrylate in implantation of a port-catheter system for hepatic arterial infusion chemotherapy with the fixed-catheter-tip method: is it necessary? AJR Am J Roentgenol. 2008;191(5): 1523–9.
24. Hamada A, Yamakado K, Nakatsuka A, et al. Repeated hepatic arterial infusion chemotherapy using an implanted port system in patients with unresectable malignant liver neoplasms: significant factors affecting early hepatic arterial occlusion. Oncol Rep. 2003;10(6):1821–7.
25. Wood BJ, Ramkaransingh JR, Fojo T, et al. Percutaneous tumor ablation with radiofrequency. Cancer. 2002;94(2):443–51.
26. Nahum Goldberg S, Dupuy DE. Image-guided radiofrequency tumor ablation: challenges and opportunities—part I. J Vasc Interv Radiol. 2001;12(9):1021–32.
27. Rachbauer F, Mangat J, Bodner G, et al. Heat distribution and heat transport in bone during radiofrequency catheter ablation. Arch Orthop Trauma Surg. 2003;123(2–3):86–90.
28. Dupuy DE, Goldberg SN. Image-guided radiofrequency tumor ablation: challenges and opportunities—part II. J Vasc Interv Radiol. 2001;12(10): 1135–48.
29. Lau WY, Leung TW, Yu SC, et al. Percutaneous local ablative therapy for hepatocellular carcinoma: a review and look into the future. Ann Surg. 2003;237(2):171–9.
30. Allgaier HP, Galandi D, Zuber I, et al. Radiofrequency thermal ablation of hepatocellular carcinoma. Dig Dis. 2001;19(4):301–10.
31. Rossi S, Buscarini E, Garbagnati F, et al. Percutaneous treatment of small hepatic tumors by an expandable RF needle electrode. AJR Am J Roentgenol. 1998;170(4):1015–22.
32. Haemmerich D, Wright AW, Mahvi DM, et al. Hepatic bipolar radiofrequency ablation creates coagulation zones close to blood vessels: a finite element study. Med Biol Eng Comput. 2003;41(3):317–23.
33. Baere TD, Denys A, Wood BJ, et al. Radiofrequency liver ablation: experimental comparative study of water-cooled versus expandable systems. AJR Am J Roentgenol. 2001;176(1):187–92.
34. Kettenbach J, Kostler W, Rucklinger E, et al. Percutaneous saline-enhanced radiofrequency ablation of unresectable hepatic tumors: initial experience

in 26 patients. AJR Am J Roentgenol. 2003;180(6):1537–45.
35. Livraghi T, Solbiati L, Meloni MF, et al. Treatment of focal liver tumors with percutaneous radio-frequency ablation: complications encountered in a multicenter study. Radiology. 2003;226(2):441–51.
36. McGrane S, McSweeeney SE, Maher MM. Which patients will benefit from percutaneous radiofrequency ablation of colorectal cancer metastases ? A critically appraised topic. Abdom Imaging. 2008;33:48–53.
37. Solbiati L, Livrhagi T, Goldberg SN, et al. Percutaneous radiofrequency ablation of hepatic metastases from colorectal cancer: long-term results in 117 patients. Radiology. 2001;221:159–66.
38. Siperstein A, Berber E, Ballerm N, Rikesh T. Survival after radiofrequency ablation of colorectal metastases: 10-year-experience. Ann Surg. 2007;246: 559–67.
39. Veltri A, Sacchetto P, Tosetti I, et al. Radiofrequency ablation of colorectal liver metastases: small size favorably predicts technique effectiveness and survival. Cardiovasc Intervent Radiol. 2008;31:948–56.
40. Ruers T, van Coevorden F, Pierie JPJ, et al. Radiofrequency ablation (RFA) combined with chemotherapy for unresectable colorectal liver metastases (CRC LM): interim results of a randomized phase II study of the EORTC-NCRI CCSG-ALM Intergroup 40004 (CLOCC). J Clin Oncol. 2008, ASCO annual meeting proceedings; 2008, 26:4012.
41. Livraghi T, Solbiati L, Meloni F, et al. Percutaneous radiofrequency ablation of liver metastases in potential candidates for resection: the "test-of-time approach". Cancer. 2003;97:3027–35.
42. Kokudo N, Miki Y, Sugai S, et al. Genetic and histological assessment of surgical margins in resected liver metastases from colorectal carcinoma: minimum surgical margins for successful resection. Arch Surg. 2002;137:833–40.
43. Pawlik TM, Scoggins CR, Zorzi D, et al. Effect of surgical margin status on survival and site of recurrence after hepatic resection for colorectal metastases. Ann Surg. 2005;241:715–22.
44. Mulier S, Ni Y, Jamart J, et al. Local recurrence after hepatic radiofrequency coagulation: multivariate meta-analysis and review of contributing factors. Ann Surg. 2005;242:158–71.
45. Oka M, Hazama S, Suzuki M, et al. Depression of cytotoxicity of nonparenchymal cells in the liver after surgery. Surgery. 1994;116:877–82.
46. Wissniowski TT, Hansler J, Neureiter D, et al. Activation of tumor-specific T lymphocytes by radiofrequency ablation of the VX2 hepatoma in rabbits. Cancer Res. 2003;63:6496–500.
47. Zerbini A, Pilli M, Penna A, Pelosi G, et al. Radiofrequency thermal ablation of hepatocellular carcinoma liver nodules can activate and enhance tumor specific T cell responses. Cancer Res. 2006;66:1139–46.
48. Oshowo A, Gillams A, Harrison E, et al. Comparison of resection and radiofrequency ablation for treatment of solitary colorectal liver metastases. Br J Surg. 2003;90(10):1240–3.
49. Abdalla EK, Vauthey JN, Ellis LM, et al. Recurrence and outcomes following hepatic resection, radiofrequency ablation, and combined resection/ablation for colorectal liver metastases. Ann Surg. 2004;239(6):818–25.
50. Mulier S, Ni Y, Jamart J, et al. Radiofrequency ablation versus resection for respectable colorectal liver metastases: time for a randomized trial? Ann Surg Oncol. 2008;15:144–57.

19 Prevention of Postoperative Liver Metastasis by Preoperative Interventional Chemotherapy in Colorectal Cancer

Jianmin Xu, Yunshi Zhong, Dexiang Zhu, and Qingyang Feng

19.1 Incidence of Liver Metastasis After Radical Resection of Colorectal Cancer

A community-based research in Europe [1] was carried out in a community of one million population in France. During the period of 1976–2000, 3,655 cases of colorectal cancer patients were subject to the radical surgery, of which postoperative liver metastasis occurred in 467 cases of patients (12.8 %) within 5 years, and the rates of postoperative liver metastasis within 1 year, 3 years, and 5 years were 4.3 %, 12.0 %, and 16.5 %, respectively. The relation between different clinical pathological characteristics and postoperative liver metastasis was shown in Table 19.1. The multivariate analysis showed that the patients of women (OR 0.82, 95 % 0.68–0.99, $P=0.036$), earlier staging of TNM (stage II OR 3.28, 95% CI 2.24–4.82, $P<0.001$; stage III OR 8.30, 95 % CI 5.67–12.14, $P<0.001$), and fungiform tumors (ulcer fungiform or ulcer infiltration type of patients, OR 1.35, 95 % CI 1.06–1.71, $P=0.012$) have a lower incidence of postoperative liver metastasis.

J. Xu (✉) • Y. Zhong • D. Zhu
Q. Feng
Zhongshan Hospital, Fudan University,
180 fengling road, Xuhui district,
Shanghai 200032, China
e-mail: xu.jianmin@zs-hopital.sh.cn;
xujmin@aliyun.com

19.2 Prevention of Postoperative Liver Metastasis of Colorectal Cancer by Neoadjuvant Therapy (Preoperative Interventional Chemotherapy)

19.2.1 Advantages of Neoadjuvant Therapy

The neoadjuvant chemotherapy is a systematic chemotherapy applied for the treatment of cancer, before radical surgery or radiotherapy, also known as preoperative chemotherapy. Since 1982, Frei firstly proposed the concept of neoadjuvant chemotherapy, and thereafter its clinic effect and value were recognized gradually. According to the theory of first-order kinetics of Skipper [2], administration of a certain amount of anticancer drugs can only kill a certain percentage of cancer cells, which is not associated with the number of cancer cells existing in the treatment, that is, it is not a fixed number of cells, which provided the basis for the preoperative chemotherapy. Therefore, administration of sufficient large dose of anticancer drugs within the tolerance range of the patients is allowed. The proportion of the proliferating cells among the tumor cell is called growth fraction (GF). During the early stage, there are fewer tumor cells, GF is greater, and the time of growth is short, relatively sensitive to the cell-cycle-specific drugs. And in the advanced tumor, the number of the

X. Qin et al. (eds.), *Multidisciplinary Management of Liver Metastases in Colorectal Cancer*,
DOI 10.1007/978-94-017-7755-1_19

Table 19.1 Relation between different clinicopathological features and postoperative delayed liver metastasis

	Number of cases	First year (%)	Third year (%)	Fifth year (%)	P
All patients	3,655	4.3	12.0	14.5	
Gender					0.0253
Male	1,994	4.8	13.8	16.5	
Female	1,661	4.7	11.4	13.7	
Age					0.0281
<75	2,152	4.4	13.2	15.7	
≥75	1,501	4.1	10.1	12.5	
Tumor site					NS
Right colon	953	4.7	10.4	11.6	
Left colon	1,290	4.6	13.0	16.6	
Site of intersection of the rectum and sigmoid colon	611	3.8	12.1	14.5	
Rectal ampullas	798	3.6	12.2	14.3	
Diagnosis time					0.0010
1976–1980	510	5.0	16.7	19.8	
1981–1985	663	5.3	13.3	15.7	
1986–1990	815	5.0	12.8	15.9	
1991–1995	779	3.8	9.5	11.2	
1996–2000	888	2.9	10.0	12.2	
Staging					<0.0001
I	1,058	0.1	2.2	3.7	
II	1,589	3.7	10.6	13.3	
III	1,008	9.9	26.5	30.4	
General type					
Fungiform	1,303	1.8	6.0	8.0	<0.0001
Ulcer fungiform or ulcer infiltration type	2,263	5.9	15.9	18.7	
Tumor size					<0.0001
<3 cm	599	1.0	4.8	6.9	
3–6 cm	2,434	5.1	14.1	16.5	
≥6 cm	555	4.8	12.5	15.7	

tumor cells increases, GF decreases, and the time of growth extends, which reduces the sensitivity to the cell-cycle-specific drugs, but at this time, the use of a large dose of cell-cycle-specific drugs may reduce the volume of the tumor cells and promote the increase of the GF, and the sensitivity of the cell-cycle-specific drugs will increase. Therefore, before resection of primary foci of the tumor, administration of chemotherapy drugs is sensitive and effective to the treatment of small cancer foci; besides, it also has killing effect on the primary focus. Therefore, theoretically the earlier the chemotherapy is given, the less the drug-resistant cell strains. Moreover, many animal model tests showed that after the tumor resection, the stimulating factors to promote the cancer cell growth would be induced to accelerate the metastasis focus growth, inducing the cancer cells to form the clones with the anti-chemotherapy drug characteristics. In addition, through the preoperative chemotherapy, the number of the tumor cells reduces, thus inhibiting the production of such growth-stimulating factor and slowing down the growth of the metastasis foci. Compared with postoperative chemotherapy, the advantages of the neoadjuvant chemotherapy are as follows:

1. Prevent the change of the postoperative tumor blood supply from affecting the chemotherapeutic effect. After the surgery, the vascularity of the primary lesions is changed, and the scar and the changed vascularity cannot achieve an effective concentration of residual lesions after chemotherapy. But preoperative chemotherapy has no such problems. Schuhmacher CP et al. discovered that [3] the patients who have complete remission from the neoadjuvant chemotherapy have a significant improvement on the survival rate. And it is believed that the preoperative chemotherapy can realize the cytotoxic drugs to access to the tumor through the complete tumor blood vessels, thus avoiding the reduction of the concentration of chemotherapeutic drugs in the residual tumor tissues due to the destruction of tumor blood vessels after surgery.
2. Control and kill the small clinical or subclinical metastases and reduce the postoperative recurrence and metastasis [3].
3. Most of the preoperative patients can tolerate the higher doses of chemotherapeutic drugs, and the acute toxicity reactions can be reduced.
4. Reduce the clinical staging, shrink the primary focus, and increase the surgery opportunity.
5. The observation of the pathological results of the surgical specimens can help to understand the sensitivity of the tumor on the chemotherapeutic drugs and help the selection of the postoperative chemotherapy drugs.
6. Rule out the patients that are not suitable for surgery. Some tumors of poor biological actions advance rapidly and during the chemotherapy period, the wide local infiltration and remote metastasis may occur. For such patients, even if surgical resections are conducted, they can relapse rapidly.

For the patients of non-metastases of colorectal cancer, whether or not they should accept the neoadjuvant chemotherapy, the "guidelines of diagnosis and comprehensive treatment of liver metastases of colorectal cancer draft" (2009 edition) specifies that "generally, the stage III preoperative patients, if they have no bleeding, obstruction or perforation, etc., can accept the neoadjuvant chemotherapy, with the regimens of FOLFOX, capecitabine alone or 5-FU/LV and the recommended time is 1–3 months before the surgery" [4, 5].

However, there are no EBM evidences for the patients of non-metastases of colorectal cancer for whether or not to accept the neoadjuvant chemotherapy (intravenous chemotherapy). But as recommended by the NCCN Guidelines of Colon Cancer in 2010, these patients are not applicable to accept the neoadjuvant chemotherapy (intravenous chemotherapy), but directly accept the surgery.

Since the higher recurrence rate and demanding for continuing the physiological functions after radical resection of rectal cancer, the neoadjuvant therapy of rectal cancer mainly focuses on the combined therapy of preoperative local radiotherapy and chemotherapy, to enhance the R0 operative resection rate and reduce the local recurrence rate. But there is no great significance of improving the patients' overall survival [6–9].

19.3 Local Artery Infusion Chemotherapy (Interventional Chemotherapy) Can Enhance the Local Drug Concentration, and the Drugs Flowing Back to the Liver Can Reduce the Incidence of Liver Metastasis

How to further improve the efficacy and targeting of neoadjuvant chemotherapy is an urgent issue to be solved. The traditional intravenous injection was applied earlier, easy to do but with great side effect, and the effective concentration cannot be met in the local part of the tumor and easy to produce drug resistance. Therefore, people try to find more effective chemotherapy drugs and better chemotherapy regimen to enhance the effect of the intravenous chemotherapy. With the progress of the interventional radiology techniques, the chemotherapy drugs can be delivered to the major feeding arteries of the primary tumor or tumor metastases directly through the selective arterial cannula, that is, preoperative interventional chemotherapy, which is featured by strong selection, centralized drug administration, and high concentration of drug in the foci as well as small systematic toxicity reaction. Clinically, the femoral artery puncture (Seldinger method) is generally adopted for the preoperative intervention. The chemotherapy drugs are injected to the major feeding arteries through the superselective arterial catheterization. For patients whose tumor's nutrition blood vessels cannot be judged directly, the tumor staining method can be adopted to judge the sources of the major blood supply and then superselective arterial catheterization is adopted. In addition, intraperitoneal chemotherapy is a highly selective local drug treatment method, with significant pharmacokinetic advantages compared with the venous chemotherapy. The high concentration of chemotherapy drugs in the enterocoelia is absorbed through the peritoneum, after through the portal vein system and the retroperitoneal lymphatic system, that involves the blood circulation, which consists of the blood dissemination and lymphatic metastasis paths of the digestive tumors. The preoperative intraperitoneal chemotherapy can improve the concentration and the action time of the chemotherapy drugs of the peritoneum, tumor tissue, and the related lymph nodes, which can help to reduce the intraoperative iatrogenic cancer cell dissemination, eliminate the subclinical or small peritoneal metastases, and has better curative effect of control over the postoperative peritoneal recurrence, lymph node metastasis, and reduction of liver metastasis [10].

Compared with traditional intravenous chemotherapy drug application, the intervention chemotherapy can realize the onetime administration of drugs through the major nutrition artery of the tumors, and over two thirds of the drugs will produce effect in the local tumors. The pharmacokinetic studies have shown that there is obvious dose-effect relationship between the drugs and the toxicity of tumor cells, that is, concentration dependence. When the local concentration of the chemotherapeutic drugs increases by one time, the killing effect on the tumor cells can be increased by ten times. Therefore, under the same drug doses, the killing effect of the intervention chemotherapy on tumor cells can be increased significantly. In addition, the arterial injection of chemotherapy drugs can enter the systemic circulation again, which have certain effect on the systematic clinical or subclinical metastases, and flow back to the tumor site through the venous return to realize the secondary chemotherapy [11]. Studies have shown that after intervention chemotherapy, the tumor necrosis foci are mainly at the tumor center surrounding the blood vessels, with the necrotic rate up to 80 %, medium to severe necrosis rate of 60 %, while after the systematic intravenous injection of drugs, the tumor necrosis is mainly located at the shallow layer of the tumor with the necrosis rate of about 40 %, mostly mild to moderate necrosis. After the intervention chemotherapy, varying degree of vascular inflammation and microvascular thrombosis will occur for the tumor-feeding vessels, which also delayed the growth of tumors to a certain degree [12].

In addition, due to the particularity of colorectal blood supply, the arterial infusion of chemotherapy drugs can flow back to the liver through the portal vein system, which also has an "infusion chemotherapy" effect on the micrometastasis in the liver.

19.3.1 Reasons for the Hepatic Artery Administration of Drugs

The injection of the chemotherapy drugs in the hepatic artery for preoperative interventional therapy is mainly based on the following: (1) the multiplication rate of the tumors – for the patients with delayed liver metastasis after the radical operation, their livers have the "small metastasis" that cannot be discovered through the existing imaging techniques before operation; after surgical removal of primary foci, the inhibited factor of blood vessels are removed, which activates the growth of the dormant micrometastatic tumor and causes the occurrence of distant metastasis [13, 14]; (2) the blood supply of the micrometastasis with the diameter of 0.5–3 mm in the liver is mainly from the hepatic artery, and this micrometastasis is just the target of preoperative intervention therapy [15].

19.3.2 Why Choose the Stage III Colorectal Cancer Patients

Sadahiro from the University of Tokyo firstly reported the randomized controlled trial of preoperative preventative hepatic artery intervention therapy of colorectal cancer in 2004. There were 305 cases of stage II and stage III colorectal cancer patients involved in this study, and no preoperative liver metastasis has been discovered for the patients. The 305 patients were divided into two groups randomly: 119 cases of preoperative hepatic artery intervention group (3-week perioperative 5-FU continuous observation of hepatic artery chemotherapy) and 186 cases of surgery alone group. The results showed that, for the stage III patients, the preoperative intervention therapy can reduce the postoperative recurrence rate by 60 % (95 % CI 0.24–0.64; $P=0.0002$), mortality rate 63 % (95 % CI 0.21–0.67; $P=0.0009$), and liver metastasis rate 62 % (95 % CI 0.22–0.66; $P=0.0005$), but no effect for the metastasis of other organs. There is no curative effect for the stage II patients [16].

The General Surgery Department, Zhongshan Hospital affiliated to Fudan University firstly carried out the clinical study of prophylactic hepatic and regional arterial infusion chemotherapy (PHRAIC) in China and obtained the preliminary results. The PHRAIC group of patients were firstly subject to the prophylactic hepatic and regional arterial infusion chemotherapy: infusion of the fluorodeoxyuridine 500 mg, MMC 10 mg, and oxaliplatin 50 mg, respectively, to the hepatic artery and the major feeding arteries of the tumor; after 7 days of chemotherapy, the patients accepted the radical surgery of colorectal cancer; the control group of patients were directly accepted of the radical resection of colorectal cancer. The results showed that in stage III patients, PHRAIC group was significantly better than the control group in 3-year liver metastasis rate (12.7 % vs. 28.3 %, $P=0.001$), 3-year tumor-free survival rate (82.3 % vs. 58.7 %, $P=0.0096$), overall survival rate (87.7 % vs. 75.7 %, $P=0.002$), and median survival time (40.1 vs. 36.3 months, $P=0.03$). The preoperative intervention would not increase the incidence of the postoperative complications. These clinical results were published in Annals of Surgery in 2007 (IF=7.678) [17]. For the patients of stage II, there was no significant difference between the two groups.

19.4 Application of Neoadjuvant Regional Infusion Chemotherapy (Intervention Therapy) in the Stage III Colorectal Cancer

19.4.1 Method

Choose the regimen of fluorodeoxyuridine (FUDR) + oxaliplatin + MMC of short half-life and high proportion of first dose after intervention infusion (>90 %).

19.4.1.1 Dose

Oxaliplatin	75 mg/m^2
FUDR	650 mg/m^2
MMC	8 mg/m^2

19.4.1.2 Method

The femoral artery puncture (Seldinger method) is adopted for the preoperative intervention. The half dose of chemotherapy drug (FUDR + MMC + oxaliplatin) is injected to the major feeding arteries through the superselective arterial catheterization. And then the other half (FUDR + MMC + oxaliplatin) is injected from the superselective artery to the hepatic artery (Fig. 19.1). After the surgery, the puncture site should be compressed for 12 h, and the antibiotics, acid inhibition, and liver protection infusion should be carried out.

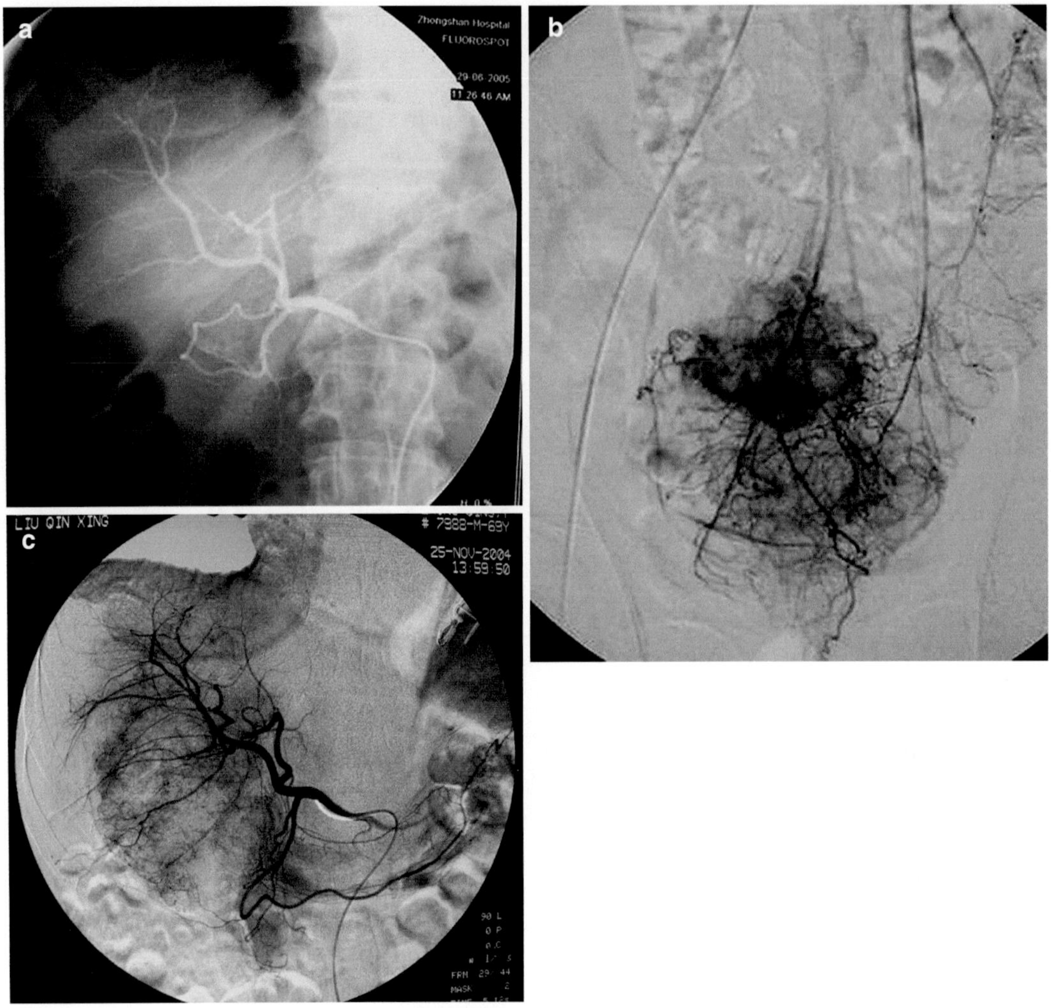

Fig. 19.1 Preoperative interventional chemotherapy. (**a**) Hepatic artery infusion chemotherapy; (**b**) rectal arterial infusion chemotherapy; (**c**) hepatic flexure cancer infusion chemotherapy

The oxaliplatin must be dissolved in 150–200 ml of 5 % glucose solution; FUDR and mitomycin must be dissolved in 150–200 ml of normal saline; the injection duration of each chemotherapy drug should not be less than 15 min.

The design of the addition of platinum drugs in the neoadjuvant chemotherapy is based on the platinum drugs study. In 2004, Professor De Gramont [18] reported the 3-year follow-up results of MOSAIC study on the 2004 ASCO Conference; 2,246 stage II (40 %) or stage III (60 %) of postoperative colon cancer patients after radical surgery from 148 centers and 20 countries were enrolled and randomly divided into two groups. The patients would be subject to 5-FU/LV or FOLFOX4 chemotherapy every 2 weeks, 12 cycles in total. For the FOLFOX4 group, the 3-year disease-free survival (DFS) was significantly superior to that of the 5-FU/LV group (78.2 % vs. 72.9 %, HR 0.77, 95 % CI 0.65–0.90), but no significant difference in overall survival rate. Professor De Gramont reported the 6-year follow-up results of MOSAIC study in the 2007 conference [19]: the stage III colon cancer patients were subject to the chemotherapy with FOLFOX4; the 6-year overall survival rate was 72.9 %, while in the 5-FU/LV group, the 6-year overall survival rate was 68.3 %

(HR 0.80, 95 % CI 0.66–0.98), i.e., for the stage III colorectal cancer patients, after receiving the FOLFOX4 chemotherapy after radical surgery, the relative risk of mortality can be dropped by 20 %. For the stage II patients, there is no significant difference of the FOLFOX4 for the DFS or overall survival rate.

19.4.2 Selection of Surgery Time After Intervention

The selection of surgery time after intervention chemotherapy depends on the onset time of chemotherapy drugs. If the time is too short (<4 days), the cytotoxicity of chemotherapy drugs is not complete yet. If the time is too long (>10 days), the necrotic tumor will regenerate the neovasculature and tumor regeneration, and the proliferating cell nuclear antigen (PCNA) will be higher than that before treatment. Five to 9 days after the intervention therapy, the tumor necrosis is most significant, and the vascular microembolization is most significant, suitable for surgery [20, 21].

19.4.3 Safety Evaluation of Preoperative Intervention

The preoperative intervention chemotherapy has small trauma, which can be used in the patients as long as the patients have no serious cardiopulmonary dysfunction and no serious bleeding tendency with normal liver functions. The main toxic reactions are gastrointestinal reactions; a few patients may have slight elevation of the total bilirubin, alanine aminotransferase, or creatinine. In addition, some patients have fever, mostly low fever, which will generally occur 3 days after the intervention surgery, possibly resulted from the endogenous pyrogen generated from possible tumor necrosis, particularly obvious for the patients who undergo embolization of liver metastasis. In addition, the vascular injury can be caused by interventional operation. To prevent the complications, repeating operations in the artery should be avoided for intervention chemotherapy; to avoid the vascular spasm and intimal injury, the chemotherapy drugs should be diluted and injected slowly; after treatment, appropriately use some vasodilators.

After the preoperative intervention, the patients' hematopoietic mechanism and liver functions are affected. The postoperative blood system and liver function abnormality evaluation indicators refer to the evaluation criteria of NCI [22]. The grading is based on the serious item of various indicators.

19.4.3.1 Impact of Preoperative Intervention on the Liver Functions

There are 256 cases in the intervention group and 253 cases in the control group enrolled in the study of Zhongshan Hospital affiliated to Fudan University. Before enrollment, the various indicators of liver functions of the two groups of patients (total bilirubin (TB), conjugated bilirubin (CB), alanine aminotransferase (ALT), aspartate transaminase (AST), alkaline phosphatase (ALP), and γ-glutamyl GGT (γ-GT)) have no significant statistical difference.

In the intervention group, 7 days after the intervention (before surgery), the proportions of the abnormal liver function of grade 0, grades I–II, grade III, and grade IV were, respectively, 54.3 % (139/256), 42.6 % (109/256), 3.1 % (8/256), and 0, which could be improved through drug treatment, and none of the cases were affected thereby.

The grading of 7-day postoperative abnormal liver functions of the intervention group and the control groups, respectively, was shown in Fig. 19.2. The proportion of grade I–III abnormal liver function in the intervention group was as high as 29.9 % (77/256), significantly higher than 11.9 % (31/253) of the control group ($\chi^2=5.21$, $P<0.05$).

19.4.3.2 Impact of the Preoperative Intervention on the Hematopoietic Functions

Before enrollment, there was no significant difference of the level of the blood routine test (including hemoglobin (Hgb), white blood cell (WBC), and platelets (Plt)) between the two groups.

Leukopenia The proportion of grades 0, I–II, III, and IV of leukopenia 7 days after intervention (before surgery) in the intervention group were, respectively, 56.2 % (144/256), 38.3 % (98/256), 5.5 % (14/256), and 0. Their clinical symptoms could be improved through medication, and none of the cases thereby were affected for the surgery. The grading of leukopenia in the 7 days after surgery of the intervention group and the control group was, respectively, shown in Fig. 19.2. In the intervention group, the grade I–II leukopenia was 24.5 % (63/256), significantly higher than 5.7 % (14/253) of the control group ($\chi^2=4.17$, $P<0.05$).

Anemia The proportion of grades 0, I–II, III, and IV of anemia 7 days after intervention (before surgery) in the intervention group was, respectively, 14.5 % (37/256), 78.1 % (200/256), 7.4 % (19/256), and 0. Their clinical symptoms could be improved through medication, and none of the cases thereby was affected for the surgery. The proportions of grades 0, I–II, III, and IV of anemia 7 days after surgery of the intervention group and the control group were, respectively, 12.1 % (31/256), 13.4 % (34/253), 65.2 % (167/256), 61.7 % (156/253), 22.7 % (58/256), 24.9 % (63/253), and 0. There was no significant statistical difference.

Thrombocytopenia The proportions of grades 0, I–II, III, and IV of thrombocytopenia 7 days after intervention (before surgery) in the intervention group were, respectively, 80.5 % (206/256), 12.9 % (33/256), 6.6 % (17/256), and 0. Their clinical symptoms can be improved through medication, and none of the cases thereby were affected for the surgery. The grading of thrombocytopenia in the 7 days after surgery of the intervention group and the control group was, respectively, shown in Fig. 19.2. In the intervention group, the grade I–II thrombocytopenia was 16.9 % (43/256), significantly higher than 3.8 % (10/253) of the control group ($\chi^2=6.05$, $P<0.05$).

19.4.3.3 Postoperative Complications and Average Length of Stay

The incidences of postoperative complications in the intervention group and the control group were, respectively, 9.8 % (25/256) and 8.3 % (21/253), and there was no significant statistical difference ($\chi^2=1.86$, $P>0.05$). The ratio of cases of the poor wound healing, lung infection, anastomotic fistula, and cardiac complications in the intervention group and the control group was, respectively, 12:10, 5:6, 2:1, and 6:4.

The total average length of stay in the intervention group was 14.6 ± 2.5 days and that of the control group was 7.6 ± 1.8 days ($\chi^2=4.05$, $P<0.05$). The length of stay after surgery in the PHRAIC group was 7.9 ± 3.1 days, compared with that of the control group (6.5 ± 1.9 days); there was no statistical difference ($\chi^2=3.01$, $P>0.05$).

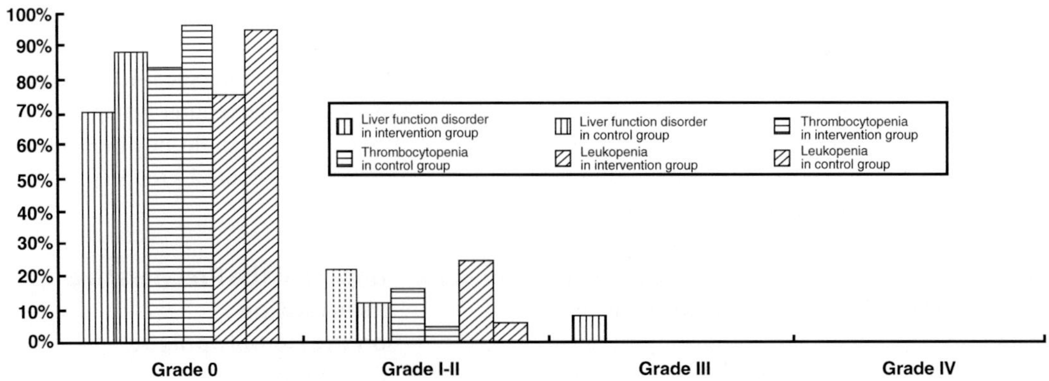

Fig. 19.2 Comparison of the postoperative liver function, blood routine test, and platelet abnormalities of the seventh day between the intervention group and the control group

19.4.4 Impact of Preoperative Intervention Chemotherapy on the Tumor Proliferation and Apoptosis

The interventional chemotherapy may function through the following four aspects:

1. Induction of the apoptosis of tumor cells: after interventional therapy, the apoptosis is a continuous process, at the peak 24 h after treatment. With the increase of apoptotic cells, tumor growth gradually slows down.
2. Inhibition of cell proliferation: in the period of 7–10 days after the intervention chemotherapy, it has the most significant cell proliferation inhibition effect.
3. Promotion of the pathological necrosis of tumors: the joint action of chemotherapy drug itself, tumor cell apoptosis, and microembolism of feeding blood vessels.
4. Inhibition of tumor angiogenesis: after intervention chemotherapy, the microvessel count, vascular endothelial growth factor (VEGF), and platelet-derived growth factor expression in endothelial cells in the tumor cells were significantly decreased [21, 23–27].

Tumor Necrosis The individual pathologists randomly selected five high-power microscope fields of vision to evaluate the percentage of the necrosis, which were divided into the following five grades according to the average value: 0 (0–20 %), + (21–40 %), ++ (41–60 %), +++ (61–80 %), and ++++ (81–100 %).

There was no statistical difference for the percentage of the degree of necrosis of the pathological specimens between the control group and the PHRAIC group before intervention ($P>0.05$). In the PHRAIC group, after intervention, the +++ in the pathological specimens accounted for 22.7 %, and ++++ accounted for 13.5 %, compared with the preoperative +++ (3.1 %) and ++++ (0 %); there was no statistical difference ($P<0.05$, Table 19.2, Fig. 19.3).

Assessment of Positive Rates of Ki67, P16, Bax, bcl-2, and Survivin The positive rate of

Table 19.2 Impact of PHRAIC on the tumor necrosis degree

	0	+	++	+++	++++
Control group (253)	52.2 % (132)	26.5 % (67)	21.3 % (54)	0 (0)	0 (0)
Before intervention of PHRAIC group (256)	47.6 % (122)	30.5 % (78)	18.8 % (48)	3.1 % (8)	0 (0)
After intervention	21.1 % (54)	27.0 % (69)	15.6 % (40)	22.7 % (58)	13.5 % (35)

There was no statistical difference of the degree of necrosis of the preoperative pathological specimens between the control group and the PHRAIC group ($P>0.05$)

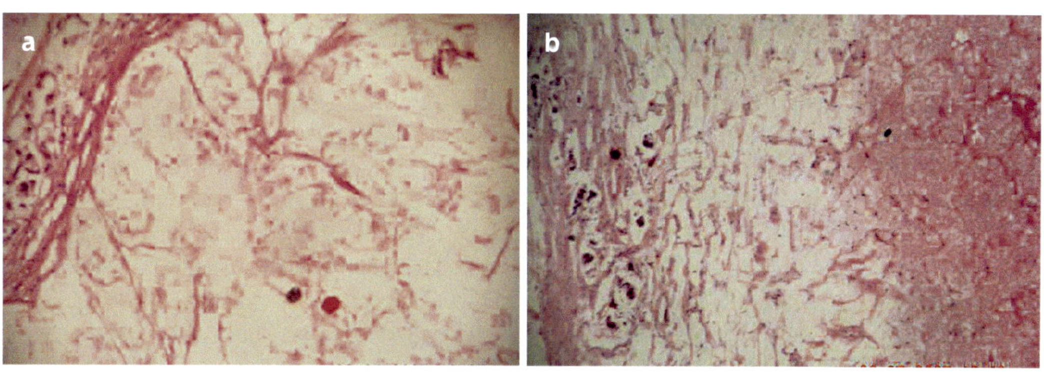

Fig. 19.3 Surgery of 7 days after the preoperative intervention chemotherapy. Large area of necrosis of primary tumor (**a**) and large area of necrosis of lymph node metastasis (**b**)

Ki67 was expressed by the labeling index, i.e., the average value of percentages of five high magnification views of positive cells.

The positive rates of P16, Bax, bcl-2, and survivin were used to evaluate the percentage and staining degree of the positive cells and scored by the percentage of the positive cells among the tumor cells – <5 %, 0; 5–25 %, 1; 26–50 %, 2; 51–75 %, 3; and >75 %, 4 – and then scored according to the staining degree of the positive cells, negative 0, light yellow 1, brown yellow 2, and brown 3, and finally the scores of both were added. The score was evaluated for five times, and the final result was the average value. <2, negative (−); 2–3, weakly positive (+); 4–5, moderately positive (++); and 6–7, strongly positive (+++), of which −~+ as the low expression and ++~+++ as the overexpression.

Impact of PHRAIC on Tumor Proliferation (Ki67) The Ki67 labeling index of pathological specimens before intervention of the control group and the PHRAIC group was, respectively, 52.6±21.5 and 48.6±17.1 (P>0.05). The Ki67 labeling index of pathological specimens after intervention of the PHRAIC group was 38.4±13.3, compared with that before intervention, with significant statistical difference (P<0.05).

Impact of PHRAIC on Tumor Apoptosis (Bax, P16, bcl-2, and Survivin) The overexpression rates of P16 before and after intervention in the control group and the PHRAIC group, respectively, were 47.4 %, 41.4 %, and 42.6 % (P>0.05). The overexpression rates of BAX, bcl-2, and survivin in the pathological specimens before intervention in the control group and the PHRAIC group, respectively, were 52.6 % and 48.0 %, 72.0 % and 75.0 %, and 55.3 % and 52.0 % (P>0.05); the overexpression rates of BAX, bcl-2, and survivin in the pathological specimens after intervention in the PHRAIC group were, respectively, 77.0 %, 43.0 %, and 31.6 %, compared with that before intervention; there was statistically significant difference (P<0.05).

Judgment of the Apoptosis Index The positive substance is located in the nucleus, stained yellow, and scattered in the cytoplasm. Five high-power microscope fields of visions were randomly selected, and the average value of the percentage of the positive cells among the total gland cells is the apoptosis index. The apoptosis rates of the pathological specimens before intervention for the control group and the PHRAIC group were, respectively, 5.2±3.9 % and 4.3±2.2 % (P>0.05). The apoptosis rate of the pathological specimens before intervention for the PHRAIC group was 16.7±6.4 %, compared with that before intervention; there was no statistical difference (P<0.05). The ratios of G0–G1, S, G2-M in the pathological specimens of the control group were, respectively, 38.2±15.1 %, 42.2±9.3 %, and 19.6±5.1 %, compared with the ratios of G0–G1 (35.1±12.1 %), S (42.1±11.2 %), G2-M (21.8±9.7 %), with no statistical difference (P>0.05). In the PHRAIC group, the ratio of the S stage of the pathological specimens after invention was 21.8±10.7 %, significantly lower than that before intervention (P<0.05); the ratio of G0–G1 was 57.1±18.1 %, higher than that before intervention (P<0.05).

19.4.5 Influence of Preoperative Intervention on the Survival of Patients

19.4.5.1 Postoperative Liver Metastasis and Other Distant Metastases

Among the patients in the PHRAIC group, there were 36 cases of liver metastasis, 7 cases of lung metastasis, 2 cases of bone metastasis, and 7 cases of local recurrence, while in the control group, there were 50 cases of liver metastasis, 7 cases of lung metastasis, 5 cases of bone metastasis, 6 cases of local recurrence, and 3 cases of supraclavicular lymph node metastasis; there was statistical difference between them (P<0.01).

The 3-year liver metastasis rates in the PHRAIC group and the control group were, respectively, 10.0 % and 19.2 % (Fig. 19.4), and the relative risk was 0.52 (95 % CI 0.42–0.67,

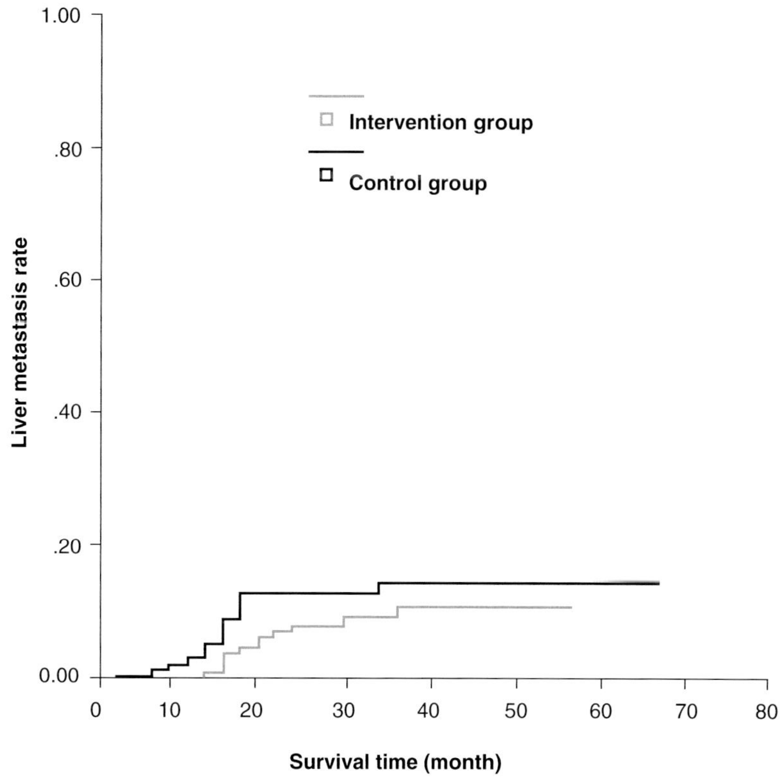

Fig. 19.4 The postoperative 3-year liver metastasis rate of stage II and stage III patients ($P=0.07$)

$P=0.001$), that is, the preoperative PHRAIC therapy could reduce the risk of postoperative liver metastasis by 48 %. Further analysis showed that the postoperative liver metastasis rate has no significant difference among the stage II patients ($P>0.05$, Fig. 19.5), but has significant difference among the stage III patients ($P<0.01$, Fig. 19.6). The 3-year liver metastasis rates in the PHRAIC group and the control group were 12.7 % and 28.3 %, respectively, and the relative risk was 0.45 (95% CI 0.38–0.57, $P=0.001$), that is, the preoperative PHRAIC treatment for the stage III patients could reduce the risk of postoperative liver metastasis by 55 %, as shown in Table 19.3.

19.4.5.2 Disease-Free Survival

The disease-free survival is defined as no postoperative metastasis or recurrence. The 3-year disease-free survival rates of the stage II patients in the PHRAIC group and the control group were, respectively, 89.4 % and 84.5 % ($P>0.05$), and the 3-year disease-free survival rates of the stage III patients in the PHRAIC group and the control group were, respectively, 82.5 % and 61.2 % ($P<0.05$); the relative risk was 0.44 (95 % CI 0.23–0.67, $P=0.03$); that is, the preoperative PHRAIC treatment of stage III patients can reduce the risks of postoperative metastasis and recurrence by 56 % (Figs. 19.7, 19.8, and 19.9).

19.4.5.3 Overall Survival Rate

The overall 3-year survival rates of the stage II patients in the PHRAIC group and the control group were, respectively, 92.0 % and 90.0 % ($P>0.05$), while the overall 3-year survival rates of the stage III patients in the PHRAIC group were, respectively, 87.7 % and 75.7 % ($P<0.05$, Figs. 19.10, 19.11, and 19.12).

19.5 Prospect

In 2008, funded by the Clinical Key Subject Program of the Ministry of Health (2007–2009), the Zhongshan Hospital affiliated to Fudan

Fig. 19.5 The postoperative 3-year liver metastasis rate of stage II patients ($P=0.21$)

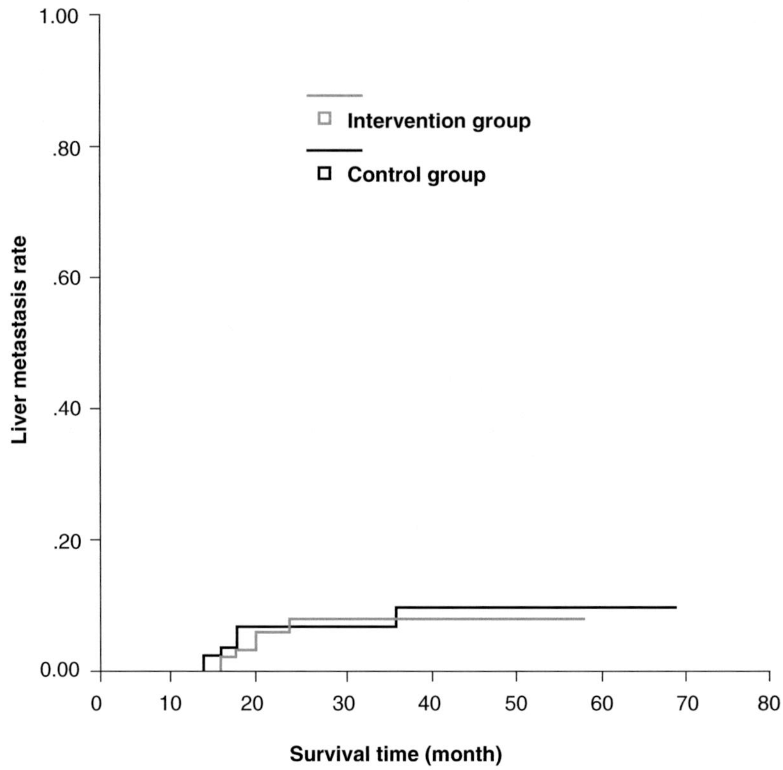

Fig. 19.6 The postoperative 3-year liver metastasis rate of stage III patients ($P=0.04$)

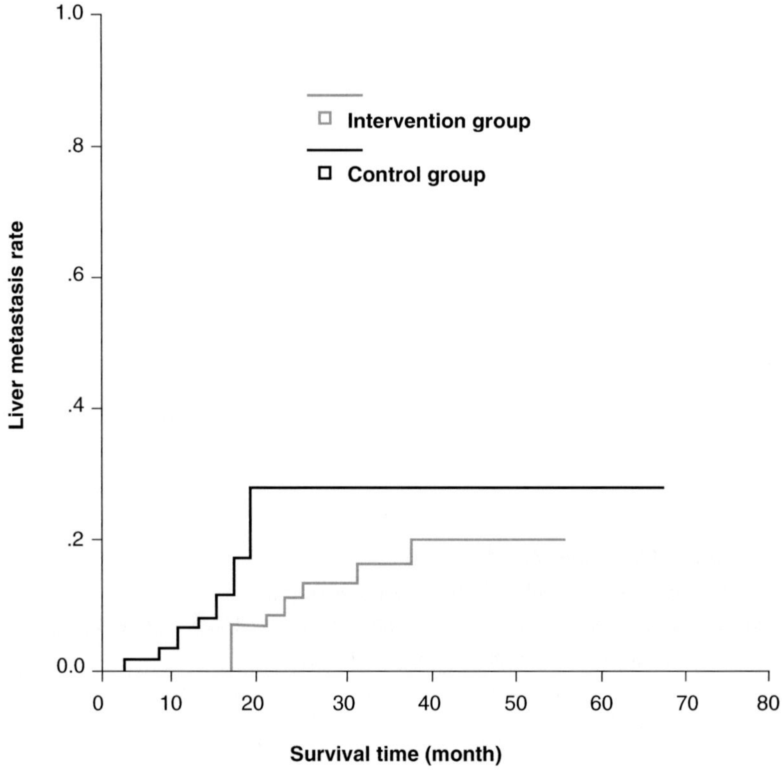

Table 19.3 Influence of PHRAIC on survival

	Stage II		Stage III	
	Intervention group	Control group	Intervention group	Control group
Total 5-year survival rate	91.3 %	89.6 %	81.0 %	60.4 %
Intermediate survival term (months)	63	58	45	40
Metastasis and recurrence rate	15.6 % (17)	14.5 % (15)	26.3 % (39)	38.0 % (57)
Liver	7.4 % (8)	8.7 % (9)	18.9 % (28)	27.3 % (41)
Lung	2.8 % (3)	1.9 % (2)	2.7 % (4)	3.3 % (5)
Bone	1.8 % (2)	1.0 % (1)	0 % (0)	2.7 % (4)
Local recurrence	1.8 % (2)	1.0 % (1)	3.4 % (5)	3.3 % (5)
Other	1.8 % (2)	1.9 % (2)	1.3 % (2)	1.4 % (2)

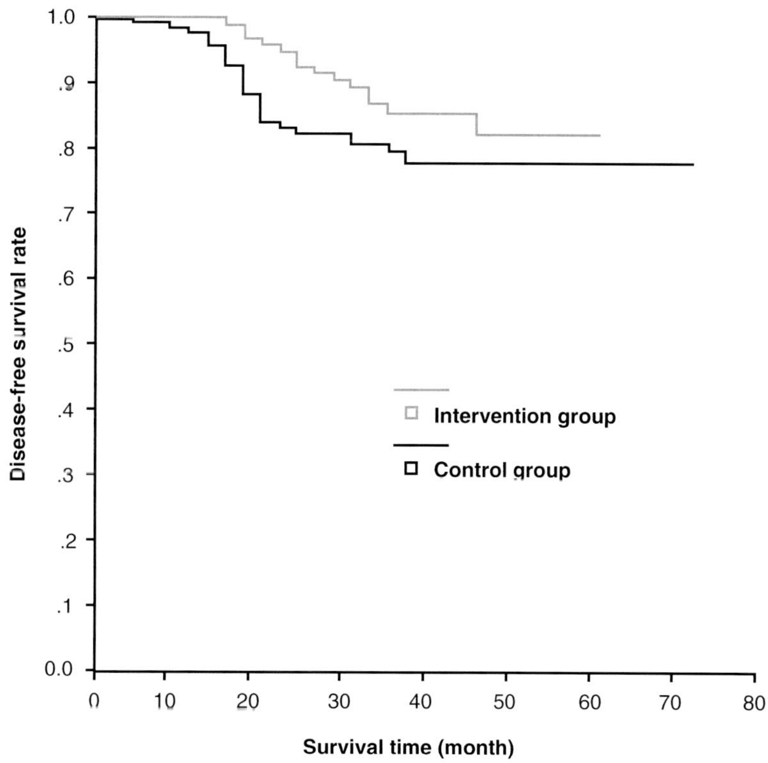

Fig. 19.7 Disease-free survival rate of stage II and stage III patients ($P=0.08$)

University (Party A), as the head, with the Ruijin Hospital affiliated to Jiaotong University, the Ninth People's Hospital affiliated to Jiaotong University, Second Hospital affiliated to Zhejiang Medical University, First Hospital affiliated to Nanjing University, etc., carried out the multicenter, prospective, randomized controlled study – "Study of preoperative intervention chemotherapy of oxaliplatin in combination with oxygen floxuridine and mitomycin on the prevention of postoperative liver metastasis of colorectal cancer." It is anticipated to provide a basis for more accurate evaluation of the value of the preoperative intervention.

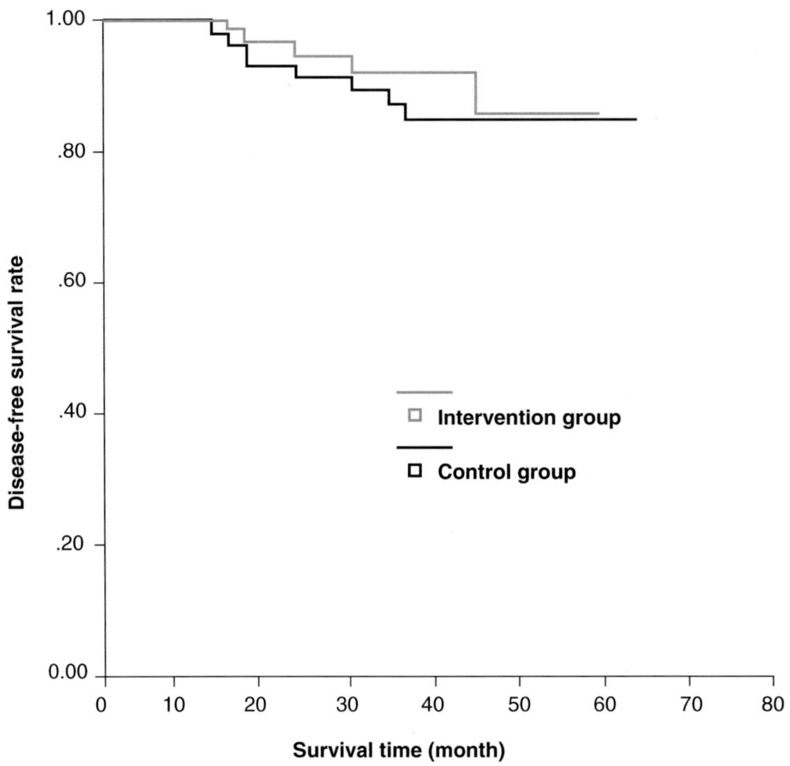

Fig. 19.8 Disease-free survival rate of stage II patients ($P = 0.09$)

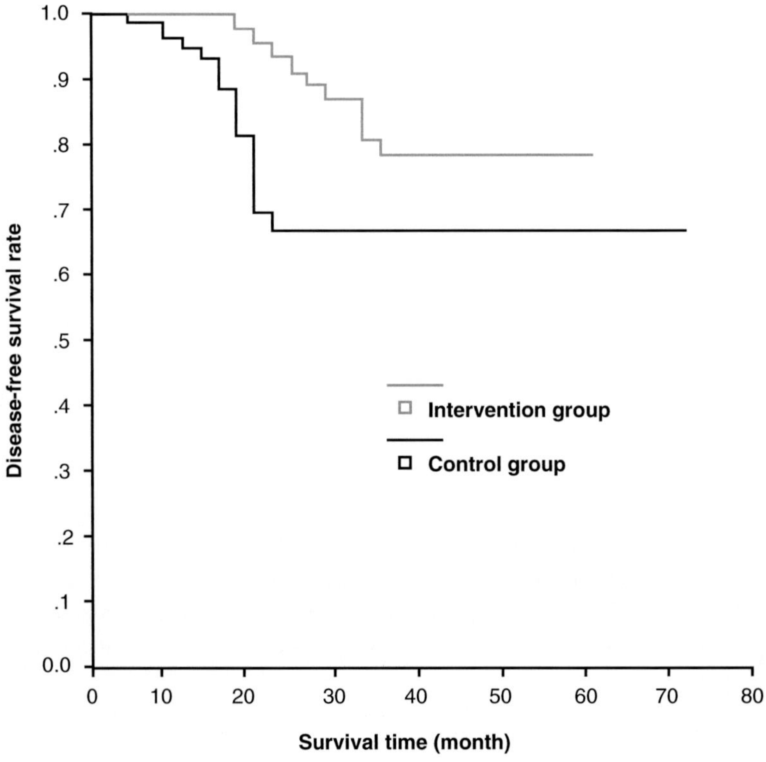

Fig. 19.9 Disease-free survival rate of stage III patients ($P = 0.01$)

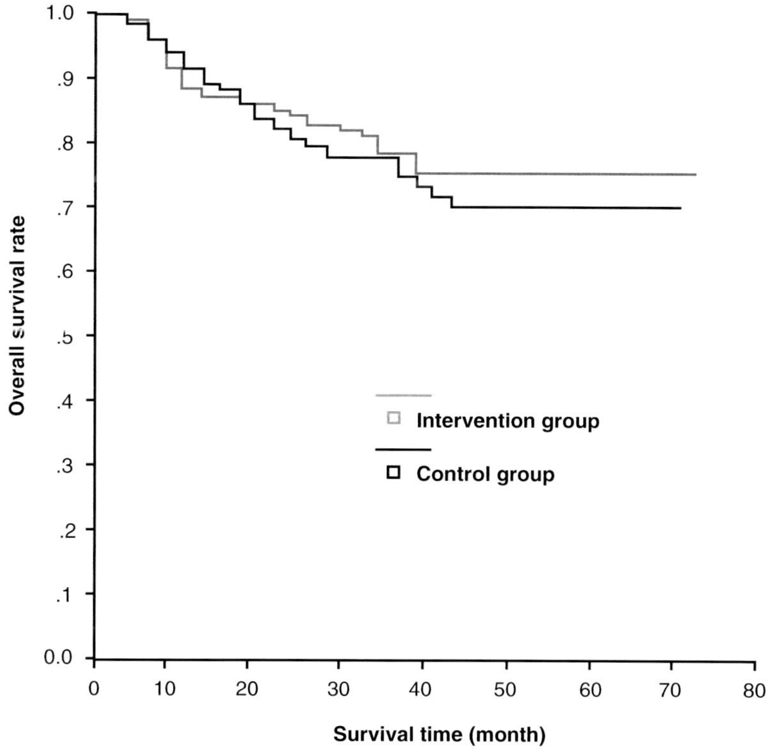

Fig. 19.10 Overall postoperative survival rate of stage II and stage III patients ($P=0.09$)

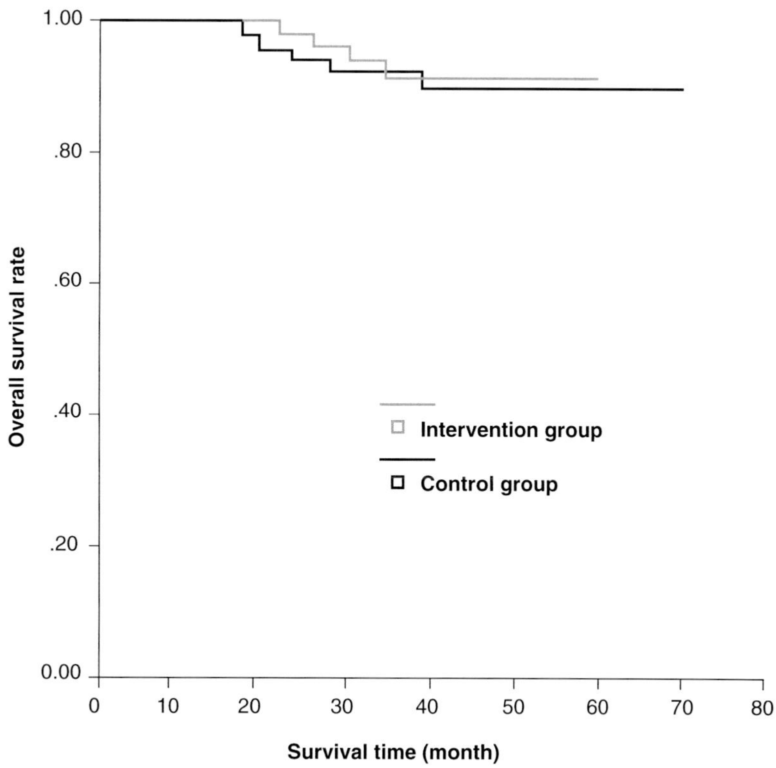

Fig. 19.11 Overall postoperative survival rate of stage II patients ($P=0.12$)

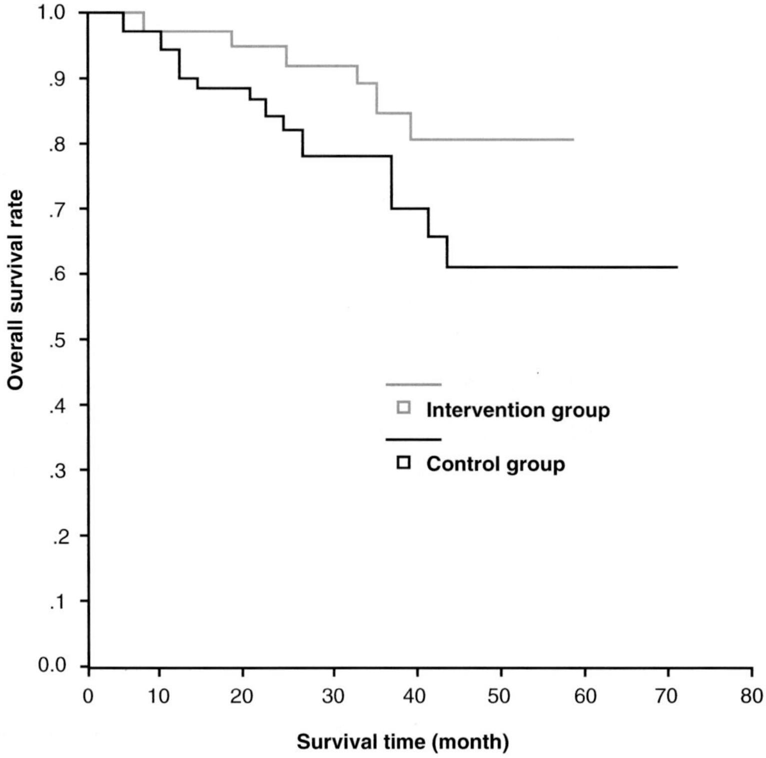

Fig. 19.12 Overall postoperative survival rate of stage III patients ($P = 0.025$)

References

1. Manfredi S, Lepage C, Hatem C, et al. Epidemiology and management of liver metastases from colorectal cancer. Ann Surg. 2006;244(2):254–9.
2. Crookes P, Leichman CG, Leichman, et al. Systemic chemotherapy for gastric carcinoma followed by post-operative intraperitoneal therapy: a final report. Cancer. 1997;79(9):1767–75.
3. Schuhmacher CP, Fink U, Becker K, et al. Neoadjuvant therapy for patients with locally advanced gastric carcinoma with etoposide, doxorubicin, and cis-platinum. Closing results after 5 years of follow-up. Cancer. 2001;9(5):918–27.
4. Chinese Society for Surgery, Gastrointestinal Surgery Group, Anal Colorectal Cancer Surgery Group and the China Association of Professional Committee of Colon Cancer. Liver metastasis diagnosis and comprehensive treatment guidelines of colorectal cancer (draft). Chin J Gastrointest Surg. 2008;11(5):501–5.
5. Chinese Society for Surgery, Gastrointestinal Surgery Group, Anal Colorectal Cancer Surgery Group and the China Association of Professional Committee of Colon Cancer. Liver metastasis diagnosis and comprehensive treatment guidelines of colorectal cancer (draft). Chin J Gastrointest Surg. 2008;11(6):597–603.
6. Fernández-Martos C, Pericay C, Aparicio J, et al. Phase II, randomized study of concomitant chemoradiotherapy followed by surgery and adjuvant Capecitabine Plus Oxaliplatin (CAPOX) compared with induction CAPOX followed by concomitant chemoradiotherapy and surgery in magnetic resonance imaging-defined, locally advanced rectal cancer: Grupo Cancer de Recto 3 Study. J Clin Oncol. 2010;28(5):859–65.
7. Minsky BD. Is preoperative chemoradiotherapy still the treatment of choice for rectal cancer? J Clin Oncol. 2009;27(31):5115–6.
8. Gérard JP, Conroy T, Bonnetain F, et al. Preoperative radiotherapy with or without concurrent fluorouracil and leucovorin in T3-4 rectal cancers: results of FFCD 9203. J Clin Oncol. 2006;24(28):4620–5.
9. Bosset JF, Collette L, Calais G, et al. Chemotherapy with preoperative radiotherapy in rectal cancer. N Engl J Med. 2006;355(11):1114–23.
10. Speryer JL. The rationale behind intraperitoneal chemotherapy in gastrointestinal malignancies. Semin Oncol. 1985;12(1):23–5.
11. Bonnen M, Crane C, Vauthey JN, et al. Long-term results using local excision after preoperative chemoradiation among selected T3 rectal cancer patients. Int J Radiat Oncol Biol Phys. 2004;60(4):1098–105.
12. Tao HQ, Zou SC. Effect of preoperative regional artery chemotherapy on proliferation and apoptosis of gastric carcinoma cells. World J Gastroenterol. 2002;8(3):451–4.
13. Kemeny MM, Adak SA, Gray B, et al. Combined-modality treatment for resectable metastatic colorectal carcinoma to the liver: surgical resection of hepatic

metastases in combination with continuous infusion of chemotherapy- an intergroup study. J Clin Oncol. 2002;20:1499–505.
14. Kemeny N, Huang Y, Cohen AM, et al. Hepatic arterial infusion of chemotherapy after resection of hepatic metastases from colorectal cancer. N Eng J Med. 1999;341:2039–48.
15. Archer SG, Gray BN. Vascularization of small liver metastases. Br J Surg. 1989;76:545–8.
16. Sadahiro S, Suzuki T, Ishikawa K, et al. Prophylactic hepatic arterial infusion chemotherapy for the prevention of liver metastasis in patients with colon carcinoma: a randomized control trial. Cancer. 2004;100(3):590–7.
17. Xu JM, Zhong YS, Niu WX, et al. Preoperative hepatic and regional arterial chemotherapy in the prevention of liver metastasis after colorectal cancer surgery. Ann Surg. 2007;245(4):583–90.
18. André T, Boni C, Mounedji-Boudiaf L, et al. Oxaliplatin, fluorouracil, and leucovorin as adjuvant treatment for colon cancer. N Engl J Med. 2004;350(23):2343–51.
19. André T, Boni C, Navarro M, et al. Improved overall survival with oxaliplatin, fluorouracil, and leucovorin as adjuvant treatment in stage II or III colon cancer in the MOSAIC trial. J Clin Oncol. 2009;27(19):3109–16.
20. Xu Z, Shou LJ, Liu FK, et al. Selection of preoperative arterial chemotherapy for rectal cancer. Chin J Surg. 1999;37(3):174–6.
21. WeiSu L, Liu FK, Chen ZH, et al. Influence of intervention chemotherapy colon cancer cell proliferation, apoptosis and angiogenesis. J Gen Surg. 2002;17(4):245–6.
22. Xu JM, Zhong YS, Niu WX, et al. Preoperative hepatic and regional arterial infusion chemotherapy in the prevention of liver metastasis after colorectal cancer surgery. Chin Med J. 2006;86:88–92.
23. Kimura H, Konishi K, Kaji M, et al. Apoptosis, cell proliferation and expression of oncogenes in gastric carcinomas induced by preoperative administration of 5-fluorouracil. Oncol Rep. 2000;7(5):971–6.
24. Huang W, Zhao Y, Luo L. Pathology analysis of preoperative interventional chemotherapy for gastric cancer. J Third Milit Med Univ. 2003;25(18):1659–61.
25. Ishii HH, Gobe GC, Pan W, et al. Apoptosis and cell proliferation in the development of gastric carcinomas: associations with c-myc and p53 protein expression. J Gastroenterol Hepatol. 2002;17(9):966–72.
26. Jin G, YiFan P, Pei L, et al. Influence of preoperative regional intra- arterial infusion chemotherapy on the platelet-derived endothelial cell growth factor expression in the tissues of colorectal cancer. Pract Oncol. 2001;16(6):388–90.
27. Xiao EH, Li JQ, Huang JF. Effects of p53 on apoptosis and proliferation of hepatocellular carcinoma cells treated with transcatheter arterial chemoembolization. World J Gastroenterol. 2004;10(2):190–4.

20 Establishment of Postoperative Follow-Up and Database of Colorectal Cancer

Desen Wan and Xiaojun Wu

The colorectal cancer is the most likely curable and preventable gastrointestinal cancer. However, the incidence and mortality rate of the colorectal cancer are still soaring in the world. In 2007, there are nearly 1.2 million new cases of colorectal cancer worldwide, and 630,000 deaths, respectively, increased by 27 and 28 % compared with that in 2000, with an average increase of 3.9 and 4 % [1, 2]. In the recent four decades, there is no significant improvement on the treatment, and the prognosis improvement is also not ideal. The postoperative survival rate in different countries or regions, or even different places in the same country, varies greatly and one of the important reasons for that is implementation of follow-up.

20.1 Significance and Objective of Postoperative Follow-Up

In the 1960s, Professor Xie Zhiguang ever pointed out that special follow-up group should be established for the establishment of South China Tumor Hospital (the Affiliated Tumor Hospital of Sun Yat-sen University); otherwise, the hospital should not be opened. In foreign countries, as early as the 1950s, follow-up of the tumor patients was proposed in Germany to monitor the postoperative condition; early find the recurrence, metastasis, and multiple primary tumor; and enhance the probability of radical surgery.

20.1.1 Significance and Necessity of Postoperative Follow-Up

20.1.1.1 Early Detection of Recurrence and Metastasis After Resection of Colorectal Cancer

The recurrence or metastasis will occur in about 30–50 % patients after the surgery of colorectal cancer, particularly liver metastasis. In the process of colorectal cancer diseases, about over half of patients will have liver metastasis. Local recurrence of rectal cancer is quite common, McCall et al. (1997) collected 52 papers in Western countries including 10,640 cases of rectal cancer, and the postoperative local recurrence rate is 3–50 % (median 18.5 %) [3]. The recurrence and metastasis forms of colon and rectal cancers are also different; for the rectal cancer, the pelvic recurrence is the first site, and its risk is twice as that of the colon cancer (30 % vs 15 %); for colon cancer, liver metastasis is the first site, and its risk compared with the rectal cancer is 36 % vs 25 %. In addition, many clinical data concluded that

D. Wan (✉) • X. Wu
Department of Colorectal Surgery, Sun Yat-Sen University Cancer Center, Guangzhou, Guangdong, China
e-mail: wds@medmail.com.cn

X. Qin et al. (eds.), *Multidisciplinary Management of Liver Metastases in Colorectal Cancer*,
DOI 10.1007/978-94-017-7755-1_20

80–90 % of postoperative recurrence after radical resection of colorectal cancer is at the 2–3 years after surgery and less than 5 % at 5 years later, and the early recurrence period is generally independent; if it can be completely resected, 35 % of them can be cured (including local recurrence, liver metastases, lung metastases, etc.) [4]. It is particularly important to be aware of this. After we know that the high rate of metastasis and recurrence of colorectal cancer patients within the 2–3 years after surgery and early discovery and treatment of them, we can obtain better effects and attach importance to the close follow-up patients. Many prospective follow-up results showed that the close follow-up can help to early discovery of recurrence, with higher resection success rate, lower 5-year mortality rate, and higher 5-year survival rate. Andrew analyzed five clinical trials with a total of 1,342 cases of colorectal cancer. The discovery of recurrence of the follow-up group was 8.5 months earlier than that of the control group, and the isolated local recurrence was higher [5]. Goldberg et al. reported there were 548 cases of postoperative recurrence of 1,247 cases of stage II or stage III colon cancer, of which 109 cases underwent a second curative resection, and the postoperative 5-year survival rate was 23 %. Among the 109 cases, 77 % of them were discovered through the regular test of serum CEA or CT scan [6]. Catells et al. reported that among the 56 cases of recurrence of follow-up, 18 cases can be resected (32.1 %), but among the symptomatic treatment of 28 patients, only 3 cases can be resected (10.7 %); in addition, the mortality rate within 5 years for the patients of regular follow-up was 31% and that of the patients of no regular follow-up was 51 % [7].

Therefore, strengthening the follow-up can help to discover the recurrence and metastasis in the early stage and implement the early re-excision and other treatments, so as to obtain good curative effect.

20.1.1.2 Discovery of More MPCC

Since Czerny (1880) firstly reported the multiple primary colorectal cancer (MPCC), there were relevant reports and papers, which reported that the MPCC was about 2–10 % among the colorectal cancer. The MPCC includes the synchronous MPCC and asynchronous MPCC; the synchronous MPCC mainly relies on the careful preoperative examination; asynchronous MPCC is about 1–4 % among the colorectal cancer patients, mainly relying on the postoperative follow-up. According to the reports, the interval between the first cancer and the second cancer is about 8.7 years; the longer the follow-up time, the more the MPCC. We have discovered four times of successive asynchronous MPCC (at different sites), all of which could be cured. Except for the multiple primary colorectal cancers, the extra-colorectal cancer should also be noted. The hereditary nonpolyposis colorectal cancer (HNPCC) can be divided into two types: Lynch I syndrome (also known as hereditary site-specific colorectal cancer, non-intestinal tumor) and Lynch II syndrome (also known as cancer family syndrome, intestinal tumor). The incidence rates of the synchronous MPCC and asynchronous MPCC of the former were, respectively, 18.1 % and 24.2 %, and for the latter, in addition to colorectal cancer, there were tumors of other organs, such as endometrial cancer, gastric cancer, small intestine, ureter, and renal pelvis cancer, ovarian cancer, brain tumors, etc. [8–10].

20.1.1.3 Timely Implementation of Salvage Therapy

Almost all surgeons unanimously believe that the reoperation should be carried out for the patients of recurrence of colorectal cancer with better results. The 5-year survival rate of liver metastasis of colorectal cancer patients is as high as 25–58 %, and the 10-year survival rate is 22–26 % [11]. The 5-year survival rate of patients' resection of postoperative local recurrence of rectal cancer is about 27 %, and if unresectable for reoperation, the patients can be subject to high dose (20 Gy) of brachytherapy or labeling and external beam radiotherapy, to obtain the ease effect. Rodriguez-Moranta et al. reported the prospective multicenter randomized trial results and strengthened follow-up to benefit the stage II rectal cancer and all rectal cancer patients. The overall survival rate was higher than that of the control group (ordinary follow-up); the reason is that the early discovery of recurrence has higher resection rate [12].

20.1.1.4 Improvement of Treatment Methods

The insufficient resection of rectal cancer is the main reason for the local recurrence. In the past, people generally focused on whether the bowel resection is sufficient. To meet 3–5 cm of safety margin, many patients have to accept Miles surgery, but actually after follow-up, it was discovered that the postoperative recurrence rate between Miles surgery and sphincter-preserving Dixon surgery has no significant difference. The British doctor Heald (1982) firstly discovered that the mesorectum micrometastasis was extensive than that of the intestinal wall expansion; even if reverse expansion along the intestinal wall is within 0.5 cm, the distal metastasis of mesorectum micrometastasis can reach below 4 cm; therefore, he proposed to total mesorectal excision (TME) of the middle and lower rectal cancer, or at least the mesorectum 5 cm from the tumor lower edge should be resected. The follow-up results showed that the local recurrence rate of rectal cancer according to the TME principle was less than <10 %, far less than those patients who were not subject to TME ($p<0.0001$), and the 5-year survival rate was relatively higher (71 % vs 50 %, $p<0.0001$) [3, 13]. The Dixon surgery following TME principle can not only preserve the sphincter but also reduce local recurrence, obviously superior to the traditional Miles surgery, which is from the obvious improvement of the treatment method of the middle and lower part of rectal cancer through a large number of follow-up data.

20.1.1.5 Improving the Living Quality of Patients

1. Psychological support to "reduce pressure" for patients. From the discovery, diagnosis, and treatment, the patients have suffered anger, fear, worry, sadness, depression, and pains, and they have great psychological pressure in the cancer-fighting process. The follow-up can allow them to feel delighted; warm and strong support greatly reduce the mental pressure. Taking rectal cancer radical surgery (Miles surgery) as an example, the patients with the artificial anus will have no regular defecation, and their sexual function is impaired, so many patients are afraid to face others, even their relatives and family members. As early as 1985, the psychologist Nordstrom believed that the colostomy would produce great psychological effect on patients more than the physiological effect, and 25 % colostomy patients suffered from persistent clinical depression, of which 5 % was more serious and even suicidal. Fortunately, the colostomy patients have received people's attentions; in many places, the colostomy patient club or association was organized, and the colostomy therapist will offer assistance and guidance. Since 1993, the first Saturday of October every 3 years is set as the World Ostomy Day, to arouse the whole society's attentions to the colostomy patients and allow them to be more confident to communicate with others [14, 15].
2. Discovery of the complications after treatment and offering guidance. With the extension of the follow-up, many complications after treatment such as hernia, prolapse, stenosis, and dermatitis will occur, with the incidence rate as high as 21–71 %. The incidence of incisional hernia within 5 years after surgery is nearly 50 %; all these complications will seriously affect the quality of life of the patients; through follow-up and guidance, the patients can be treated timely [15].

20.1.1.6 Evaluate the Treatment Effect and the Medical Care Quality

The most effective index for evaluation of treatment of cancer is disease-free survival and overall survival. Therefore, the follow-up should be strengthened in a planned way for treatment of cancers. For instance, which method is the best for treatment of colorectal liver metastases? Can resection cure it? Recently, it was reported that the 5-year survival rate after resection of colorectal liver metastases is as high as 30 % from a large number of literatures [11]. Tomlinson et al.

carried out a long-term continuous follow-up of 612 cases of patients with colorectal cancer liver metastasis; among them, 34 % of patients with 5 years of survival were subject to tumor-related death; and among the 102 cases of actual survival of 10 years or more, only one case had disease-specific death. Therefore, we believe that the 10 years of survival after the resection of colorectal liver metastases can be regarded as cured [16].

In recent years, through analysis on the curative effect of rectal cancer, including the local recurrence rate, it was concluded that it was associated with the technical level of the surgeons; generally the colorectal surgeons are better than the nonspecialist physicians for the colorectal surgery. Martling et al. reported that the postoperative recurrence rate of rectal cancer of patients whose surgery was conducted by a TME-trained colorectal surgeon reduced by 50 % [17]. In addition to the trained surgeons, the hospital size and number of surgery will also affect the technological level of surgeon and the postoperative recurrence rate of the rectal cancer [18, 19]. There have been two reports on the comparison of the surgical quality of the colorectal surgeons and general surgeons. In Swedish Ersta hospital, 18 general surgeons conducted radical surgery of rectal cancer for 72 patients and 52 % of them need the colostomy (the local recurrence rate of 18 %, the lowest anastomosis level of 8 cm), while two colorectal surgeons conducted radical surgery of rectal cancer for 180 patients and 33 % of them need the colostomy (the local recurrence rate of 3 %, the lowest anastomosis level of 4 cm). In Spain Valencia hospital, 14 general surgeons conducted radical surgery of rectal cancer for 94 patients, of which 25.8 % had Miles surgery, with the local recurrence rate 30 % and 5-year survival rate of 61 %; after trained, four colorectal surgeons conducted surgery of rectal cancer for 108 patients, of which only 16.7 % had Miles surgery, with the local recurrence rate 9 %and 5-year survival rate of 87 % [20].

As shown above, the close follow-up can help to evaluate the effect of the treatment method, which provides criterion for the selection of treatment method and for the elevation of medical quality and technological level of the hospitals and physicians.

20.1.2 Purpose of Postoperative Follow-Up

Through understanding of the significance and necessity of the postoperative follow-up of colorectal cancer, we can understand its purpose, summarized as follows:

(i) Early discovery of recurrence and metastasis for early re-excision.
(ii) Discover the asynchronous MPCC and treat it in the early period.
(iii) Identify and deal with various complications during treatment, such as postoperative intestinal obstruction, side effects of chemotherapy, radiation enteritis, incisional hernia, stoma complications, etc.
(iv) Give patient care, psychological support treatment, to better ensure the quality of life of patients.
(v) Evaluate the treatment effect and quality of medical care, sum up experience, and learn lessons.
(vi) Track the family members through follow-up and discover familial genetic diseases.

20.2 Postoperative Follow-Up Method of Colorectal Cancer

There are three ways for follow-up: one is follow-up clinic (the patients regularly come to the hospital for outpatient visit); second is petition letter, by letters, e-mail, telephone and fax, etc.; third is periodic meeting (the physician organizes 10–20 patients to have an informal discussion to understand the patient's feeling and reactions to the treatment method, seek their opinions on the hospital and medical staff, etc.). However, all of the follow-up must be recorded in the medical records and archived in the follow-up column of the database.

The postoperative follow-up methods include medical history, physical examination, laboratory examination, fiber colonoscopy and imaging examination, and so on.

20.2.1 Medical History and Physical Examination

The postoperative recurrence and metastasis of colorectal cancer are often accompanied by clinical symptoms, possibly some nonspecific symptoms such as weight loss, whole body discomfort, fatigue, night sweats, and so on; local symptoms such as pain in the right upper abdomen (liver metastasis), perineal pain (pelvic recurrence), and blood in the stool (anastomotic recurrence or multiple primary carcinoma); or other symptoms such as unilateral edema of lower extremities (deep vein thrombosis), chest pain and cough (lung metastasis), claudication (bone metastasis), and so on. Clinicians must be patient to listen to the patient's chief complaints, carefully analyze his/her symptoms, and carefully conduct body check. The anal digital rectal examination must be included in the routine examination item. The detailed inquiry of medical history and careful physical examination are the most basic methods for early discovery of recurrence and metastasis.

20.2.2 Laboratory Examination

20.2.2.1 Fecal Occult Blood Test, FOBT

FOBT is convenient and economical, which have great value for the discovery of the colorectal cancer, but it is of little value for the recurrent cases, and its positive rate is only about 10 % [21].

20.2.2.2 Liver Function Test

Liver is the most common site for the metastasis of colorectal cancer. As early as 1940, Gutman reported that ALP is the best and noninvasion indicator for the judgment of liver metastasis, and its sensitivity is 77 %, but the false-positive rate is also as high as 34 % and false negative of 4 %. The ALP combined with serum carcinoembryonic antigen (CEA) detection can enhance the sensitivity to 88 % and reduce the false-positive rate to 12 %. In the follow-up, it can be used as a screening indicator [21].

20.2.2.3 Tumor Marker

CEA (carcinoembryonic antigen) can be expressed in a variety of human epithelial tissues, endoderm-derived tissues and related diseases, but highest expression in the colorectal cancer and the positive rate varied 60–90 % [22, 23]. The serum CEA level of 245 cases of colorectal cancer in Cancer Hospital, Sun Yat-sen University, in 2002 increased by 42 % (≥5 ng/ml), respectively, 27.9 %, 36.0 %, 39.3 %, and 85 % in Dukes A–D stages. Therefore, about over half of patients, particularly at the early stage of diseases, have no increase in serum CEA. As early as 1977, the International CEA Association proposed that the serum CEA cannot be used as an early diagnosis indicator of tumor, but it has considerable value for the prediction of prognosis, efficacy monitoring, and postoperative recurrence and metastasis. For instance, if the CEA is higher before treatment and decreases after treatment, it shows that the treatment is effective, otherwise, not effective. According to the reports, if the CEA half-life is 8.6 ± 3.4 days after colon cancer surgery, there is fewer postoperative recurrence and metastasis, and if the CEA half-life exceeds 23.7 days, there is very high opportunity of postoperative recurrence and metastasis; the postoperative-elevated CEA level suggests the possible recurrence or metastasis, and further examination is required.

Other tumor markers such as tissue polypeptide antigen (TPA), carbohydrate antigen CA19-9, tumor-associated glycoproteins TAG-72, CA50, CA724, CA242, etc. have no advantages compared with CEA. But if tested by CEA combined with CA199 and TAG-72, the positive rate can be increased to 84 % [24].

20.2.3 Fiber Colonoscopy

The fiber colonoscopy has two functions in the postoperative follow-up of colorectal cancer: (1) confirm the tumor recurrence (especially anastomotic recurrence) and (2) discover the metachronous colorectal neoplasms, including the benign and malignant neoplasms. However, since most recurrence starts from the outer enteric cavity, the colonoscopy, as a means of detection of recurrence, is not sensitive. According to most reports, only 3–4 % patients can obtain the first evidence of recurrence through colonoscopy, and Audisio reported it was no more than 1 %. In addition, the incidence of metachronous colorectal carcinoma after surgery is about 0.6–9 %, and the colonoscopy detection rate is 0.2–3.1 % [25]. There is at least 5 years from adenoma to cancer (generally 10–15 years) [26]; for the patients who are subject to radical resection, the pathological data of tumor are not likely to be available in the first 3 years after resection through the colonoscopy; however, in the follow-up of 4 years, more than 14 % of patients can be discovered of adenomas every year, so most physicians prefer the colonoscopy. But according to the study of Andrew, regardless of the frequency of colonoscopy, recurrence and metachronous cancer can be discovered only in a minority of them.

20.2.4 Imaging

Most of postoperative metastasis and recurrence of colorectal cancer happen outside the enteric cavity; therefore, the follow-up imaging is particularly important.

20.2.4.1 X-Ray Examination

The chest X-ray can be used to detect the asymptomatic lung lesions; further slices or chest CT examination can help to diagnose or discover the multiple lesions. For the patients of postoperative lung metastasis of colorectal cancer, the postoperative 5-year survival rate after resection can be up to 21–64 % [27, 28].

The barium enema, as the colonoscopy, is mainly used to detect the lesion recurrence and metachronous colorectal neoplasms in the intestine (multiple primary cancers or adenoma) for orientation effect. The air-barium double-contrast examination can help to observe the lesions of 1 cm in diameter, which is superior to the colonoscopy for the observation of lesions of the right half colon and outside of the intestines, but the pathological tissues cannot be available.

20.2.4.2 Scanning

Ultrasound (US), CT, and MRI

The scanning can help to obtain the data of local recurrence and distant metastasis in the follow-up. More information of the inside and outside of the intestinal walls, liver, pelvic, and retroperitoneal lymph node can be available through US, and the recurrence and metastasis of one half of patients can be discovered through US examination. The special probes can be used to guide puncture to obtain the pathological data. The rectal ultrasound can accurately detect the local recurrence of lesions. There is no great difference in the sensitivity and accuracy for the discovery of recurrent lesions through the techniques of US, CT, and MRI, but the latter both are more sensitive to the pelvic lesions; MRI is superior for the detection of the lesion depth and length.

Monoclonal Antibody Imaging or Radioimmunoscintigraphy (RIS), Positron Emission Tomography (PET), and Positron Emission Computed Tomography (CT-PET)

The main difficulty for US, CT, and MRI used in the diagnosis of local recurrence is unable to identify the postoperative change (such as formation of fibrous scar) or a tumor recurrence, while RIS, PET, and CT-PET can identify the scar tissue and malignant tissue from the functional or metabolic differences and, moreover, understand the metastasis conditions of the whole body. The monoclonal antibodies, including TAG-72 or B72-3 antigens for colon, ovarian, and breast cell surfaces and the CEA antigens of colon cancer expression, are labeled by indium (^{111}In), iodine (^{125}I), or ^{99}Te isotopes, which have more precise positioning effect on the small lesions, particularly for the positioning of the occult recurrent metastasis of lesions.

New Techniques

The up-to-date CT virtual colonoscopy (CTVC) and magnetic resonance virtual colonoscopy (MRVC) are exciting new techniques, which combine CT, MRI, and advanced imaging software to produce the 3D (three-dimensional) and 2D (two-dimensional) images of the colons to form the simulation images of the enteric cavity and the images of the intestinal canal, combination with the cross-sectional image, and thus diagnosed. From multiple perspectives, the overall observed lesions, combined with internal and external surface reconstruction and cross-sectional images, the bowel wall thickening, swollen lymph nodes, intestinal fat, pelvic wall invasions, etc. can be observed. Although there are many advantages, these techniques are expensive, which are difficult to be applied in the regular follow-up.

20.3 Evaluation of Postoperative Follow-Up of Colorectal Cancer

20.3.1 Study of Follow-Up Plan

Since the 1990s, there are great differences on strengthening the follow-up strategy after radical surgery of colorectal cancer. Generally it is believed that the active follow-up is conducive to the early diagnosis of recurrence, metastasis, or metachronous cancer (second primary cancer) and increase the resection rate to enhance the survival, and the necessity of the follow-up is also questioned, "no evidence" or "not worth it"; from the perspective of efficacy and costs, the implementation of follow-up is of controversy.

20.3.1.1 Follow-Up and Recurrence

Most studies showed that there was no difference of the recurrence between the follow-up group and non-follow-up group, and between the intensive follow-up group and controlled follow-up group.

Andrew [5] conducted a meta-analysis of five groups of clinical trials [29–33] (Table 20.1), 1,342 patients in total, and discovered that there was no difference of the recurrence rate of all sites between the intensive group and the controlled follow-up group: the intensive follow-up group 212/666 (32 %) and the control group 224/676 (33 %). However, the recurrent time was 8.5 months earlier than that of the intensive follow-up group (Table 20.2). The intensive follow-up was closely associated with the discovery of the isolated local recurrence.

Since the diagnostic examination methods for follow-up of all clinical trials are different, i.e., CT or frequent serum detection method CEA or both of them, they possibly have greater impact on the improvement of the survival of the patients with colorectal cancer compared with the direct examination of mucosal lesions (such as colonoscopy) strategy for the early detection of recurrence outside the mucosa (i.e., local pelvic recurrence and isolated liver metastases). The results of subgroup analysis are consistent.

20.3.1.2 Follow-Up and Survival Rate

Whether the intensive follow-up can improve the survival rate of the patients with colorectal cancer is controversial. Sugarbaker et al. [34] and Safi and Beyer [35] strongly supported that the intensive follow-up and early intervention can reduce the number of deaths of patients. Cochrane et al. [36] and Ballantyne et al. [37] questioned about the value of the follow-up. But they are not proven by randomized clinical trials. Until 1994, Bruinvels et al. [38, 39] provided rational data through meta-analysis of seven nonrandomized studies (more than 3,000 cases). The study showed that in the intensive follow-up group, there were more cases of asymptomatic recurrence and re-resection, but there was no difference in the survival rate between the two groups. But in the test including carcinoembryonic antigen (CEA) analysis, the 5-year survival rate in the intensive follow-up group increased by 9 %, and the author was cautious to explain these data and believed there may be deviation in values. Some studies [40, 41] showed that the intensive follow-up was ineffective and costly.

Table 20.1 Five randomized controlled trials of intensive follow-up after radical resection of colorectal cancer

Author	Year	Number of cases	Test items and frequency of the intensive follow-up group	Test items and frequency of the control group
Makela et al.	1995	106	Visit one time every 3 months for the first 2 years and then one time every 6 months later: examine the body, whole blood, fecal occult blood test (FOBT), CEA level, and chest X-ray film. Colonoscopy every year, sigmoidoscope examination every 3 months for the sigmoid colon and rectal cancer patients, and liver ultrasound every 6 months. All the patients will be followed up for 5 years	Visit one time every 3 months for the first 2 years and then one time every 6 months later: examine the body, whole blood, fecal occult blood test (FOBT), CEA level, and chest X-ray film. Barium enema every year. Rigid sigmoidoscope examination every 3 months for the rectal cancer patients. All patients were followed up for 5 years
Ohlsson et al.	1995	107	Visit one time every 3 months for the first 2 years and then one time every 6 months later: examine the body, rigid sigmoidoscopy, liver function tests, fecal occult blood test (FOBT), CEA level, and chest X-ray film. Colonoscopy at the third, fifth, 30th, and 60th months; CT examination in the third, sixth, 12th, 18th, and 24th months; all patients were followed up for 5 years	No systematic follow-up. Guide the patient to leave the specimens for fecal occult blood test every 3 months at the first 2 years, once every year. all the records of patients will be kept for 5 years
Schoemaker et al.	1998	325	Visit one time every 3 months for the first 2 years and then one time every 6 months later: examine the body, whole blood, liver function, fecal occult blood test II. Annual chest X-ray inspection and liver CT. Colonoscopy every year The CEA test, but not used to start further examination. 94 % of the patients were followed up for 5 years	Visit one time every 3 months for the first 2 years and then one time every 6 months later within 5 years: examine the body, whole blood, liver function, fecal occult blood test (FOBT). The CEA test, but not used to start further examination. 94 % of the patients were followed up for 5 years
Pietra et al.	1998	207	Visit one time every 3 months for the first 2 years and then one time every 6 months in the following 3 years and then once every year; physical examination, liver ultrasound, and CEA level. Annual chest X-ray inspection and CT and colonoscopy. All patients were followed up for 5 years	Visit one time every 6 months for the first year and then one time every year: physical examination, liver ultrasound, CEA level. Annual chest X-ray inspection and colonoscopy. All patients were followed up for 5 years

(continued)

Table 20.1 (continued)

Author	Year	Number of cases	Test items and frequency of the intensive follow-up group	Test items and frequency of the control group
Kjeldsen et al.	1997	597	Psychical examination, digital rectal examination, gynecological examination, occult blood test II, whole blood, ESR, liver function, chest X-ray, colonoscopy; visit one time every 6 months for the first 3 years and then one time every 12 months in the following 2 years and then once every year; 79 % of the patients were followed up for 5 years	Psychical examination, digital rectal examination, gynecological examination, occult blood test II, whole blood, ESR, liver function, chest X-ray, colonoscopy in the fifth and tenth years. 73 % of patients were followed up for 5 years

Table 20.2 The average time of initial recurrence of the colorectal cancer patients in the intensive follow-up group and the control group (months)

Researcher	Year	Intensive follow-up group	Control group
Makela et al.	1995	10.0	15.0
Ohlsson et al.	1995	20.4	24.0
Schoemaker et al.	1998	–	–
Pietra et al.	1998	10.3	20.2
Kjeldsen et al.	1997	17.7	26.5

Northover et al. [42] randomly divided the patients after radical surgery into the intensive follow up group and the control group and tested the CEA. In the intensive follow-up group, if the CEA level is elevated, further observation should be conducted; and after an appropriate period, patients should receive another examination. Through the preliminary analysis, there was no difference of the survival rate between two groups.

The studies conducted by Makela et al. [29], Ohlsson et al. [30], Schoemaker et al. [31], and Kjeldsen et al. [33], respectively, showed that the recurrence rate between the two groups was similar. The tumor recurrence in the intensive follow-up group was 9 months earlier on average, and more patients underwent the secondary radical surgery; but there was no difference of the overall survival rate or tumor-related survival rate between the two groups.

But Andrew et al. concluded that the intensive follow-up can improve the 5-year survival rate after systematic review and meta-analysis on the five groups of randomized clinical trials, although the past clinical trials cannot determined that due to too small samples. They believed that the mortality of patients with the modern follow-up program (including CT or regular serum CEA or both for the detection of recurrence outside of the mucous membrane, i.e., local pelvic recurrence and isolated liver metastasis) was absolutely decreased by 9–13 % compared with the direct examination of mucosal lesions (such as the use of colonoscopy). In contrast, this improvement is more beneficial to the patients of adjuvant chemotherapy in the stage of Dukes C that reduces the mortality rate of 5 %, and it is applicable to different stages of colorectal cancer.

As early as 1999, Howell et al. [43] also believed that the tests conducted by Makela et al., Ohlsson et al., and Schoemaker et al. may be based on a wrong premise, that is, the intensive follow-up can discover the recurrent tumor in the following radical surgery. However, the above tests showed that although the intensive follow-up can help to observe more asymptomatic recurrence and has more opportunities for surgical resection, there was no difference in the survival rate or the tumor-related survival rate. Howell et al. suggested that since the most frequent part of recurrence and metastasis of the colorectal cancer is the liver, it is necessary to strengthen the follow-up of the liver imaging in the first 3 years in addition to the observation of the local and regional recurrences, so as to discover the effective liver metastasis that can be resected and chemotherapy, to enhance the survival rate.

Therefore, the multidisciplinary treatment of colorectal cancer is strengthened at present, including extensive application of liver resection, the pelvic exenteration for the pelvic cavity recurrence, and the combined therapy for the advanced diseases. All these methods will affect the survival, and on the basis of them, it is more beneficial to strengthen the follow-up.

20.3.2 Develop the Follow-Up Program

The development of the follow-up program of the colorectal cancer patients should be based on the staging, prognosis factors, and whether or not accept postoperative auxiliary treatment. The frequent follow-up will not only waste the medical resources but also increase the psychological burden of patients. So what kind of follow-up is useful?

20.3.2.1 Basis for the Development of the Follow-Up Program

To develop an ideal follow-up plan for the colorectal cancer patients, the physicians shall be aware of (1) which type(s) of colorectal cancer patients are mostly likely to occur recurrence and metastasis, (2) which period that these patients are most likely to occur recurrence and metastasis, and (3) the most likely sites for recurrence and metastasis (see the relevant chapters).

Second, it is required to identify the following: (1) Can the local recurrence and early discovery of metastasis increase the probability of cure (this has been confirmed from the above)? (2) Can the treatment after the follow-up reduce the colorectal cancer mortality or overall mortality? (3) Which kind of examination method is required to achieve the above purpose? Is the costs and efficiency reasonable? (4) To answer the above questions, how does one determine the moral baseline for the design of the control group, particularly under the conditions that the current studies support to improve the living through intensive follow-up?

20.3.2.2 The Development of the Follow-Up Plan

The development of the follow-up plan is easily affected by the individual subjective thinking. Kievet and Bruinvels [4] proposed four conditions for the practicality of routine follow-up:

1. At least some lesions can be limited and of curative treatment. The recurrence process includes no lesions observed, subclinical lesions that can be observed, curable symptoms, palliative resection, and unresectable lesions. But the recurrence of curable colorectal cancer is not usually a time-dependent process.
2. The follow-up should be able to discover the curable recurrence and, under the ideal situation, do not wait until the incurable stage.
3. Follow-up should help to improve life expectancy and have more curable resection. The follow-up should not produce worthless findings that are incurable, do not improve the mortality rate, and are false-positive results by the re-surgery.
4. Cost-efficiency ratio should be of assistance for the adjustment of the conventional follow-up methods.

The development of the most effective follow-up plan should refer to a large number of literatures and be based on the multicenter randomized controlled clinical trials. The follow-up contents, intensity, costs, etc., should be described in details, and different results should be compared to obtain the best follow-up plan, but the benefits from the follow-up and excessive unnecessary financial burden of patients should be avoided.

20.3.2.3 Establishment of the Follow-Up Frequency and System

After the initial treatment of colorectal cancer, the discovery of the recurrence through the follow-up still lacks of sufficient and ideal proofs. To obtain follow-up, the efficiency results of effective plan, different methods and intensities, and the multicenter randomized clinical trials should be conducted.

In the early period of postoperative follow-up of colorectal cancer, it is necessary to focus on the postoperative rehabilitation and further treatment plan (including possible adjuvant therapy and stoma treatment), and at this time, patients should receive spiritual comfort and practical medical support. For the patients of colorectal cancer, the importance of the psychological factors remains unclear. But for the patients who underwent Miles and pelvic resection, the acceptance of the artificial anus or urethrostomy will affect the effect of further treatment; at this time, the psychological support is absolutely vital. Besides, the patients should receive the knowledge about the symptoms associated with the tumor recurrence so that they can be treated at the time of relevant symptoms. The patients should also be aware that the risk of recurrence will rapidly drop 2 years after treatment and very small 5 years after treatment; in this way, the patients are comforted in the mind and minimize their psychological pressure.

The implementation of the follow-up work should be completed by the physicians and patients. The doctors are obliged to remind the patients of reexamination, and the patient's compliance is also very important. In the early postoperative period, since they need further treatment, most patients can observe the follow-up, but as the time passes, some patients will be slack, not pay attention, and believe to be good; at this time, it is necessary to remind and urge the patients to visit timely. The establishment of the follow-up system is crucial. We are now at an information age; the large hospitals at the provinces and cities have implemented the information management on the cases, which lays foundation for the establishment of the follow-up system. The follow-up group should determine whether or not to remind the patients of visit according to the operation time and the last visit time recorded on the cases database through the most effective means – mail, e-mail, and telephone.

Although the most effective follow-up plan has not been established or not unified, we suggest regular follow-up of the patients of colorectal cancer who underwent radical surgery. The recommended follow-up program by referring to NCCN Colorectal Clinical Practice Guidelines (first edition 2009) and clinical practice guidelines developed by Professional Committee of China's Colorectal Cancer (in print) are as follows: ① follow-up once every 3–6 months in 2 years after surgery, then once every 6 months, and then once every year after 5 years. Particularly the first time of follow-up should be within the 3 months after the surgery, so that there are comparative data for the future follow-up. The items for follow-up include the medical history; detailed physical examination; serum CEA; blood routine examination; liver function test; fecal occult blood test; chest X-ray examination and the liver, retroperitoneal lymph nodes, and pelvic B-ultrasound scanning. ② One time of fiber colonoscopy within 1 year after the surgery to discover the metachronous multiple primary neoplasms and anastomotic recurrence. If the preoperative fiber-optic colonoscopy and barium enema examination are not conducted, select one of them for examination in 6 months after surgery. If there is any abnormality, recheck within 1 year, and if no abnormality is discovered, recheck within 3 years and then recheck once in the future every 5 years. ③ One time of CT examination, 5 years in total. ④ For patients who receive postoperative adjuvant chemotherapy, the examination of CEA and liver and kidney functions should be conducted one time every 1 or 2 months. If any abnormality is discovered in the follow-up, implement detailed examination to discover the recurrence and metastasis lesions in the early stage. The check of the blood cell count should be more regular, and for the patients of DPD enzyme deficiency or applied with bone marrow suppression drugs, check at least once every week.

20.4 Establishment of Database of Colorectal Cancer

Currently China has not established a sound and unified cancer statistical system, and it is difficult to obtain the latest and accurate data for the colorectal cancer incidence and mortality, diagnosis, treatment, and prognosis. The establishment and improvement of the national colorectal cancer registration system, further monitoring of the colorectal cancer progress, and dynamic observation of the treatment and prevention results can provide timely feedback for the prevention, screening, and treatment of colorectal cancer and lay a foundation of the development of the prevention and treatment strategies of colorectal cancer.

The two elements for the establishment of the database of colorectal cancer are contents and the software, both of which are important. The software is the "framework" and the contents are the "fresh." The database will be useless if it lacks any one of them. The contents should be accurate and detailed, and the software should be easy to learn and operate, to meet the remote input. Besides, after the database is output, they can directly be converted to SPSS, SAS, and other statistical software. We here give a brief description of the database of colorectal cancer. The contents include the basic information and the follow-up information data.

20.4.1 Basic Information Data

The basic data should be the information for the first time of diagnosis, generally including the basic information of patients, symptoms and signs, laboratory tests, imaging studies, complications, accompanied diseases, treatment program, operation conditions and pathological staging, etc.

20.4.1.1 Basic Information of Patients

Name, sex, age, date of birth (or ID number), address, zip code, telephone number, hospital number, pathology number, admission date, discharge date, length of hospital stay, and surgery date are the basic information, which are for the data classification and query and for providing the contact information for follow-up.

The blood type, blood transfusion, and surgical blood transfusion are the factors that affect the prognosis. The family history is essential for the statistics of hereditary colorectal cancer.

20.4.1.2 Information of Symptoms and Signs

These information of symptoms and signs are necessary for the database: the length of the course of disease, first symptom, tumor location, the distance of tumor lower margin from anal edge, rectal tumor location, the total lumen perimeter of rectal tumor, maximum diameter of tumor, whether there is intestinal obstruction, intestinal perforation, severe anemia (Hb <90 g/L), and other complications.

20.4.1.3 Information of Laboratory Test

Preoperative and postoperative tumor markers CEA, CA19-9 test, are the most important, which are associated with the postoperative efficacy and monitoring of the recurrence and metastasis. Where permitted, the examination of the bile of preoperative duodenoscopy or intraoperative puncture of common bile duct for check of CEA is helpful for the judgment of the liver metastasis. For the immune system, including cellular and humoral immune functions, generally check the T-lymphocyte subsets and IgA, IgG, and IgM. The testing of DPD and TP enzymes is helpful to remind the drug dose during the chemotherapy period and observe the side effect closely.

20.4.1.4 Imaging

Actually the basis for the preoperative localization and staging, especially judgment of the tumor level and infiltration, ranges through endoscopic ultrasound, endosonography, CT, and MRI. It is recommended before and after treatment, especially before and after concurrent chemoradiotherapy, to test all the items to compare the curative effect.

20.4.1.5 Accompanied Diseases

Diabetes, heart disease, and high blood pressure are the common accompanied diseases of colorectal cancer. The treatment of them is directly associated with the selection of the curative means and the success of surgery. The incidence of the multiple primary cancer is also increasing.

20.4.1.6 Treatment Protocol

The main means for colorectal cancer is surgery. The registration of the patient is of significance for the prognosis. The specific preoperative and postoperative chemoradiotherapy protocol should be recorded. The biological treatment is the supplement of the three treatment programs, which cannot be missed. The specific items of surgery include the nature of surgery, tumor condition in surgery, metastasis condition, surgical method, operative mortality, and whether or not to use the anastomat, anti-adhesive, and intraoperative chemotherapy technique. Of which, the location of the rectal cancer is closely associated with the T staging.

20.4.1.7 Staging of Pathological Tissues

Staging of pathological tissues usually records the tumor type, histological type, tumor grade, bowel wall infiltration, lymph node metastasis (number of inspection/ metastasis), Dukes staging, and TNM staging. The distance between the lower tumor margins to the distant cutting edge (dentate line for the Miles' surgery) must be recorded, especially for the rectal cancer below the peritoneal fold. The status of these biomarkers should also be recorded, including the tissues ER, PR, CEA, p53, PCNA, c-erbB2/neu, K-ras, maspin, Ck19, Ck20, osteopontin, PRL3, SNC, nm23, etc., of which the ER, PR, c-erbB2/neu, and K-ras have been confirmed to be of great help for the selection of the treatment.

20.4.2 Follow-Up Information Data

They provide data for the survival rate, disease-free survival rate, and the treatment program and efficacy after metastasis and recurrence. They are preferred to register according to the follow-up interval, including the follow-up time, signs and symptoms, examination items, whether or not there is recurrence and metastasis, date of recurrence and metastasis, basis for postoperative metastasis and recurrence, locations of metastasis and recurrence and solution, and outcome (cause of death). Pay attention to the registration of the postoperative complications. The stoma complications are more common, which directly affect the quality of life of patients.

Annex: Registration Form of Database Information of Colorectal Cancer

(i) Basic Information

Name: **H: Hospitalization No.** **P: Pathological No.**

Address: **Zip code:_** **Tel:**

Family history: **HNPCC: _** **FAP:**

( ) Nx: Sex Male = 0, female = 1 ( ) Nx: age (years)

( ) Nx: Date of birth : ID number: __

( ) BG: blood group A = 1, B = 2, AB = 3, O = 4

Nx: Hospital blood transfusion __ml Nx: Blood transfusion for operation _ ml

Nx: Admission date __ day__ month__ year Nx: Date of discharge __ day__ month__ year

Nx: length of hospital stay___ Nx: Date of operation __ day__ month__ year

( ) Nx: Time for resection of colorectal tumor __

( ) Nx: course of disease __months, 1 month or less = 1, unknown = 0

( ) Nx: first symptom Mucus bloody stool = 1, abdominal pain = 2, change in bowel habits (frequent, constipation, diarrhea, alternative diarrhea and constipation) = 3, thinner defecation = 4, abdominal mass = 5, anemia = 6, other = 7, asymptomatic (physical examination found) = 0

( ) Nx: Tumor location ileocecal site = 1, appendix = 2, ascending colon = 3, hepatic flexure colon =4, transverse colon = 5 , splenic flexure colon = 6, descending colon = 7 sigmoid colon = 8, rectum = 9, anal canal = 10, entire colon = 11, entire colorectal part = 12

( ) Nx: distance between the lower margin of rectal cancer and the anal verge __ cm, colon = 0, unknown = 99

( ) Nx: rectal tumor location anterior = 1, posterior = 2, left wall = 3, right wall = 4, circumference= 5, unknown = 9, colon = 0

( ) Nx: circumference of rectal cancer accounted for enteric cavity 1 / 4 = 1, 1 / 2 = 2, 3 / 4 = 3, ring = 4, unknown = 9, colon = 0

( ) Nx: maximum tumor diameter___ cm, unknown = 99

() Nx: preoperative / intraoperative metastasis none = 0, liver metastasis = 1, local infiltration = 2, abdominal / pelvic plantation = 3, lung metastases = 4, bone metastases = 5, other distant metastases = 6

( ) Nx: preoperative complications None= 0, intestinal obstruction= 1, intestinal perforation = 2, severe anemia (Hb <90 g / L) = 3, Other = 4

( ) Nx: accompanied diseases None=0, diabetes = 1, heart disease = 2, high blood pressure = 3, Other = 4

( ) Nx: accompanied with multiple primary cancer None = 0, multiple primary colorectal cancer = 1, parenteral cancer = 2, multiple intestinal polyps=3, intestinal polyposis = 4

( ) Nx: preoperative treatment None = 0,, surgery = 1, chemotherapy = 2, radiotherapy = 3, Chinese medicine = 4, Other = 5

Nx: chemotherapy protocol None= 0, 5-Fu / CF = 1, oxaliplatin = 2, CPT-11 = 3, HCPT = 4, xeloda = 5, S1 = 6, toremifene = 7, intraperitoneal chemotherapy = 8, other = 9

Nx: preoperative chemotherapy regimen __

Nx: radiotherapy plan ___

O: Surgeon (fill in the first surgeon)

( ) Nx: the nature of surgery radical = 1, palliative resection = 2, palliative surgery = 3, exploratory surgery = 4

( ) Nx: intraoperative findings ascites= 1, bowel obstruction = 2, tumor activity limitation = 3 tumor activity= 4, tumor fixation= 5

( ) Nx: type of surgery, open surgery= 1, simple laparoscopy= 2, hand-assisted laparoscopy = 3

( ) Nx: surgical means right half = 1, transverse colon resection = 2, left half= 3, sigmoid colon resection = 4, total colectomy = 5, Miles operation = 6, Dixon surgery = 7, Bacon surgery = 8, Park surgery = 9, posterior pelvic exenteration =10, total pelvic exenteration = 11, local resection through anus=12, Hartmann = 13, enterostomy = 14, bowel resection = 15, Other = 16

( ) Nx: The distance between the lower margin of tumor and the distant resection margin (dentate line for the Miles operation)__ cm (Subject to the measurement of the postoperative dissection)

( ) Nx: combined organ resection None= 0, liver = 1, bladder = 2, vaginal = 3, ovary = 4, lung = 5, Other = 6

( ) Nx: operative mortality No= 0, yes = 1

( ) Nx: anastomat None = 0, single- anastomat = 1, double anastomat = 2

( ) Nx: anti-stick agent none = 0, low molecular weight dextran = 1, sodium hyaluronate = 2, Other = 3

( ) Nx: Intraoperative chemotherapy No = 0 , intestine = 1 (), abdominal cavity = 2 ( ), portal vein = 3 ( )

( ) Nx: gross tumor type Proliferation type = 1, ulcer type = 2, infiltration type = 3, unknown = 9

( ) Nx: = tissue type adenocarcinoma =1, mucinous adenocarcinoma (including signet ring cell carcinoma) = 2, undifferentiated carcinoma= 3, adenoma = 4, squamous cell carcinoma = 5, Other = 6

( ) Nx: pathological grade grade I = 1, grade II = 2, grade III = 3

( ) Nx: bowel wall infiltration mucosa = 1, superficial muscular layer = 2, deep muscular layer = 3, serosa = 4, outer serosa infiltration= 5

( ) Nx: lymph node metastasis None= 0, intestinal side = 1, intermediate = 2, central = 3,

( ) Nx: submission of __ LNM

( ) Nx: Number of LN metastases __

( ) Nx: Dukes staging A = 1, B = 2, C = 3, D = 4

( ) Nx: T stage T__ (1 ~ 4) ( ) Nx: preoperative T stage T__ (1 ~ 4)

( ) Nx: N stage N ___(0 ~ 2) ( ) Nx: Preoperative N stage N __ (0 ~ 2)

( ) Nx: M stage M___ (0 ~ 1) ( ) Nx: preoperative M stage M__ (0 ~ 1)

= 0, + = 1, + + = 2, + + + = 3 ,++++ = 4

( ) Nx: Tissue ER ( ) Nx: Tissue PR ( ) Nx: tissue CEA

( ) Nx: Tissue p53 ( ) Nx: Tissue PCNA ( ) Nx: Tissue c-erbB2/neu

( ) Nx: Tissue K-ras ( ) Nx: Tissue maspin ( ) Nx: Tissue Ck19

( ) Nx: Tissue Ck20 ( ) Nx: Tissue osteopontin ( ) Nx: Tissue PRL3

( ) Nx: Tissue SNC ( ) Nx: Tissue nm23

( ) Nx: determination method of rectal infiltration CT = 1, MRI = 2, endoscopic ultrasound = 3, intracavity B ultrasound-= 4

( ) Nx: rectal surgery / before /radiotherapy infiltration level mucosa = 1, submucosa = 2, muscularis mucosa = 3, superficial muscle= 4, deep muscle = 5, subserosa= 6, serosa = 7, outside serosal = 8, lymph node metastasis = 9

( ) Nx: rectal surgery / radiotherapy mucosal invasion level = 1, submucosa = 2, muscularis mucosa = 3 = 4 superficial muscle, deep muscle = 5 = 6 subserosa, serosa = 7, plasma extracellular = 8, lymph node metastasis = 9

( ) Nx: treatment after surgery None=0, chemotherapy = 1, radiotherapy= 2, biological therapy = 3, Chinese medicine = 4, combined therapy = 5, unknown = 9

( ) Nx: postoperative complications, None = 0, intestinal obstruction = 1, anastomotic leakage = 2, bleeding = 3, infection = 4, Other = 5

( ) Nx: stoma complications, None = 0, edema = 1, necrosis = 2, hemorrhage = 3 dermatitis around =4, infection = 5, prolapse = 6, shrink = 7, narrow = 8, hernia = 9 , around the fistula = 10, stoma enteritis = 11, mucous membranes - skin separation = 12, ischemia = 13, Other = 14

Laboratory data:

Blood CEA Nx: preoperative__ ng / ml Nx: postoperative___ ng / ml Nx: recurrence ___ng / ml

Bile CEA Nx: preoperative___ ng / ml Nx: postoperative__ ng / ml Nx: recurrence___ ng / ml

Serum CA19-9 Nx: preoperative__ u / ml Nx: postoperative __ u / ml Nx: recurrence __u / ml

( ) Nx: DPD enzyme__ () Nx: TP enzyme ___

( ) Nx: CD3 ___ () Nx: CD8___ () Nx: CD44 ___

( ) Nx: IgA__ () Nx: IgM___ () Nx: IgG ____

(ii) follow-up information data:

Nx: follow-up time __ day__ month__ year

( ) Nx: metastasis / recurrence None= 0, exist = 1, suspicious = 2, unknown = 3

Nx: metastasis / recurrence date__ day__ month__ year :

( ) Nx: metastasis / recurrence basis pathological = 1, CT = 2, BUS = 3, X ray = 4, ECT = 5, serology= 6, clinical = 7, PET = 8, endoscope = 9, other = 10, unknown = 99

( ) Nx: recurrence / site anastomosis = 1, cut = 2, perineum = 3, pelvic = 4, abdominal = 5, unknown = 9

( ) Nx: metastatic sites, liver = 1, lung = 2, bone = 3, abdominal= 4, pelvic = 5, lock LN = 6, inguinal LN = 7, Other = 8, unknown = 9

( ) Nx: treatment of recurrence / metastasis None = 0, chemotherapy = 1, surgery = 2, radiotherapy = 3, biological treatment = 4, Chinese medicine = 5, comprehensive treatment = 6, Other = 7, unknown = 9

Nx: Date of last visit __ day__ month__ year

( ) Nx: conclusion survival = 0, tumor death = 1, non-tumor deaths = 2, cause of death unknown = 3

Memo： ______________________________

____

____

***N=A~Z， x=1~n**

***Memo：The content should be no more than 50 Chinese characters.**

References

1. Steward BW, Kleihues P, editors. World cancer report. Lyon: IARC Press; 2003. p. 198–202.
2. American Cancer Society. Global cancer facts & figures 2007. Atlanta: American Cancer Society; 2007. p. 12–3.
3. Søreide O, Norstein J, editors. Rectal cancer surgery. Berlin: Springer; 1997. p. 3–45.
4. Abeloft MD, Armitage JD, Lichter AS, Niederhuber JE, editors. Clinical oncology, vol. 2. 2nd ed. Beijing: Harcourt Publishers Limited; 2001. p. 1611–60.
5. Andrew GR, Matthias E, Mark PS, et al. Impact on survival of intensive follow-up after curative resection for colorectal cancer: systematic review and meta-analysis of randomized trials. BMJ. 2002;324:813–6.
6. Goldberg RM, Fleming TR, Tangen CM, et al. Surgery for recurrent colon cancer: strategies for identifying respectable recurrence and success rates after resection. Ann Inter Med. 1998;129:27.
7. Castells A, Bessa X, Daniels M. Value of postoperative surveillance after radical surgery for colorectal cancer: results of a cohort study. Dis Colon Rectum. 1998;41:714.
8. Fitzgibbons RJ, Lynch HT. Recognition and treatment of patients with hereditary nonpolyposis colorectal cancer. Ann Surg. 1987;206:289–95.
9. Yuan Y, Zheng S. Hereditary nonpolyposis colorectal cancer treatment. J Pract Oncol. 1998;13(4):253–5.
10. Xu Y, Cai SJ, Mo SJ, et al. Clinical features and diagnostic principles of hereditary nonpolyposis colorectal cancer. Chin J Digest Med. 2002;22:157–9.
11. Lupinacci R, Penna C, Nordlinger B. Hepatectomy for resectable colorectal cancer metastases – indicators of prognosis, definition of resectability, techniques and outcomes. Surg Oncol Clin N Am. 2007;16(3):493–506.
12. Rodrignez-Moranta F, Saló J, Arcusa A, et al. Postoperative surveillance in patients with colorectal cancer who have undergone curative resection: a prospective, multicenter, randomized, controlled trial. J Clin Oncol. 2006;24(3):386–93.

13. Barabouti DG, Wing WD. Current management of rectal cancer: total mesorectal excision (nerve sparing) technique and clinical outcome. Surg Oncol Clin N Am. 2005;14:137–55.
14. Hoffman KE, McCarthy EP, Recklitis CJ, et al. Psychological distress in long-term survivors of adult-onset cancer: results from a national survey. Arch Intern Med. 2009;169(14):1274.
15. Wan DS. Pay attention to the stoma rehabilitation. Guangdong Med. 2009;30(8):1025–6.
16. Tomlinson JS, Jarnagin WR, Demetteo RP, et al. Actual 10-year survival after resection of colorectal liver metastases defines cure. J Clin Oncol. 2007;25(29):4575–80.
17. Martling AL, Holm T, Rutqvist LE, et al. Effect of a surgical training program on outcome of rectal cancer in the country of Stockholm. Lancet. 2000;356(9224):93–6.
18. Meyerhardt JA, Tepper JE, Niedzwiecki D, et al. Impact of hospital procedure volume on surgical operation and long-term outcomes in high-risk curatively resected rectal cancer: findings from the Intergroup 0114 study. J Clin Oncol. 2004;22:166–74.
19. Harling H, Bulow S, Moller LN, et al. Hospital volume and outcome of rectal cancer surgery in Denmark 1994–1999. Colorectal Dis. 2005;7:90–5.
20. Renzulli P, Laffer UT. Learning curve: the surgeon as a prognostic factor in colorectal cancer surgery. In: Buchler MW, editor. Rectal cancer treatment. Berlin: Springer; 2005. p. 86–104.
21. Kelly C, Daly J. Colorectal cancer. Principles of postoperative follow-up. Cancer. 1992;70(5):1397–408.
22. Jiang XM. Tumor antigen. In: Jiang XM, Zheng S, editors. Tumor biology. Hangzhou: Zhejiang Science and Technology Press; 1990. p. 262–3.
23. Gold P, Freedman SC. Demonstration of tumor-specific antigens in human colonic carcinomata by immunological tolerance and absorption technique. J Exp Med. 1995;121:439.
24. Dhuchi N, Taira Y, Sakai N, et al. Comparison of serum assays for TAG-72, CA199 and CEA in gastrointestinal carcinoma patients. Jpn J Clin Oncol. 1989;3:242–8.
25. Audisio R, Setti-Carraro P, Segala M, et al. Follow-up in colorectal cancer patients: a cost-benefit analysis. Ann Surg Oncol. 1996;3:349–57.
26. Zheng S. Colorectal cancer. In: Wang J, editor. Gastrointestinal surgery. Beijing: People's Medical Publishing House; 2000. p. 920–39.
27. Ogata Y, Matono K, Hayashi A, et al. Repeat pulmonary resection for isolated recurrent lung metastases yields results comparable to those after first pulmonary resection in colorectal cancer. World J Surg. 2005;29:363–8.
28. Ike H, Shimadu H, Ohki S, et al. Results of aggressive resection of lung metastases from colorectal carcinoma detected by intensive follow-up. Dis Colon Rectum. 2002;45:468–73.
29. Makela JT, Laitinen SO, Kairaluoma MI. Five-year follow-up after radical surgery for colorectal cancer. Results of prospective randomized trial. Arch Surg. 1995;130:1062–7.
30. Ohlsson B, Breland U, Ekberg H, et al. Follow-up after curative surgery for colorectal carcinoma. Randomized comparison with no follow-up. Dis Colon Rectum. 1995;38:619–26.
31. Schoemaker D, Black R, Giles L, et al. Yearly colonoscopy, liver CT, and chest radiography do not influence 5-year survival of colorectal cancer patients. Gastroenterology. 1998;114:7–14.
32. Pietra N, Sarli L, Costi R, et al. Role of follow-up in management of local recurrences of colorectal cancer: a prospective, randomized study. Dis Colon Rectum. 1998;41:1127–33.
33. Kjeldsen BJ, Kronborg O, Fenger C, et al. A prospective randomized study of follow-up after radical surgery for colorectal cancer. Br J Surg. 1997;84:666–9.
34. Sugarbaker PH. A simplified plan for follow-up of patients with colon and rectal cancer and rectal cancer supported by prospective studies of laboratory and radiological test results. Surgery. 1987;102:79–87.
35. Safi F, Beyer HG. The value of follow-up after curative surgery of colorectal carcinoma. Cancer Detect Prev. 1993;17:417–24.
36. Cochrane J, Williams JT, Faber R, et al. Value of outpatient follow-up after curative surgery for carcinoma of the large bowel. BMJ. 1980;280:593–5.
37. Ballantyne GH, Modlin IM. Postoperative follow-up for colorectal cancer: who are we kidding? J Clin Gastroenterol. 1988;10:359–64.
38. Bruinvels DJ, Stiggelbout AM, Kievit J, et al. Follow-up of patients with colorectal cancer. A meta-analysis. Ann Surg. 1994;219:174–82.
39. Bruinvels DJ, Stiggelbout AM, Klaassen MP, et al. Follow-up after colorectal cancer: current practice in the Netherlands. Eur J Surg. 1995;161:827–31.
40. Biggs CG, Ballantyne GH. Sensitivity versus cost effectiveness in postoperative follow-up for colorectal cancer. Curr Opin Gen Surg. 1994:94–102.
41. Vigo KS, Wade TP, Longo WE, et al. Surveillance after curative colon cancer resection: practice patterns of surgical subspecialists. Ann Surg Oncol. 1995;2:472–85.
42. Northover J, Houghton J, Lennon T. CEA to detect recurrence of colon cancer. JAMA. 1994;272:31.
43. Howell JD, Wotherspoon H, Leen L, et al. Evaluation of a follow-up programme after curative resection for colorectal cancer. Br J Cancer. 1999;79(2):308–10.

MIX
Papier aus verantwortungsvollen Quellen
Paper from responsible sources
FSC® C105338

If you have any concerns about our products,
you can contact us on
ProductSafety@springernature.com

In case Publisher is established outside the EU,
the EU authorized representative is:
Springer Nature Customer Service Center GmbH
Europaplatz 3, 69115 Heidelberg, Germany

Printed by Libri Plureos GmbH
in Hamburg, Germany